Richard R. Heuser • Markus Schlaich
Horst Sievert

Editors

Renal Denervation

A New Approach to Treatment of Resistant Hypertension

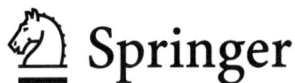 Springer

Editors
Richard R. Heuser
St. Luke's Medical Center
Phoenix, AZ
USA

Markus Schlaich
Baker IDI Heart and Diabetes Institute
Melbourne, VIC
Australia

Horst Sievert
CardioVascular Center Frankfurt
Sankt Katharinen
Frankfurt
Germany

ISBN 978-1-4471-7076-1   ISBN 978-1-4471-5223-1   (eBook)
DOI 10.1007/978-1-4471-5223-1
Springer London Heidelberg New York Dordrecht

Preface

In the Western world, 30–40 % of the adult population suffers from hypertension. The prevalence is expected to increase with the aging population. Sixty-five percent of patients over 60 years of age are affected by hypertension. It is thought to be the greatest risk factor for cardiovascular disease. Renal sympathetic efferent and afferent nerves are recognized as critical in the hypertensive disease process and represent an important therapeutic target. From the 1930s to 1950s, investigators performed surgical interruption of the sympathetic pathway and effectively lowered the pressure significantly in patients, but there were complications that precluded the continued application of this technique at the same time that effective drug regimens evolved.

Recently, renal denervation has been reborn as a catheter technique utilizing the proximity of the renal nerves to the renal arteries utilizing various forms of energy or injections. This technique has been effective in treating resistant hypertension in as many as 85 % of patients. The ability to perform this transcatheter technique has the potential to cause a paradigm shift in cardiovascular care. Resistant hypertension is defined as blood pressure persistently above goal despite the use of antihypertensive medications from ≥3 drug classes. These patients face worse cardiovascular outcomes and systemic hypertension-related complications, for which there is no viable treatment option. For example, poorly controlled hypertension can increase stroke rate by 50 %.

The new percutaneous approach, based on the concept of an old surgical technique, may be a true game changer for treating patients with not only hypertension but also renal insufficiency, congestive heart failure, diabetes mellitus, obesity, sleep apnea, and glucose intolerance. Given the enormous market for this treatment approach and the rapidly compounded annual growth rate, an estimated 60 companies are pursuing technologies to achieve RDN with equivalent or superior approaches. This treatment is moving so quickly and has been thought effective enough in its early stages that the European Society of Cardiology (ESC) has issued a consensus statement describing patients that are appropriate to be screened for this therapy. The whole field of renal arterial based renal denervation dealt a serious blow with the publication of the Symplicity HTN-3 6-month data. This blinded trial did not show significant reduction of systolic blood pressure in patients with resistant hypertension 6 months after renal-artery denervation as compared with a sham control (Funded by Medtronic: SYMPLICITY HTN-3 ClinicalTrials.gov, number, NCT01418261) [1]. After 6 months, office systolic blood pressure decreased from baseline to a similar extent in the renal-denervation and sham-procedure groups ($P<0.001$) for both comparisons of the change from baseline); the difference in the change in blood pressure between the two groups was a paltry −2.39 mmHg. In addition, a prespecified difference in 24-h ambulatory systolic pressure of only 2 mmHg was not met. Thus, in the SYMPLICITY HTN-3 STUDY, renal denervation had no significant effect on office or 24-h ambulatory systolic blood pressure, findings that contradict most published data on renal denervation. While renal denervation lowered blood pressure by an average of 14.1 mmHg, it was not statistically significant when compared to the sham treatment. Patients receiving no treatment may experience Hawthorne effect, believing they had received the treatment, resulting in an 11.7 mmHg reduction. The trial used the first-generation Medtronic Symplicity catheter, which uses a single electrode that must be maneuvered into specific positions for ablations that last about a minute each. The procedure is similar to cardiac ablations to isolate arrhythmia-causing cardiac tissue. Electrophysiology ablations are sometimes difficult to perform or have mixed outcomes, depending on several factors, including catheter pressure applied, duration of the ablation and the ability of the operator to connect all the dots between ablation points to prevent the transmission of electrical signals across the scarred areas. Further studies in rigorously designed trials will be needed to confirm the results of the earlier trials. The 5-year results of this study will be fascinating and some groups had a near significant benefit compared to medical therapy. Results were maintained in prespecified subgroup analysis, although non–African Americans tended to benefit from renal denervation more so than African Americans ($P=0.09$). A number of limitations were identified by the study's authors, and also reviewed by the discussion panel after the presentation. Blood levels of antihypertensive medications were not obtained, so drug adherence was not directly measured. The large and significant change over time in both groups may have been related to the placebo effect, or it may be that study participants in both arms achieved improved medication compliance after enrollment in the study. Further, there is no commonly accepted and easily obtained measure of denervation of the renal sympathetic system, so it is possible that renal denervation did not occur, although the study authors could confirm that the appropriate energy had been delivered by the device.

Experts have weighed in as to why this study showed different results than other studies, particularly in Europe. A large concern was operator's inexperience with denervation (they were all experienced interventional cardiologists) another flaw in the trial design was that no method was used to monitor the efficacy of each denervation procedure, an easy decision because there is still no proven way to measure denervation efficacy during the procedure. In the first clinical study of renal denervation, in a series of 45 patients treated at five centers in Australia and Europe reported just 5 years ago (*Lancet* 2009;373:1275–81), Dr. Esler, a lead investigator for that study, and his associates carefully tested the efficacy of denervation in ten patients by measuring the direct effect of successful denervation and reduction of renal norepinephrine spillover. They reported that, in those ten patients, renal denervation cut norepinephrine spillover by an average of 47 %, which correlated with an average reduction in systolic blood pressure of 22 mmHg after 6 months.

Because of the aging of the population and rising rates of obesity, hypertension is increasing in prevalence worldwide. Approximately 10 % of patients with diagnosed hypertension have resistant hypertension, defined as a systolic blood pressure of 140 mmHg or higher despite adherence to at least three maximally tolerated doses of antihypertensive medications from complementary classes, included a diuretic at an appropriate dose. The sympathetic nervous system – in particular, sympathetic cross-talk between the kidneys and the brain – appears to play an important role in resistant hypertension.

In spite of this recent published study, very limited data has been published on preclinical and clinical experiences with these new devices, and the future of this field is controversial. Other new approaches, including less invasive and outpatient-based therapies, may or may not be effective. Unfortunately, during the last 10 years, very few new antihypertensive agents have reached the market and no new therapeutic class has really emerged if one considers renin inhibitors as members of drugs inhibiting the renin-angiotensin system (RAS). Thus, the actual strategy to control blood pressure in hypertension relies on the use of three major classes of antihypertensive drugs, i.e., blockers of the RAS, calcium channel blockers (CCBs), and diuretics (D) as reported in the last 2013 hypertension guidelines of the European Society of Hypertension and European Society of Cardiology. One very important issue with any study of hypertensive patients, including HTN-3, is that there was no confirmation of medication adherence. More than 50 % of patients with resistant hypertension are known to be nonadherent to medications. There was no direct measurement to confirm that the renal nerves were in fact denervated by the procedure, because there is no test that can be easily performed in a large trial. However, the Symplicity catheter system allowed confirmation of energy delivery, and the presence of angiographic notching indicated a biologic effect of energy delivery on the artery. Finally, the results of this trial are specific to the catheter tested and cannot necessarily be generalized to other denervation systems. We shall await further data. This textbook is aimed to provide an overview of the field, to describe the preclinical and clinical experiences with the most prominent technologies in the pipeline, and to provide insights regarding the possible directions this field may be heading.

I was pleased to have been introduced to Victoria John from Springer Publishing who agreed with me that a textbook describing this new treatment would be a welcome addition. My co-editors are two world renowned leaders in the field including Horst Sievert from Germany and Markus Schlaich from Australia. We have attempted to pull together the experts in the field in our textbook and are proud to say everyone we invited to contribute agreed to be represented in the textbook. We have described most of the current devices and approaches, and we hope to give the reader a snapshot of where things are available at this time.

I would like to thank Victoria and my co-editors Horst Sievert and Markus Schlaich, along with our co-authors without which the textbook would not have been possible. As with other textbooks I have edited, I will donate all my royalties to Johns Hopkins Hospital where I trained. I also wish to dedicate this book to the Phoenix Heart Center, St. Luke's Medical Center and my daughter Alexandra and wife Shari. Special thanks to Peggy Layman for putting up with everything she needs to deal with not only this publication, but everything involved with interacting with me.

We hope the reader will find this textbook a springboard for study and advancement of this new, exciting field.

Phoenix, AZ, USA   Richard R. Heuser

Reference

1. Bhatt DL, Kandzari DE, O'Neill WW, et al. A controlled trial of renal denervation for resistant hypertension. N Eng J Med. 2014;370:1393–401.

Contents

Contributors

Nevin C. Baker, DO Department of Interventional Cardiology, MedStar Washington Hospital Center, Washington, DC, USA

Israel M. Barbash, MD Department of Interventional Cardiology, MedStar Washington Hospital Center, Washington, DC, USA
Interventional Cardiology Department, Sheba Medical Center, Tel Aviv University, Ramat Gan, Israel

Stefan C. Bertog, MD, FACC, FSCAI CardioVascular Center Frankfurt, Frankfurt, Germany

Deepak L. Bhatt, MD, MPH, FACC, FAHA, FSCAI, FESC Interventional Cardiovascular Programs, Brigham and Women's Hospital Heart and Vascular Center, Harvard Medical School, Boston, MA, USA

Michael Böhm, MD Klinik für Innere Medizin III, Kardiologie, Angiologie und Internistische Intensivmedizin, Universitätsklinikum des Saarlandes, Homburg/Saar, Germany

Terrence J. Buelna Verve Medical Inc., Peoria, AZ, USA

Sandeep Chopra, MBBS, MD, DM Department of Cardiology, Royal Perth Hospital, Perth, WA, Australia

Leslie A. Coleman, DVM, MS ReCor Medical Inc., Palo Alto, CA, USA

Randy I. Cooper, MD Department of Nephrology, Southwest Vascular Center/Southwest Kidney Institute, Tempe, AZ, USA

Justin E. Davies, MBBS, BSc, MRCP, PhD Department of Cardiology, Hammersmith Hospital, Imperial College London, London, UK

Mihir Desai, MD Department of Urology, University of Southern California, USC Institute of Urology, Los Angeles, CA, USA

Michalis Doumas, MD Aristotle University, Thessaloniki, Greece
Department of Cardiology/Hypertension, Department of Veterans Affairs Medical Center, Washington, DC, USA

Michael Evans, BS Palo Alto, CA, USA
Northwind Medical, San Jose, CA, USA

Sebastian Ewen, MD Klinik für Innere Medizin III, Kardiologie, Angiologie und Internistische Intensivmedizin, Universitätsklinikum des Saarlandes, Homburg/Saar, Germany

Charles Faselis, MD Veteran Affairs Medical Centre and George Washington University, Washington, DC, USA

Department of Internal Medicine/Hypertension, Department of Veterans Affairs Medical Center, Washington, DC, USA

Tim A. Fischell, MD, FACC Heart Institute at Borgess Medical Center, Kalamazoo, MI, USA

Ablative Solutions, Inc., Kalamazoo/Menlo Park, MI/CA, USA

Darrel P. Francis, MA, MB BChir, FRCP International Centre for Circulatory Health, National Heart and Lung Institute, Imperial College London, London, UK

Marat Fudim, MD Internal Medicine, Vanderbilt Medical Center, Nashville, TN, USA

Kristine Fuimaono, BS Cordis Corporation/Biosense Webster, Inc., Diamond Bar, CA, USA

Sameer Gafoor, MD CardioVascular Center Frankfurt, Frankfurt, Germany

Vartan E. Ghazarossian, PhD Ablative Solutions Inc., Kalamazoo/Menlo Park, MI/CA, USA

Adam Gold, MSME Verve Medical, Inc., Peoria, AZ, USA

David G. Harrison, MD Medicine and Pharmacology, Vanderbilt Medical Center, Nashville, TN, USA

Richard R. Heuser, MD Department of Cardiology, St Lukes Medical Center, Phoenix, AZ, USA

Ilona Hofmann, MD CardioVascular Center Frankfurt, Frankfurt, Germany

James P. Howard, MA, MB BChir, MRCP International Centre for Circulatory Health, National Heart and Lung Institute, Imperial College London, London, UK

Michael Joner, MD CVPath Institute, Inc., Gaithersburg, MD, USA

Jacek Kądziela, MD, PhD Department of Interventional Cardiology and Angiology, Institute of Cardiology, Warsaw, Poland

Frank D. Kolodgie, PhD CVPath Institute, Inc., Gaithersburg, MD, USA

A. Srinivasa Kumar Cardiology Department, Continental Hospitals, Hyderabad, AP, India

Elena Ladich, MD CVPath Institute, Inc., Gaithersburg, MD, USA

Dominik Linz, MD, PhD Department of Cardiology, University Hospital of Saarland, Homburg/Saar, Germany

Felix Mahfoud, MD Department of Internal Medicine, University Hospital of Saarland, Homburg/Saar, Germany

Aung Myat, BSc (Hons), MBBS, MRCP The Rayne Institute, British Heart Foundation of Research Excellence, St Thomas' Hospital, King's College London, London, UK

William E.L. Ormiston, MBChB Department of Radiology, Auckland City Hospital, Auckland, New Zealand

John A. Ormiston, MBChB, FRACP, FRACR Department of Mercy Angiography, Mercy Hospital, Auckland, New Zealand

University of Auckland School of Medicine, Auckland, New Zealand

Cardiology, Auckland City Hospital, Auckland, New Zealand

Fumiyuki Otsuka, MD CVPath Institute, Inc., Gaithersburg, MD, USA

Vasilios Papademetriou, MD Veteran Affairs Medical Center and Georgetown University, Washington, DC, USA

Department of Interventional Cardiology/Hypertension, Department of Veterans Affairs Medical Center, Washington, DC, USA

Atul Pathak, MD, PhD, DACLAM Clinical Pharmacology and Cardiovascular Medicine, University Hospital and Faculty of Medicine, Toulouse, France

C. Venkata S. Ram, MD, MA, CP, FACC Apollo Institute for Blood Pressure Management, Apollo Blood Pressure Clinics, Apollo Hospitals, Hyderabad, AP, India

Texas Blood Pressure Institute, Medical School, University of Texas Southwestern, Dallas, TX, USA

Rahul R. Rao, P.E. BSc Verve Medical, Inc., Peoria, AZ, USA

Claire E. Raphael, MA, BSc, MRCP Department of Cardiology, Royal Brompton and Harefield NHS Foundation Trust, London, UK

Helen L. Reeve, PhD ReCor Medical BV, Herengracht 124-128, 1015 BT Amsterdam, The Netherlands

Krishna J. Rocha-Singh, MD Department of Cardiology, Prairie Heart Institute at St. John's Hospital, Springfield, IL, USA

Austin R. Roth, BS, MS ReCor Medical, Palo Alto, CA, USA

Kenichi Sakakura, MD CVPath Institute, Inc., Gaithersburg, MD, USA

Marc Sapoval, MD, PhD Interventional Radiology, Hopital Européen Georges Pompidou, Paris, France

Yusuke Sata, MD Neurovascular Hypertension and Kidney Disease Laboratory, Baker IDI Heart and Diabetes Institute, Melbourne, VIC, Australia

Markus P. Schlaich, MD, PhD Neurovascular Hypertension and Kidney Disease Laboratory, Baker IDI Heart and Diabetes Institute, Melbourne, VIC, Australia

Sharad V. Shetty, MBBS, MD, FRACP Department of Cardiology, Royal Perth Hospital, Perth, WA, Australia

Matthew J. Shun-Shin, MA, MB BChir, MRCP International Centre for Circulatory Health, National Heart and Lung Institute, Imperial College London, London, UK

Horst Sievert, MD, FESC, FACC, FSCAI CardioVascular Center Frankfurt, Frankfurt, Germany

Paul A. Sobotka, MD Division of Cardiology, Department of Medicine, The Ohio State University, West St. Paul, MN, USA

Christodoulos Stefanadis, MD, FESC, FACC First Department of Cardiology, Athens Medical School, Hippokration Hospital, Athens, Greece

Emily Stein, PhD San Leandro, CA, USA

Northwind Medical, San Jose, CA, USA

Andreas Synetos, MD, FACC First Department of Cardiology, Athens Medical School, Hippokration Hospital, Athens, Greece

Konstantinos Toutouzas, MD First Department of Cardiology, Athens Medical School, Hippokration Hospital, Athens, Greece

Costa Tsioufis, MD Kapodistrian University, Athens, Greece

Department of Interventional Cardiology/Hypertension, Department of Veterans Affairs Medical Center, Washington, DC, USA

Christian Ukena, Dr. med Department of Internal Medicine, University Hospital of Saarland, Homburg/Saar, Germany

William G. Van Alstine, DVM, PhD, DACVP Department of Veterinary Medicine, Purdue University, Lafayette, IN, USA

Laura Vaskelyte, MD CardioVascular Center Frankfurt, Frankfurt, Germany

Félix Vega, VMD Preclinical Consultants, San Francisco, CA, USA

K.T. Venkateswara Rao, PhD Northwind Medical, San Jose, CA, USA

Renu Virmani, MD CVPath Institute, Inc., Gaithersburg, MD, USA

Ron Waksman, MD Department of Interventional Cardiology, MedStar Heart Institute/MedStar Washington Hospital Center, Washington, DC, USA

Mark H. Wholey, MD UPMC Shadyside, Pittsburgh Vascular Institute, Pittsburgh, PA, USA

Northwind Medical, San Jose, CA, USA

Adam Witkowski, MD, PhD, FESC Department of Interventional Cardiology and Angiology, Institute of Cardiology, Warsaw, Poland

Kazuyuki Yahagi, MD CVPath Institute, Inc., Gaithersburg, MD, USA

Thomas Zeller, MD Department Angiology, Universitäts-Herzzentrum Freiburg – Bad Krozingen, Bad Krozingen, Germany

Pathophysiology: The Target for Renal Denervation

Michael Böhm, Dominik Linz, Christian Ukena,
and Felix Mahfoud

Introduction

In 1842 the first description of sympathetic nerves surrounding the renal artery was provided in the thesis in Latin by Carl Ludwig [1]. Since then the field became a matter of ongoing scientific interest. Mechanosensitive baroreceptors, volume sensors and chemoreceptors regulate afferent signaling to various nuclei in the brain stem. In the renal arteries both afferent and efferent nerve fibers are found in the adventitia, where they surround the arteries with a netlike appearance [2]. The challenge for renal denervation is to reach the adventitia from the intraluminal side and affecting both efferent and afferent nervous fibers to interrupt the interaction between sensory signals generated in the kidney and central sympathetic outflow [2] (Fig. 1.1). Sympathetic nervous outflow is regulated by the nucleus tractus solitarius located in the midbrain [3]. From there the efferent signaling reaches not only the kidney but also other peripheral structures like the heart, the vessels, the liver and other parts of the central nervous system [3].

Renal Afferent Nerve Activity

Activation of renal sensory afferent fibers derives primarily from the renal pelvis [3, 4]. Chemosensitive receptors in the renal interstitium are sensitive to ion and osmolar concentration changes, ischemia and the metabolic products of ischemia, like adenosine [2, 3]. Consistently, adenosine infusion increases the blood pressure by stimulating afferent signaling initiated by adenosine receptors located in the pelvis [4]. On the contrary, application of 100 % oxygen reduces sympathetic nerve activity in patients with renal failure [5]. The concept of direct interaction between the central nervous system and the kidney is shown by the reduction of sympathetic activity after renal nephrectomy in patients with renal failure [6]. Furthermore, the BP rise seen in rats after 5/6 nephrectomy can be prevented by dorsal thizectomy [7]. Finally, it was demonstrated that bilateral nephrectomy following successful renal transplantation reduced sympathetic activity, whereas transplantation alone did not. These data provided clear evidence to suggest that not uremia, but the remaining non-functioning kidneys via afferent signaling were the source of sympathetic overstimulation [8].

Renal Efferent Sympathetic Activity

Efferent nerve fibers from sympathetic ganglia reach the kidney as they follow the renal arteries typically within the adventitial layer of the vessel. These nerves invade all segments of the renal cortex and terminate at the arterioles of the glomeruli [9, 10]. Furthermore, the glomerular renin containing juxtaglomerular cells are targeted by efferent sympathetic nerves [11]. α1b-adrenergic receptors mediate sodium and water retention and, therefore, antidiuretic effects in the proximal tubulus, while α1a-adrenergic receptors mediate vasoconstriction and reduce renal blood flow [3]. β1-adrenergic

M. Böhm, MD (✉) • C. Ukena, Dr. med. • D. Linz, MD, PhD
F. Mahfoud, MD
Department of Cardiology, University Hospital of Saarland,
1 Kirrberger Street, 66420 Homburg/Saar, Germany
e-mail: michael.boehm@uks.eu; Christian.Ukena@uks.eu;
Dominik.linz@uks.eu; Felix.mahfoud@uks.eu

R.R. Heuser et al. (eds.), *Renal Denervation: A New Approach to Treatment of Resistant Hypertension*,
DOI 10.1007/978-1-4471-5223-1_1, © Springer-Verlag London 2015

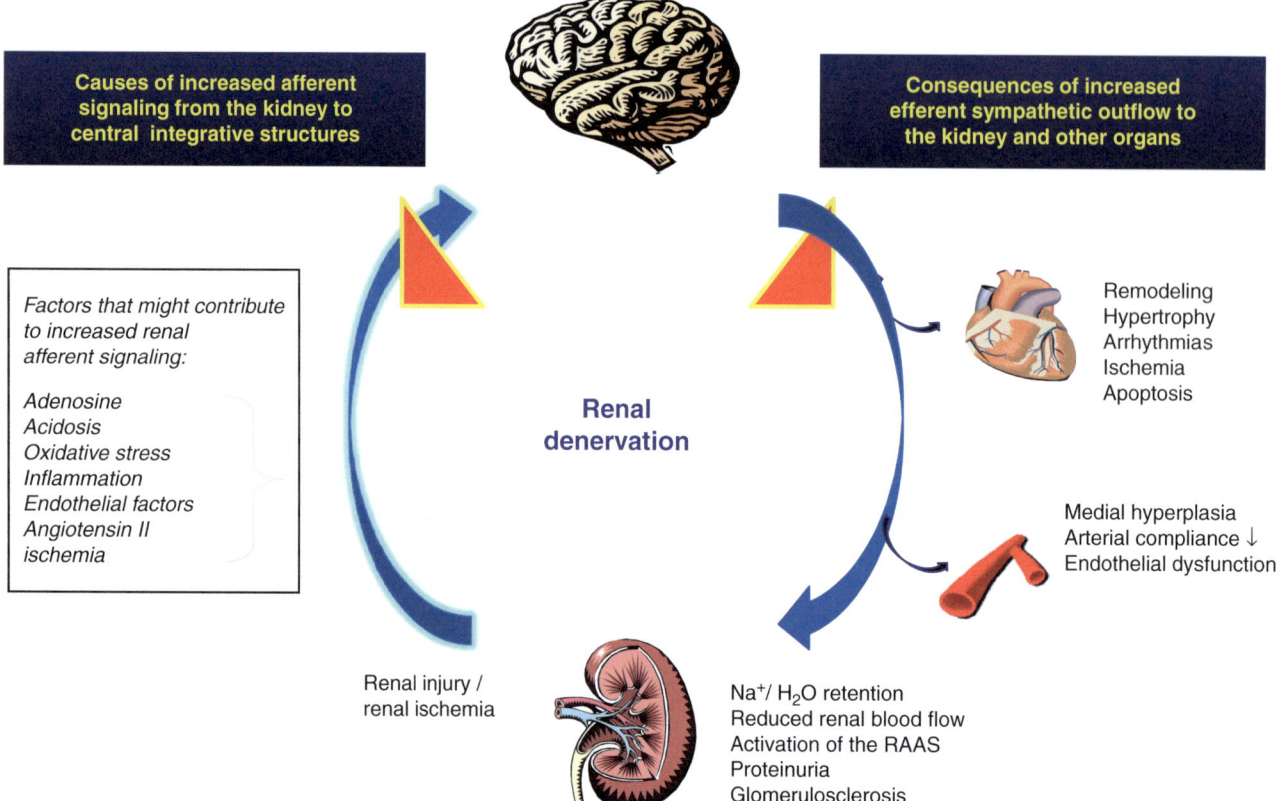

Effects of increased sympathetic tone

Causes of increased afferent signaling from the kidney to central integrative structures

Consequences of increased efferent sympathetic outflow to the kidney and other organs

Renal denervation

Factors that might contribute to increased renal afferent signaling:

Adenosine
Acidosis
Oxidative stress
Inflammation
Endothelial factors
Angiotensin II
ischemia

Remodeling
Hypertrophy
Arrhythmias
Ischemia
Apoptosis

Medial hyperplasia
Arterial compliance ↓
Endothelial dysfunction

Renal injury / renal ischemia

Na^+/ H_2O retention
Reduced renal blood flow
Activation of the RAAS
Proteinuria
Glomerulosclerosis

Fig. 1.1 Interaction between the brain and the kidney with the effect of increasing sympathetic nerve activities. Sympathetic activation is generated in the kidney, where it reaches the heart, the vessels and the kidney by efferent sympathetic nerves. Sympathetic activation activates functional and structural changes of end organs. Renal efference is activated by renal adrenergy, ischemia and impaired renal perfusion by mediation of adenosine, acidosis and others. The afferent feedback stimulation of the sympathetic nervous system further increases sympathetic activating tone. Rationale of renal denervation is to interrupt afferent and efferent nerves (depicted by *red triangles*) (Adapted by permission from Macmillan Publishers Ltd: Böhm et al. [49])

receptors stimulate renin secretion with subsequent activation of the renin-angiotensin-aldosterone system [12], again, contributing to sodium water retention and producing the right shift of the pressure natriuresis curve [2, 3, 12]. The concept is summarized in Fig. 1.1.

Interaction Between Right and Left Kidney

Interestingly, afferent stimulation of nerves in one kidney also increases norepinephrine and dopamine release from the contralateral kidney [13]. Besides these experiments in dogs [13], an increase of heart rate and blood pressure was observed by contralateral nerve stimulation in conscious rats [14]. However, the effect is highly variable in between species, because the distribution of excitatory and inhibitory

renal nerves are differently distributed among the different species [15].

Renal Denervation

Experimental Studies

Stimulation of renal sympathetic nerves increases the urinary excretion of norepinephrine, which can be inhibited by experimental renal denervation [16, 17]. Renal denervation reduces blood pressure in genetic models of hypertension [18]. In two-kidney one clip rats blood pressure was reduced [19]. In an inherited model of polycystic kidney disease, renal denervation reduced blood pressure and restored renal blood flow [20].

Radio frequency ablation

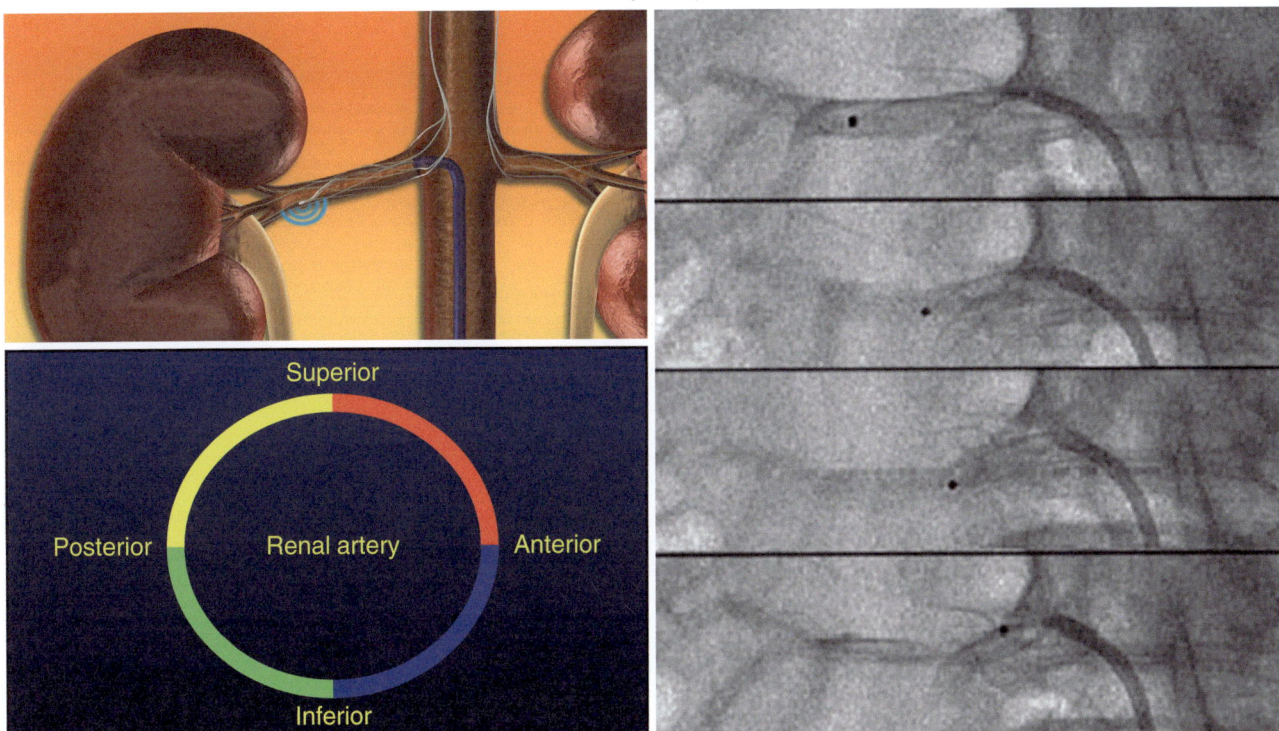

Fig. 1.2 *Upper left*: schematic illustration of sympathetic renal nerves in the adventitia of the renal artery. The high frequency electrode is positioned through a guiding catheter. The administration of high frequency energy produces heat, which is cooled by high intraluminal bloodflow, blood is sticking at the adventitia, where it damages the sympathetic nerves (©2014 Medtronic, Inc. Printed with Permission). *Lower left*: Catheter is rotationally pulled back in order to provide energy to superior, posterior, anterior and inferior part of the vessel in an attempt to provide a circumferenterial complete denervation. *Right*: The view of the investigator in four different positions of renal denervation [1–4]

In humans, the first experiences with interventional reduction of sympathetic activity were obtained by thoracolumbar splanchniectomy, which had significant effects on blood pressure in the majority but not all patients with severe hypertension and reduced cardiovascular end organ damage [21–23]. Although mortality was remarkably reduced [23], this technique had serious adverse effects and a high perioprative morbidity and mortality and was abandoned once effective antihypertensive drugs had started to emerge. More recently and applying a similar conceptin patients with resistant hypertension, catheter-based radiofrequency ablation of renal nerves (as schematically illustrated in Fig. 1.2) resulted in significant blood pressure reduction in the Symplicity HTN-1 pilot study [24] and in the randomized controlled Symplicity HTN-2 trial, in which optimal medical therapy + RDN was compared to optimal medical therapy alone ([25], Fig. 1.3). Meanwhile, Symplicity HTN-1 and Symplicity HTN-2 studies provided data to indicate that blood pressure changes that occurred were sustained up to 3 years post-procedure [26, 27]. Data from experienced centers also provided ABPM measurements showing that systolic and diastolic night time, day time and average blood pressure were significantly reduced in resistant hypertensive patients, while in pseudoresistance only office but not ABPM values were diminished [28]. In patients with moderately elevated levels of blood pressure a reduction was also observed [29], albeit the effect was less pronounced. The intriguing finding that after renal denervation not only renal spillover but also a total body spillover is reduced, is strongly arguing in favor of a significant role of both, afferent and efferent denervation [30].

Pathophysiology of Potential Adverse Effects of Renal Denervation

Exercise Tolerance and Heart Rate

Concerns were raised that renal denervation might produce a limitation in exercise tolerance through interference with the sympathetic nervous system [31].

Fig. 1.3 Changes in systolic and diastolic blood pressure at 1 month (1M), 3 months (3M) and 6 months (6M) in patients with renal denervation (*upper part*) and blood pressure changes in the control group (*lower part*) (Reprinted from Symplicity HTN-2 Investigators et al. [25] with permission from Elsevier)

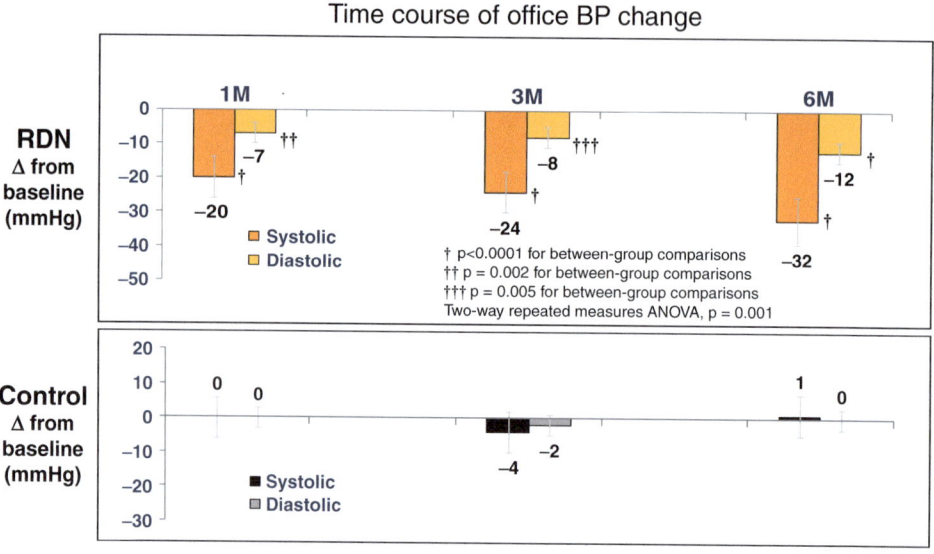

However, a systematic cardiorespiratory exercise testing revealed no evidence for chronotropic incompetence, while exercise tolerance was even slightly increased [32]. Furthermore, exercise blood pressure levels and heart rate responses and recovery were also reduced by renal denervation [32], which might explain the improved exercise tolerance. Furthermore, this finding might provide indirect evidence for potential clinical benefits, because these factors are related to cardiovascular complications including sudden cardiac death [33, 34]. Significant bradycardia was not observed [24–27], probably because heart rate reductions were only reported at higher levels of resting heart rates at baseline with no significant effects on atrioventricular conduction [35]. Interestingly, heart rate reduction and blood pressure reduction showed a dependency on baseline levels, i.e. blood pressure and heart rate effects were most pronounced in those patients with the highest the baseline values (Fig. 1.4, [35]).

Orthostatic Dysfunction

Sympathetic nervous activity regulates the increase of heart rate in vasoconstriction to maintain sufficient blood pressure after orthostatic stress. Tilting causes the transfer of thoracic blood into the venous capacitance vessels and promoted fluid filtration into the interstitium resulting in up to 1,500 ml acute volume shifting [36], which has to be counterbalanced by activation of the sympathetic nervous system. Therefore, concerns have been raised on whether hypotensive reactions might limit the clinical benefits of renal denervation [37], which is evidenced by a drop in sympathetic activity and baroreceptor function just before collapse in syncope [38–41]. However, systematic table tilt testing has not shown

significant occurrence of syncope or blood pressure drops in patients after renal denervation, in particular no difference between responders and non-responders to blood pressure reduction after renal denervation [42].

Psychological Disturbances

Hypertension is often associated with anxiety [43] involving activation of the autonomic nervous system in this condition [44]. Depression is also associated with a dysregulation of the central nervous noradrenergic process [45], but depressed individuals often have an activation of the peripheral sympathetic nervous system [46]. However, renal denervation has been reported to increase quality of life [47] and was not associated with increased depressive symptoms, rather it was associated with reduced anxiety, depression, intensity of headaches and with improved stress tolerance in patients with resistant hypertension [48].

Perspectives

Renal denervation is a promising field to improve many disease conditions by a reduction of sympathetic activity beyond hypertension with a sound pathophysiological background [49]. It might proof to be effective in renal protection [50], atrial [51] and ventricular [52] arrhythmias, sleep apnea [53], hypertrophy reduction [54] and heart failure [55] as well as in metabolic syndrome [56]. In particular, in the latter conditions prospective trials with appropriate clinical endpoints have to be evaluated in order to proof the pathophysiological concept raised by the first experiences with renal sympathetic denervation.

Fig. 1.4 Change in blood pressure (*left*) and heart rate (*right*) after 3 and 6 months according to the systolic blood pressure (*SBP*) and heart rate (*HR*) and the results at baseline. Please note that the higher SBP or heart rate at baseline were the greater were the reduction at follow-up (Reprinted from Ukena et al. [35] with permission from Elsevier)

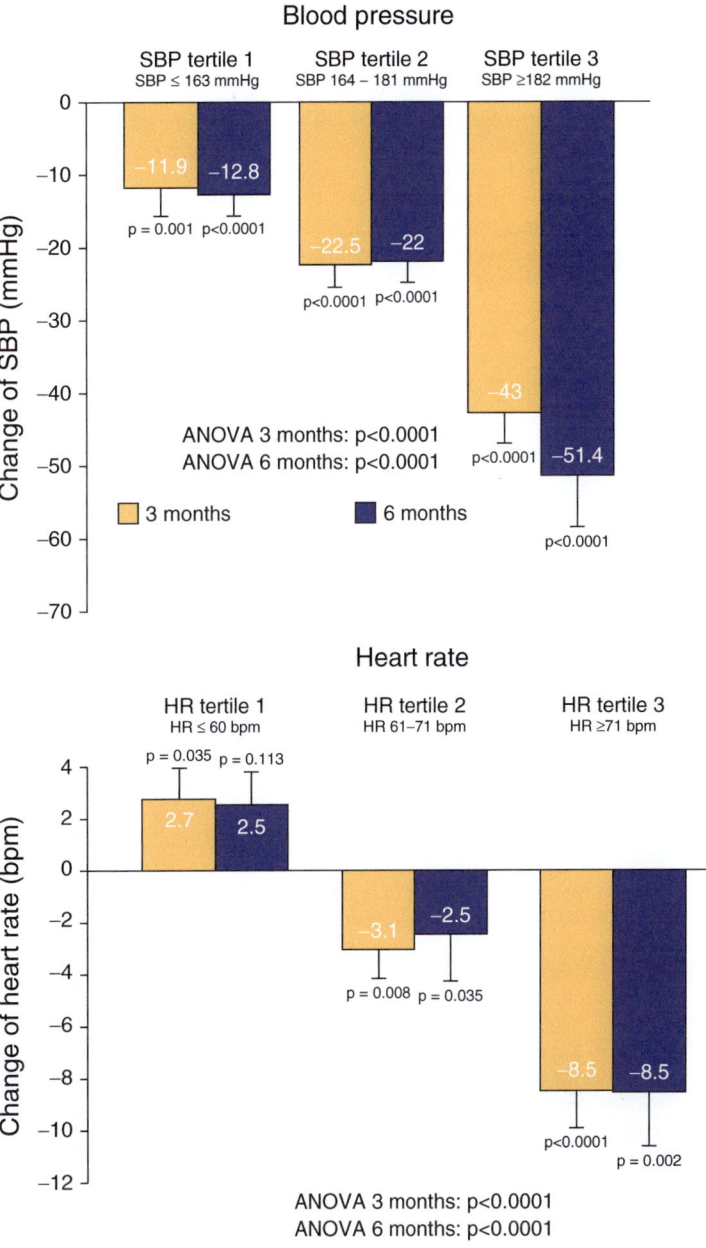

References

1. Ludwig C. De viribus physicis secretionem urinae adjuvantibus (Latin). Thesis, University of Marburg; 1842.
2. Sobotka PA, Mahfoud F, Schlaich MP, Hoppe UC, Böhm M, Krum H. Sympatho-renal axis in chronic disease. Clin Res Cardiol. 2011;100:1049–57.
3. Esler M. The 2009 Carl Ludwig lecture: pathophysiology of the human sympathetic nervous system in cardiovascular diseases: the transition from mechanisms to medical management. J Appl Physiol. 2010;108:227–37.
4. Katholi RE. Renal nerves in the pathogenesis of hypertension in experimental animals and humans. Am J Physiol. 1983;245: F1–14.
5. Hering D, Zdrojewski Z, Król E, Kara T, Kucharska W, Somers VK, Rutkowski B, Narkiewicz K. Tonic chemoreflex activation contributes to the elevated muscle sympathetic nerve activity in patients with chronic renal failure. J Hypertens. 2007;25: 157–61.
6. Converse Jr RL, Jacobsen TN, Toto RD, Jost CM, Cosentino F, Fouad-Tarazi F, Victor RG. Sympathetic overactivity in patients with chronic renal failure. N Engl J Med. 1992;327:1912–8.
7. Campese VM. Neurogenic factors and hypertension in chronic renal failure. J Nephrol. 1997;10:184–7.
8. Hausberg M, Kosch M, Harmelink P, Barenbrock M, Hohage H, Kisters K, Dietl KH, Rahn KH. Sympathetic nerve activity in end-stage renal disease. Circulation. 2002;106:1974–9.
9. Dolezel S. Monoaminergic innervation of the arteries and veins of the kidneys observed using fluorescence reaction. Folia Morphol. 1966;14:168–74.
10. Ljungqvist A, Wågermark J. The adrenergic innervation of intrarenal glomerular and extra-glomerular circulatory routes. Nephron. 1970;7:218–29.

11. Wyss JM, Carlson SH. The role of the central nervous system in hypertension. Curr Hypertens Rep. 1999;1:246–53.

12. Hering D, Esler MD, Krum H, Mahfoud F, Böhm M, Sobotka PA, Schlaich MP. Recent advances in the treatment of hypertension. Expert Rev Cardiovasc Ther. 2011;9:729–44.

13. Bradley T, Hjemdahl P. Influence of afferent renal nerve activity on contralateral renal overflow of noradrenaline and dopamine to plasma in the dog. Acta Physiol Scand. 1986;128:119–20.

14. Patel KP, Knuepfer MM. Effect of afferent renal nerve stimulation on blood pressure, heart rate and noradrenergic activity in conscious rats. J Auton Nerv Syst. 1986;17:121–30.

15. Rogenes PR. Single-unit and multiunit analyses of renorenal reflexes elicited by stimulation of renal chemoreceptors in the rat. J Auton Nerv Syst. 1982;6:143–56.

16. Bradley T, Hjemdahl P. Further studies on renal nerve stimulation induced release of noradrenaline and dopamine from the canine kidney in situ. Acta Physiol Scand. 1984;122:369–79.

17. Oliver JA, Pinto J, Sciacca RR, Cannon PJ. Basal norepinephrine overflow into the renal vein: effect of renal nerve stimulation. Am J Physiol. 1980;239:F371–7.

18. DiBona GF, Esler M. Translational medicine: the antihypertensive effect of renal denervation. Am J Physiol Regul Integr Comp Physiol. 2010;298:R245–53.

19. Katholi RE, Whitlow PL, Winternitz SR, Oparil S. Importance of the renal nerves in established two-kidney, one clip Goldblatt hypertension. Hypertension. 1982;4:166–74.

20. Gattone II VH, Siqueira Jr TM, Powell CR, Trambaugh CM, Lingeman JE, Shalhav AL. Contribution of renal innervation to hypertension in rat autosomal dominant polycystic kidney disease. Exp Biol Med. 2008;233:952–95.

21. Page IH. The effect on renal efficiency of lowering arterial blood pressure in cases of essential hypertension and nephritis. J Clin Invest. 1934;13:909–15.

22. Page IH, Heuer GJ. The effect of renal denervation on the level of arterial blood pressure and renal function in essential hypertension. J Clin Invest. 1935;14:27–30.

23. Smithwick RH, Thompson JE. Splanchnicectomy for essential hypertension; results in 1,266 cases. JAMA. 1953;152:1501–4.

24. Krum H, Schlaich M, Whitbourn R, Sobotka PA, Sadowski J, Bartus K, Kapelak B, Walton A, Sievert H, Thambar S, Abraham WT, Esler M. Catheter-based renal sympathetic denervation for resistant hypertension: a multicentre safety and proof-of-principle cohort study. Lancet. 2009;373:1275–81.

25. Symplicity HTN-2 Investigators, Esler MD, Krum H, Sobotka PA, Schlaich MP, Schmieder RE, Böhm M. Renal sympathetic denervation in patients with treatment-resistant hypertension (The Symplicity HTN-2 Trial): a randomised controlled trial. Lancet. 2010;376:1903–9.

26. Krum H, Schlaich MP, Böhm M, Mahfoud F, Rocha-Singh K, Katholi R, Esler MD. Percutaneous renal denervation in patients with treatment-resistant hypertension: final 3-year report of the Symplicity HTN-1 study. Lancet. 2013. doi:10.1016/S0140-6736(13)62192-3. pii: S0140-6736(13)62192-3.

27. Esler MD, Krum H, Schlaich M, Schmieder RE, Böhm M, Sobotka PA, Symplicity HTN-2 Investigators. Renal sympathetic denervation for treatment of drug-resistant hypertension: one-year results from the Symplicity HTN-2 randomized, controlled trial. Circulation. 2012;126:2976–82.

28. Mahfoud F, Ukena C, Schmieder RE, Cremers B, Rump LC, Vonend O, Weil J, Schmidt M, Hoppe UC, Zeller T, Bauer A, Ott C, Blessing E, Sobotka PA, Krum H, Schlaich M, Esler M, Böhm M. Ambulatory blood pressure changes after renal sympathetic denervation in patients with resistant hypertension. Circulation. 2013;128:132–40.

29. Ott C, Mahfoud F, Schmid A, Ditting T, Sobotka PA, Veelken R, Spies A, Ukena C, Laufs U, Uder M, Böhm M, Schmieder RE.

30. Schlaich MP, Sobotka PA, Krum H, Lambert E, Esler MD. Renal sympathetic-nerve ablation for uncontrolled hypertension. N Engl J Med. 2009;361:932–4.

31. Doumas M, Douma S. Renal sympathetic denervation: the jury is still out. Lancet. 2010;376:1878–80.

32. Ukena C, Mahfoud F, Kindermann I, Barth C, Lenski M, Kindermann M, Brandt MC, Hoppe UC, Krum H, Esler M, Sobotka PA, Böhm M. Cardiorespiratory response to exercise after renal sympathetic denervation in patients with resistant hypertension. J Am Coll Cardiol. 2011;58:1176–82.

33. Cole CR, Blackstone EH, Pashkow FJ, Snader CE, Lauer MS. Heart-rate recovery immediately after exercise as a predictor of mortality. N Engl J Med. 1999;341:1351–7.

34. Jouven X, Empana JP, Schwartz PJ, Desnos M, Courbon D, Ducimetière P. Heart-rate profile during exercise as a predictor of sudden death. N Engl J Med. 2005;352:1951–8.

35. Ukena C, Mahfoud F, Spies A, Kindermann I, Linz D, Cremers B, Laufs U, Neuberger HR, Böhm M, et al. Effects of renal sympathetic denervation on heart rate and atrioventricular conduction in patients with resistant hypertension. Int J Cardiol. 2013;167:2846–51. dx.doi.org/10.1016/j.iicard.2012.07.027.

36. Smit AA, Halliwill JR, Low PA, Wieling W. Pathophysiological basis of orthostatic hypotension in autonomic failure. J Physiol. 1999;519:1–10.

37. Laurent S, Schlaich M, Esler M. New drugs, procedures, and devices for hypertension. Lancet. 2012;380:591–600.

38. Jardine DL, Melton IC, Crozier IG, English S, Bennett SI, Frampton CM, Ikram H. Decrease in cardiac output and muscle sympathetic activity during vasovagal syncope. Am J Physiol Heart Circ Physiol. 2002;282:H1804–9.

39. Mosqueda-Garcia R, Furlan R, Fernandez-Violante R, Desai T, Snell M, Jarai Z, Ananthram V, Robertson RM, Robertson D. Sympathetic and baroreceptor reflex function in neurally mediated syncope evoked by tilt. J Clin Invest. 1997;99:2736–44.

40. Morillo CA, Eckberg DL, Ellenbogen KA, Beightol LA, Hoag JB, Tahvanainen KU, Kuusela TA. Diedrich AM Vagal and sympathetic mechanisms in patients with orthostatic vasovagal syncope. Circulation. 1997;96:2509–13.

41. Wallin BG, Sundlöf G. Sympathetic outflow to muscles during vasovagal syncope. J Auton Nerv Syst. 1982;6:287–91.

42. Lenski M, Mahfoud F, Razouk A, Ukena C, Lenski D, Barth C, Linz D, Laufs U, Kindermann I, Böhm M. Orthostatic function after renal sympathetic denervation in patients with resistant hypertension. Int J Cardiol. 2013;169:418–24.

43. Rafanelli C, Offidani E, Gostoli S, Roncuzzi R. Psychological correlates in patients with different levels of hypertension. Psychiatry Res. 2012;198:154–60.

44. Bajkó Z, Szekeres CC, Kovács KR, Csapó K, Molnár S, Soltész P, Nyitrai E, Magyar MT, Oláh L, Bereczki D, Csiba L. Anxiety, depression and autonomic nervous system dysfunction in hypertension. J Neurol Sci. 2012;317:112–6.

45. Brown ES, Varghese FP, McEwen BS. Association of depression with medical illness: does cortisol play a role? Biol Psychiatry. 2004;55:1–9.

46. Barton DA, Dawood T, Lambert EA, Esler MD, Haikerwal D, Brenchley C, Socratous F, Kaye DM, Schlaich MP, Hickie I, Lambert GW. Sympathetic activity in major depressive disorder: identifying those at increased cardiac risk? J Hypertens. 2007;25:2117–24.

47. Lambert GW, Hering D, Esler MD, Marusic P, Lambert EA, Tanamas SK, Shaw J, Krum H, Dixon JB, Barton DA, Schlaich MP. Health-related quality of life after renal denervation in patients with treatment-resistant hypertension. Hypertension. 2012;60:1479–84.

48. Lenski D, Kindermann I, Lenski M, Ukena C, Bunz M, Mahfoud F, Böhm M. Anxiety, depression, quality of life and stress in patients with resistant hypertension before and after catheter-based renal sympathetic denervation. EuroIntervention. 2013;9:700–8.

49. Böhm M, Linz D, Urban D, Mahfoud F, Ukena C. Renal sympathetic denervation: applications in hypertension and beyond. Nat Rev Cardiol. 2013;10:465–76.

50. Mahfoud F, Cremers B, Janker J, Link B, Vonend O, Ukena C, Linz D, Schmieder R, Rump LC, Kindermann I, Sobotka PA, Krum H, Scheller B, Schlaich M, Laufs U, Böhm M. Renal hemodynamics and renal function after catheter-based renal sympathetic denervation in patients with resistant hypertension. Hypertension. 2012;60:419–24.

51. Linz D, Mahfoud F, Schotten U, Ukena C, Hohl M, Neuberger HR, Wirth K, Böhm M. Renal sympathetic denervation provides ventricular rate control but does not prevent atrial electrical remodeling during atrial fibrillation. Hypertension. 2013;61:225–31.

52. Ukena C, Bauer A, Mahfoud F, Schreieck J, Neuberger HR, Eick C, Sobotka PA, Gawaz M, Böhm M. Renal sympathetic denervation for treatment of electrical storm: first-in-man experience. Clin Res Cardiol. 2012;101:63–7.

53. Witkowski A, Prejbisz A, Florczak E, Kądziela J, Śliwiński P, Bieleń P, Michałowska I, Kabat M, Warchoł E, Januszewicz M, Narkiewicz K, Somers VK, Sobotka PA, Januszewicz A. Effects of renal sympathetic denervation on blood pressure, sleep apnea course, and glycemic control in patients with resistant hypertension and sleep apnea. Hypertension. 2011;58:559–65.

54. Brandt MC, Mahfoud F, Reda S, Schirmer SH, Erdmann E, Böhm M, Hoppe UC. Renal sympathetic denervation reduces left ventricular hypertrophy and improves cardiac function in patients with resistant hypertension. J Am Coll Cardiol. 2012;59:901–9.

55. Davies JE, Manisty CH, Petraco R, Barron AJ, Unsworth B, Mayet J, Hamady M, Hughes AD, Sever PS, Sobotka PA, Francis DP. First-in-man safety evaluation of renal denervation for chronic systolic heart failure: primary outcome from REACH-Pilot study. Int J Cardiol. 2013;162:189–92.

56. Mahfoud F, Schlaich M, Kindermann I, Ukena C, Cremers B, Brandt MC, Hoppe UC, Vonend O, Rump LC, Sobotka PA, Krum H, Esler M, Böhm M. Effect of renal sympathetic denervation on glucose metabolism in patients with resistant hypertension: a pilot study. Circulation. 2011;123:1940–6.

Physiological Rationale for Renal Denervation Therapy in Hypertension

C. Venkata S. Ram and A. Sreenivas Kumar

Systemic hypertension is of major importance world-wide due to its significant public health implications. Hypertension is a common clinical disorder encountered not just in the western or industrialized world but also in underdeveloped and emerging countries. In most populations (at least in the western hemisphere) one in three individuals have hypertension and hence it is the largest contributor to excessive mortality and morbidity. Hypertension is a merciless killer without sparing the attributes of age, gender, and socioeconomic status. Despite remarkable advances in the physiology, and pharmacology of hypertension, blood pressure (BP) control rates are quite low globally. Whatever the reasons may be, most patients with hypertension fail to achieve recommended goal BP levels.

Even among treated patients, some exhibit "resistant hypertension" which can lead to accelerated target organ damage and serious health consequences. Thus, resistant hypertension is recognized as a special clinical entity. Patients with resistant hypertension require greater attention from the medical community and closer surveillance. While the etio-pathogenesis of resistant hypertension is complex and multi-fold, sympathetic nervous system (SNS) play a pivotal contributory role [1–4]. The importance of SNS in BP regulation has been established for many years. And a link between SNS and hypertension is an accepted interlinking mechanism. Due to the integrated connection between SNS and hypertension, the earliest anti-hypertensive drugs were all designed and developed to inhibit the activity of

C.V.S. Ram, MD, MA, CP, FACC (✉)
Apollo Institute for Blood Pressure Management, Apollo Blood Pressure Clinics, Apollo Hospitals, Hyderabad, AP, India

Texas Blood Pressure Institute, Medical School, University of Texas Southwestern, Dallas, TX, USA
e-mail: ramv@dneph.com; drram_v@apollohospitals.com

A.S. Kumar
Cardiology Department, Continental Hospitals, Hyderabad, AP, India
e-mail: arramraj@yahoo.com

SNS – either directly or indirectly. Thus, anti-sympathetic drugs have always remained as an inevitable ingredient and an cornerstone of pharmacotherapy of hypertension. Either as an initial choice or add-on option, sympathetic blocking drugs are commonly used world-wide in the long term treatment of hypertension. This chapter covers the physiological rationale of renal denervation therapy in the treatment of hypertension.

SNS and BP (Dys)regulation

Increased activity of SNS results in a parallel increase in the BP level and contributes to the development (and maintenance) of hypertension. Inappropriate or excessive stimulation of SNS causes increased cardiac output (CO), systemic vascular resistance (SVR), and sodium/fluid retention – all of which raise the level of BP. Hypertension is characterised by autonomic imbalance – ↑SNS and ↓parasympathetic tone. In the early stages of hypertension, there is a correlation between the heart rate and BP levels, providing further evidence for the role of SNS in cardiovascular homeostasis [5–7]. An increase in the heart rate is due mainly to decreased parasympathetic tone and an increase in the BP level is due mainly to increased SNS which attests to the concept of autonomic imbalance in hypertension. Increased SNS activity by causing vascular smooth muscle proliferation and remodelling increases the diastolic blood pressure. Norepinephrine (NE) spillover – an index of sympatho-effector nerve stimulation is greater in patients with hypertension than in normotensive controls which supports the theory that increased SNS activity facilitates the development and maintenance of hypertension.

The precise governing pathways of increased SNS activity in hypertension involve various chemoreflex and baroreceptor aberrations at the peripheral and central levels of neurogenic regulation [8]. Certain chemoreflex functions are altered in hypertension via enhancement of sympathetic activity; for example apnea/hypoxia augment the chemoreceptor activity and thus to exaggerated sympathetic function. A classical clinical correlate of this mechanism is hypertension in patients with obstructive sleep apnea syndrome. Baroreceptors (in the arterial tree) are reset to a higher pressure level in hypertension, compared to matched normotensive controls. The baroreceptor resetting in hypertension is mainly through neurogenic mechanisms and to some extent mediated by central actions of angiotensin-II [9]. Sympathetic stimulation in hypertension is amplified by angiotensin-II. The activity of SNS in hypertension is dictated partially by the renin-angiotensin-aldosterone system (RAAS).

Persistent stimulation of SNS in hypertension induces left ventricular hypertrophy and vascular remodelling demonstrating its direct influence on target organ damage and dysfunction. SNS also influences the release of transforming growth factor-β, fibroblast growth factor and insulin-like growth factor – all of which contribute to increased vascular resistance and decreased blood flow. Neurogenic factors, thus mediate the development of hypertension and target organ damage.

The ultimate actions of SNS on cardiovascular hemeostasis are triggered at the cell surface receptors – α and β. These two main receptors are further differentiated into various subtypes – α1, α-2, β1, β2 and β-3, etc. The process of receptor signaling is critical to the vascular actions of catecholamines. Activation or deactivation of adrenergic receptors leads to simultaneous and instant changes in the heart rate and blood pressure. Increased expression of adrenergic receptors has been noted in hypertension. Neuronal cell bodies are located lateral to the spinal cord and anterior to the vertebral column. Sympathetic afferents terminate in the spinal cord and there is a feedback system to the central nervous system (CNS). The areas of brain concerned with cardiovascular control are – nucleus tractus solitarius (NTS), rustroventrolateral medulla (RVLM), area prostrema (AP), and caudal ventrolateral medulla (CVLM). All these centers are under the tonic influence of afferent and efferent nerve traffic. Although the spinal cord components may catalyse some of the mediator functions of catecholamine, it is the higher centers in brain which contribute to the development of systemic hypertension.

Renal Sympathetic Activity: Relationship to SNS

With the recognition that sympathetic blocking drugs like phentolemine increase renal blood flow in hypertension, the role of renal sympathetic activity in hypertension has been extensively studied [10]. It is now established that renal nerve stimulation increases renal vascular resistance, decreases sodium and water excretion, and stimulates renin secretion – thus elevating the systemic blood pressure [11]. Direct assessments of function of renal sympathetic nerves have shown increased activity in hypertension; and renal denervation prevents or reverses experimental hypertension. Therefore, it has become evident that renal sympathetic activity exerts a pathogenetic role in the hypertension.

Renal sympathetic activity not only has an effect on the vasculature but also on the renal tubular functions [12]. The degree of renal sympathetic stimulation impacts renin secretion, sodium/fluid absorption, and renal blood flow; and these mechanisms raise the systemic blood pressure. It can thus be hypothesized that the SNS plays a contributory role in the development of hypertension in part mediated by renal sympathetic activity. The autonomic control of the kidney is predominantly sympathetic in nature correlated anatomically by a dense net-work of sympathetic neurons in the kidney [13].

The sympatho-renal axis defines the dual contribution of the kidney in causing neurogenic hypertension. Both the efferent and afferent neuronal signals between and kidney the central nervous system create a loop of multiple hemodynamic abnormalities raising the systemic blood pressure.

Renal Afferent Sympathetic Activity

Mechanoreceptors populating the renal pelvis and chemoreceptors populating the renal interstitium influence the central sympathetic activity. In the human model of progressive renal disease, it was shown that muscle sympathetic nerve activity (MSNA) is enhanced [14] which can be reversed by nephrectomy. In experimental models, progression of renal disease is accompanied by increased concentrations of norepinephrine in the hypothalamus. These findings are advanced by the demonstration that it is the (innervated) kidney but not the uremic environment which is responsible for excessive sympathetic activity. Ischemia/hypoxia of chronic kidney disease trigger afferent signals to the brain which in turn promote efferent signals to the kidney – with resultant hypertension. The restoration of normal blood pressure by renal denervation in the laboratory model of renovascular hypertension confirms the role of renal afferents in hypertension. Additionally, adenosine infusions (by stimulating the renal afferent activity) raise the systemic blood pressure. The chemoreceptor mediated renal afferent sympathetic activity (activated in patients with chronic kidney disease) is restored by oxygen inhalation. In polycystic kidney disease, renal ischemia occurs as a result of compression by the cysts and hypertension and in this condition is reversed by renal denervation. The aforementioned studies and data confirm the renal contribution to central sympathetic drive – a phenomenon which can be blunted by deafferentiation of the renal nerves. Decreasing the renal afferent activity reduces the "excitatory input" to the central nervous system which in turn lowers the systemic vascular resistance, the cardiac output, and the heart rate [15–18].

The unmyelinated (afferent) fibers from the kidney transmit "sensory" information to the central nervous system [19, 20]. The afferents from the kidney enter the neuronal sites at both the spinal and supraspinal levels. The cardiovascular centers in the brainstem receive the inputs directly from the renal afferent network of nerves. These renal afferents transmit the mechanoreceptor and chemoreceptor information from the kidney to the brain. The chemoreceptors are mainly found in the renal pelvis whereas the mechanoreceptors are localized in the pelvis plus the renal cortex as well. Electrical stimulation of the renal afferent nerves causes sympathoexcitation and enhancement of cardiovascular reflexes in the brain and augmentation of systemic blood pressure. Renal afferent denervation by dorsal rhizotomy prevents the onset of hypertension. Stimulation of renal afferents also enhances the central release of vasopressin and oxytocin [21] but the role of these hormones in blood pressure regulation is not known.

Renal Efferent Sympathetic Activity

Stimulation of renal efferent nerves increases renin secretion, tubular absorption of sodium and decreases the renal blood flow [16, 20]. These consequences of renal efferent function raise the systemic blood pressure. Increased release of renin (via efferent nerve activity) [22] contributes to hypertension via multiplicity of effects including angiotensin-II and aldosterone generation. The obliteration of renal efferent activity is therefore a logical therapeutic target to restore normal blood pressure. Experimental renal deefferentiation has been shown to decrease the blood pressure in various models of hypertension.

The efferent renal sympathetic nerves modulate the regional and systemic hemodynamics through the release of local neurotransmitters. It is possible that norepinephrine and neuro-peptide Y are the candidates involved in the efferent signalling pathway. Renal efferents also reduce the glomerular filtration rate (GFR) by selectively constricting the afferent arteriolar apparatus in the kidney. The renal efferent nerves form a dense web in and around the anatomical structures linked to renal cardiovascular regulation – juxtaglomerular apparatus, loop of Henle, and the renal tubules. Renal efferent stimulation stimulates protein kinase which plays a key role in the mitogenesis and hypertrophy of renal vasculature.

Renal sympathetic nerve activity (RSNA) has a pathogenetic role in the development of hypertension. Both the afferent and efferent sympathetic activities govern the factors in hypertension – SNS, renin stimulation, sodium balance, cardiac output, heart rate, and systemic vascular resistance. Support for the role of RSNA in hypertension is evidenced by the restoration of blood pressure by renal denervation [23–25]. RSNA directly or indirectly influences the fundamental mechanisms and concepts of blood pressure control. There is a sound physiological basis for the kidney – brain link through the network of efferent and afferent bidirectional anatomical pathways. Renal sympathetic nerve activity therefore plays a role in blood pressure regulation in physiological and pathophysiological conditions.

Renal Sympathetic Denervation and Blood Pressure Regulation

In the earlier years of last century, non-selective sympathectomy was shown to reduce the blood pressure dramatically in human hypertension. In many patients, crude non-selective surgical sympathetectomy provided a dramatic relief from severe hypertension [26–28]. While this procedure effectively lowered the blood pressure, it was associated with morbidity and disabling postural hypotension which impaired the patients' quality of life. The surgical experience with crude sympathetectomy reflected the pivotal role of SNS and RSNA in the genesis of hypertension. Surgical renal denervation by interrupting the sympathetic outflow and input to the kidney caused a fall in the blood pressure, inhibited renin release, and augmented natriuresis/diuresis.

The newer technique of causing renal denervation selectively with low-frequency radio-ablation applied to the endothelial lining has been shown to be safe and effective in the treatment of hypertension. The procedure involves circumferential application of radiofrequency energy in both renal arteries. Successful denervation with this technique causes a substantial drop in systemic blood pressure, presumably by intercepting the neural traffic (afferent and efferent) between the kidney and the brain. In other words, selective renal denervation (RDN) produces a systemic and renal antisympathetic effect resulting in lowering of the blood pressure).

Clinical studies [29–31] have shown a remarkable fall in blood pressure as a result of RDN in patients with resistant hypertension (Table 2.1). The anti-hypertensive effect was sustained over a period of 2 years implying the durability of RDN in the treatment of resistant hypertension. RDN therapy caused a measurable reduction in the indices of sympathetic activity includes muscle sympathetic nerve activity (RSNA).

Table 2.1 Proof of principle: related changes in underlying physiology

	Baseline	1 month	Δ (%)
Office BP (mmHg)	161/107	141/90	
Renal NE spillover (ng/min)			
Left kidney	72	37	−48
Right kidney	79	20	−75
Total body NE spillover (ng/min)	600	348	−42
Plasma renin (μg/l/h)	0.3	0.15	−50
Renal plasma flow (ml/min)	719	1,126	57%

Created using data from Schlaich et al. [31]

Conclusions

Sympathetic nervous system (SNS) plays a major role in the pathogenesis of hypertension. The activity of SNS is particularly abnormal in resistant hypertension. It is firmly established that neurogenic factors mediate the onset and progression of hypertension. The link between the kidney and the brain has the anatomic basis via renal afferent and efferent nerves, correlating with excessive SNS activity in all grades of hypertension. This pathophysiological connection between the kidney and brain is confirmed by enhanced muscle sympathetic nerve activity and non-epinephrine spill over in human hypertension. The results of RDN therapy in hypertension suggest a reduction in the SNS activity and renal nerve traffic. The pathophysiologic mechanisms discussed explain the physiological rationale for renal denervation therapy in hypertension. While the gross therapeutic consequences of renal denervation on the mechanisms of hypertension are evident, the molecular and cellular correlates of such mechanisms remain to be elucidated.

References

1. Brook RD, Julius S. Autonomic imbalance, hypertension, and cardiovascular risk. Am J Hypertens. 2000;13:112S–22.
2. Esler M, Jennings G, Korner P, Willett I, Dudley F, Hasking G, Anderson W, Lambert G. Assessment of human sympathetic nervous system activity from measurements of norepinephrine turnover. Hypertension. 1988;11:3–20.
3. Esler M, Jennings G, Lambert G, Meredith I, Horne M, Eisenhofer G. Overflow of catecholamine neurotransmitters to the circulation: source, fate, and functions. Physiol Rev. 1990;70:963–85.
4. Esler M, Jennings G, Lambert G. Noradrenaline release and the pathophysiology of primary human hypertension. Am J Hypertens. 1989;2:140S–6.
5. Esler M. The sympathetic system and hypertension. Am J Hypertens. 2000;13:99S–105.
6. Esler M, Jennings G, Biviano B, et al. Mechanism of elevated plasma noradrenaline in the course of essential hypertension. J Cardiovasc Pharmacol. 1986;8:S39–43.
7. Kim JR, Kiefe CI, Liu K, Williams OD, Jacobs Jr DR, Oberman A. Heart rate and subsequent blood pressure in young adults: the CARDIA study. Hypertension. 1999;33:640–6.
8. Mark AL. The sympathetic nervous system in hypertension: a potential long-term regulator of arterial pressure. J Hypertens Suppl. 1996;14:S159–65.
9. Chapleau MW, Hajduczok G, Abboud FM. Mechanisms of resetting of arterial baroreceptors: an overview. Am J Med Sci. 1988;295:327–34.
10. Hollenburg NK, Adams DF, Solomon H, Chenitz WR, Burger BM, Abrams HL, et al. Renal vascular tone in essential and secondary hypertension: hemodynamic and angiographic responses to vasodilators. Medicine (Baltimore). 1975;54:29–44.
11. Katholi RE. Renal nerves in the pathogenesis of hypertension in experimental animals and humans. Am J Physiol. 1983;245:F1–14.
12. Di Bona GF, Kopp UC. Neural control of renal function. Physiol Rev. 1997;77:76–155.
13. Luff SE, Hengstberger SG, McLachlan EM, Anderson WP. Distribution of sympathetic neuroeffector junctions in the juxtaglomerular region of the rabbit kidney. J Auton Nerv Syst. 1992;40:239–53.
14. Hering D, Zdrojewski Z, Krol E, Kara T, Kucharska W, Somers VK, Rutkowski B, Narkiewicz K. Tonic chemoreflex activation contributes to the elevated muscle sympathetic nerve activity in patients with chronic renal failure. J Hypertens. 2007;25:157–61.
15. Di Bona GF. Neural control of the kidney: past, present, and future. Hypertension. 2003;41:621–4.
16. Di Bona GF. Sympathetic nervous system influences on the kidney: role in hypertension. Am J Hypertens. 1989;2(Suppl):119S–24.
17. Barajas L, Liu L, Powers K. Anatomy of the renal innervation: Intrarenal aspects and ganglia of origin. Can J Physiol Pharmacol. 1992;70:735–49.
18. Barajas L, Muller J. The innervation of the juxtaglomerular apparatus and surrounding tubules. A quantitative analysis by serial section electron microscopy. J Ultrastruct Res. 1973;43:107–32.
19. Kopp UC, Cicha MZ, Smith LA. Impaired interaction between efferent and afferent renal nerve activity in SHR involves increased activation of alpha2-adrenoceptors. Hypertension. 2011;57:640–7.
20. Kopp UC. Renorenal reflexes: neural and functional responses. Fed Proc. 1985;44:2834–9.
21. Caverson MM, Ciriello J. Effect of stimulation of afferent renal nerves on plasma levels of vasopressin. Am J Physiol. 1987;252:R801–7.
22. Holmer S, Rinne B, Eckardt KU, Le Hir M, Schricker K, Kaissling B, Riegger G, Kurtz A. Role of renal nerves for the expression of renin in adult rat kidney. Am J Physiol. 1994;266:F738–45.
23. Doumas M, Faselis C, Papademetriou V. Renal sympathetic denervation and systemic hypertension. Am J Cardiol. 2010;105:570–6.
24. Hering D, Lambert EA, Marusic P, Walton AS, Krum H, Lambert GW, Esler MD, Schlaich MP. Substantial reduction in single sympathetic nerve firing after renal denervation in patients with resistant hypertension. Hypertension. 2013;61:457–64.

25. Krum H, Schlaich M, Whitbourn R, et al. Catheter-based renal sympathetic denervation for resistant hypertension. A multicentre safety and proof-of-principle cohort study. Lancet. 2009;373:1275–81.

26. Morrissey DM, Brookes VS, Cooke WT. Sympathectomy in the treatment of hypertension: review of 122 cases. Lancet. 1953;1:403–8.

27. Smithwick RH, Thompson JE. Splanchnicectomy for essential hypertension: results in 1,266 cases. JAMA. 1953;152:1501–4.

28. Smithwick RH. Hypertensive vascular disease: results of and indications for splanchnicectomy. J Chronic Dis. 1955;1:477–96.

29. Symplicity HTN-1 Investigators. Catheter-based renal sympathetic denervation for resistant hypertension: durability of blood pressure reduction out to 24 months. Hypertension. 2011;57:911–7.

30. Symplicity HTN-2 Investigators. Renal sympathetic denervation in patients with treatment-resistant hypertension. (The Symplicity HTN-2 Trial): a randomized controlled trial. Lancet. 2010;376:1903–9.

31. Schlaich MP, Sobotka PA, Krum H, Lambert E, Esler MD. Renal sympathetic-nerve ablation for uncontrolled hypertension. N Engl J Med. 2009;361:932–4. doi:10.1056/NEJMc0904179.

Preclinical Model and Histopathology Translational Medicine and Renal Denervation

Kenichi Sakakura, Elena Ladich, Fumiyuki Otsuka, Kazuyuki Yahagi, Frank D. Kolodgie, Michael Joner, and Renu Virmani

Key Points

- The swine model is frequently used for the preclinical study, since the anatomy of the renovascular system is similar to that of humans.
- A semi-quantitative ordinal grading system is useful for the evaluation of the histopathologic changes induced by renal denervation.
- Appropriate time points (acute, sub-acute, or chronic) must be selected before conducting preclinical study.

Arterial hypertension is a major health concern in the developed and developing world. More than a quarter of the world's adult population was affected by hypertension in 2000, and this proportion is expected to increase by 2025 to 29 % [1]. Hypertension is associated with an increase in the risk of myocardial infarction, heart failure, stroke, and kidney disease [2]. Each difference incremental increase in BP of 20 mmHg systolic or 10 mmHg diastolic doubles the risk of death from stroke or ischemic heart disease for individuals aged 40–69 years [3]. Although antihypertensive medications are the first-line of treatment for blood pressure control in hypertensive patients, uncontrolled hypertension rates have a high prevalence especially in older Americans, non-Hispanic blacks, diabetic individuals, and patients with chronic kidney disease [4]. Furthermore, the prevalence of resistant hypertension, which is defined as failure to achieve control of blood pressure (BP) ($\leq$150/90 in ages $\geq$60 years; $\leq$140/90 in ages <60 years) [5] despite treatment with optimal doses of three or more antihypertensive medications

(including diuretics), is as high as 12–15 % of all hypertensive patients [6–8].

Renal sympathetic denervation is a new treatment option for resistant hypertension. Catheter-radiofrequency (RF) based renal denervation has demonstrated its efficacy and safety in the SYMPLICITY-HTN1, SYMPLICITY-HTN2 and EnligHTN trials [9–11]. Furthermore, the decrease in blood pressure after RF renal sympathetic denervation has been shown to persist for 3 years in SYMPLICITY-HTN1 trial [12]. These small studies have encouraged the development of new technologies such as RF ablation with saline irrigation, extracorporeal focused ultrasound, and peri-adventitial injection of ethanol [13–16]. However, recently Medtronic, Inc. (Minneapolis, MN) announced that the SYMPLICITY-HTN3 hypertension trial failed to meet its primary efficacy endpoint [17]. The SYMPLICITY-HTN3 trial was a pivotal study designed as a prospective, randomized, masked procedure, sham controlled, single-blind trial evaluating the safety and effectiveness of catheter-based bilateral renal denervation for the treatment of uncontrolled hypertension despite compliance with at least three antihypertensive medications of different classes at maximal tolerable doses [18]. Although peer-reviewed results of SYMPLICITY HTN-3 have not published as of yet, the results of SYMPLICITY III will impact all aspect of the renal sympathetic denervation. For the moment many unanswered questions remain, however preclinical studies using different animal models may help researchers and clinicians to find answers.

Preclinical Model

Studies carried out in small rodents have assessed the effect of renal sympathetic denervation [19–21], however, the current percutaneous procedures are not applicable to small animals. Larger animals such as pig, dog, or sheep can be used for the performance of percutaneous renal sympathectomy in preclinical study. The swine preclinical model is the most

K. Sakakura, MD • E. Ladich, MD • F. Otsuka, MD • K. Yahagi, MD
F.D. Kolodgie, PhD • M. Joner, MD • R. Virmani, MD (✉)
CVPath Institute, Inc., 19 Firstfield Road,
Gaithersburg, MD 20878, USA
e-mail: rvirmani@cvpath.org

R.R. Heuser et al. (eds.), *Renal Denervation: A New Approach to Treatment of Resistant Hypertension*,
DOI 10.1007/978-1-4471-5223-1_3, © Springer-Verlag London 2015

frequently used since the anatomy of renal vasculature and sympathetic nerve distribution closely mimics that of man [22, 23]. Recently, Tellez et al. have reported the renal artery sympathetic nerve distribution in the porcine model [24]. They investigated a total of five domestic Yorkshire swine, and showed that the nerve counts were greatest in the proximal region (45.62 %) with a gradual decrease distally (mid: 24.58 %; distal: 29.79 %) [24]. Also, 52 % of all nerves were located within 2.5 mm from the arterial wall [24]. It is most important to determine the differences in nerve anatomy, between swine and human as the former is used to predict the likely outcomes in man. Atherton et al. reported the nerve distribution in nine renal arteries collected from five human cases [25]. They summarized that 90.5 % of all nerves existed within 2.0 mm of the renal artery lumen, and the number of nerves tended to increase along the length of the artery from proximal to distal segments (proximal = 216; middle 323; distal = 417) [25]. However, there were many methodological problems. The most important weakness of the study is that they measured nerves only within 2.5 mm of the ring from the lumen. Nerves beyond 2.5 mm were not included or mentioned. Also, the number of samples was too few and no perfusion fixation procedures were used to determine the variability in sampling and fixation artifacts introduced from collapse and shrinkage. We believe that more refined study methods are needed for the evaluation of human sympathetic renal nerve distribution, which must include perfusion fixation, all nerves must be assessed irrespective of distance and minimum of at least 20 individual cases must be studied.

Histologic assessment of nerve injury that will be induced during percutaneous ablation in animal models must be graded systematically and the distance from the lumen of the artery to the presence of nerves circumferentially must be determined. Similarly the extent of renal artery damage must also be graded by a well-developed and reproducible method.

How to Evaluate Histopathology in Preclinical Models

First and foremost all renal arteries must be perfusion pressure fixed at 80–100 mmHg. However, the renal artery length must be determined in vivo upon removal of tissue from the body, especially arteries which undergo shrinkage artifacts. It has been shown that the aorta undergoes marked shrinkage when removed from the body and is estimated to undergo as much as 30–40 % shrinkage but this is dependent on the age of the patient, with younger individuals showing greater shrinkage than older individuals because of loss of elasticity with age. Similarly it has been estimated that 20 % shrinkage occurs just because of fixation and dehydration used prior to sectioning in paraffin.

Semi-quantitative ordinal grading schemes are useful, when changes in the nerve, renal artery, and peri-arterial

soft tissue are evaluated following denervation [26]. When evaluating nerve damage, it is important to mention that tissue damage may affect the peri-neuronal and/or endoneuronal portions of the renal nerves. The assessment of peri-neuronal injury should include inflammation and fibrosis. Although acute-phase nerve injury may not necessarily be accompanied by peri-neuronal inflammation or fibrosis, chronic-phase nerve injury usually exhibits peri-neuronal fibrosis. Vacuolization and digestion chambers are unique findings of endoneuronal damage. Vacuolization is characterized by the presence of vacuolated areas, containing loose connective tissue with rare areas of homogenous eosinophilic staining of cell cytoplasm along with pyknotic nuclei [27]. Digestion chambers are identified by variable amounts of aggregated myelin (eosinophilic hyaline globules) and vacuolated spaces with occasional cells interspersed [27]. Since minimal or mild injury can be seen even in untreated animals form artifacts, moderate and severe injury, typically digestion chambers, frequent vacuolization, and necrosis, are considered as definite injury caused by renal denervation therapy.

Immunohistochemical stains can be used to distinguish the morphological or functional presence of neuronal markers relevant to renal sympathetic activity. However, most markers applied to date are not specific for sympathetic nerves. For example, immunoreactivity against S-100 protein, a marker for Schwann and glial cells, can be observed in all myelinated nerves [28], while neurofilament protein (NFP) as an intermediate filament serves as a marker for neurons and ganglion cells. Glial fibrillary acidic protein (GFAP) is a marker for glial cells and can be used for the recognition of nerve fascicles [29]. On the other hand, immunohistochemisty against tyrosine hydroxylase, which is the enzyme needed for converting tyrosine to DOPA (dihydroxyphenylalanine), is the most frequent marker used for efferent nerve recognition [30], and is graded as absence, very weak, moderate, and strong staining [26]. Therefore, the combination of any one axonal marker (S-100, NFP, or GFAP) and functional marker (tyrosine hydroxylase) would be important for the comprehensive evaluation of preclinical denervation therapy for efferent fiber identification. An immunostain against calcitonin gene-related peptide (CGRP), which is a neurotransmitter of sensory nerves, can be used as a marker of afferent fibers in pigs [24]. However, since the proportion of afferent nerve fibers is too little as compared to efferent nerve fibers, it would be difficult to evaluate treatment effect by using afferent nerve fibers [24]. Representative images of immunohistochemistry are shown in Fig. 3.1.

For the assessment of treatment reactions to the vascular and peri-vascular soft tissue including adjacent organs (kidney, lymph nodes, ureters, and renal veins), ordinal data can be obtained for multiple parameters including endothelial loss, arterial and venous medial injury, inflammation,

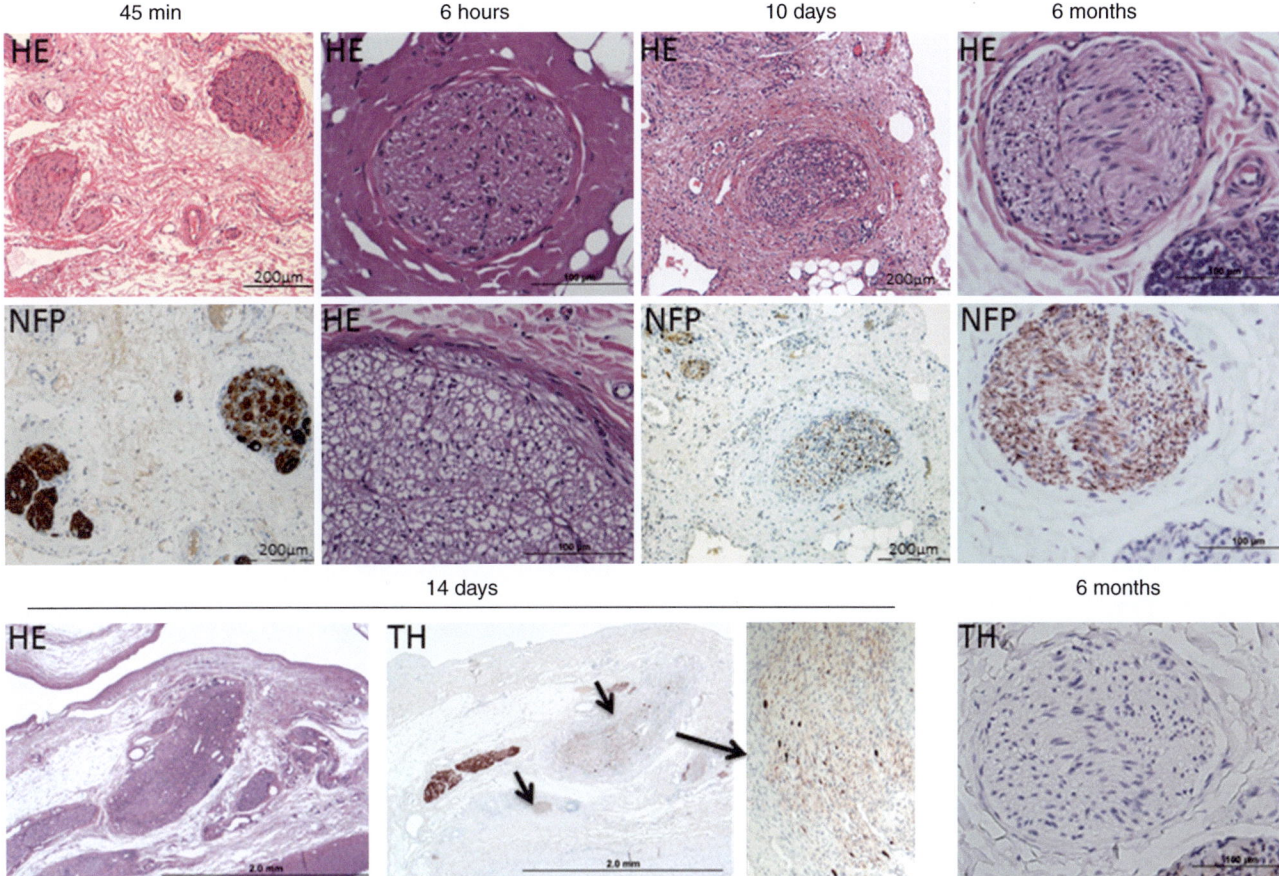

Fig. 3.1 Presentation of nerve fascicles targeted by RF energy at various time points post treatment. Nerve fascicle necrosis and vacuolisation can be found as early as 6 h after treatment using the Medtronic Symplicity™ device. Perineural delamination and fibrosis as well as moderate to severe inflammation are evident at 10 days. At this time point, nerve fascicles displayed less intense staining for neurofilament protein (*NFP*) and tyrosin hydroxylase (*TH*, *arrows*). At 6 months, NFP staining was observed while TH staining was absent (Reprinted from Ammar et al. with permission from Europa Digital & Publishing [31])

degenerative changes and necrosis. Competent endothelium is the most important luminal barrier against activation of coagulation pathways and adhesion of thrombi, it is important especially at early time points to assess its presence or absence. Acute or chronic inflammation can be a sign of irreversible tissue damage and should be evaluated in association with the presence of degenerative changes or necrosis. In addition, distances from affected tissue injury to the intimal luminal surface of the treated arterial segment can be measured with digital morphometry in histologic sections, and these measurements help determine the longitudinal depth of injury.

Histopathology of Radiofrequency Ablation Induced Lesions

RF energy is a form of alternating electrical current that produces an ablation area by two mechanisms: (1) direct resistive heating of the tissue in contact with the catheter tip, and (2) thermal conduction or passive heat transfer to deeper tissue layers [31]. While direct resistive heating in regions close to the RF current is rapid, passive heat transfer to deeper tissue layers is a slower process [32]. Since the heat transfer continues even after discontinuation of RF current delivery, ablation area may expand following RF current cessation. Both bipolar mode and unipolar mode are used for the generation of RF electrical current. RF current is delivered to the target regions through transarterial electrode catheters with a catheter tip ranging in length from 4 to 10 mm.

Steigerwald et al. reported the acute (45 min) and subacute (10 days) histopathologic changes and optical coherence tomographic (OCT) findings following RF ablation in the swine model [33]. Seven pigs underwent RF ablations of the renal arteries utilizing the Symplicity Catheter System (Medtronic Ardian, Mountain View, CA). In the acute phase, angiography showed vessel notches at the site of ablation where the catheter tip had been positioned. OCT at acute phase showed thrombotic material and a loss in signal intensity of the media wall as a result of acute cell depletion and

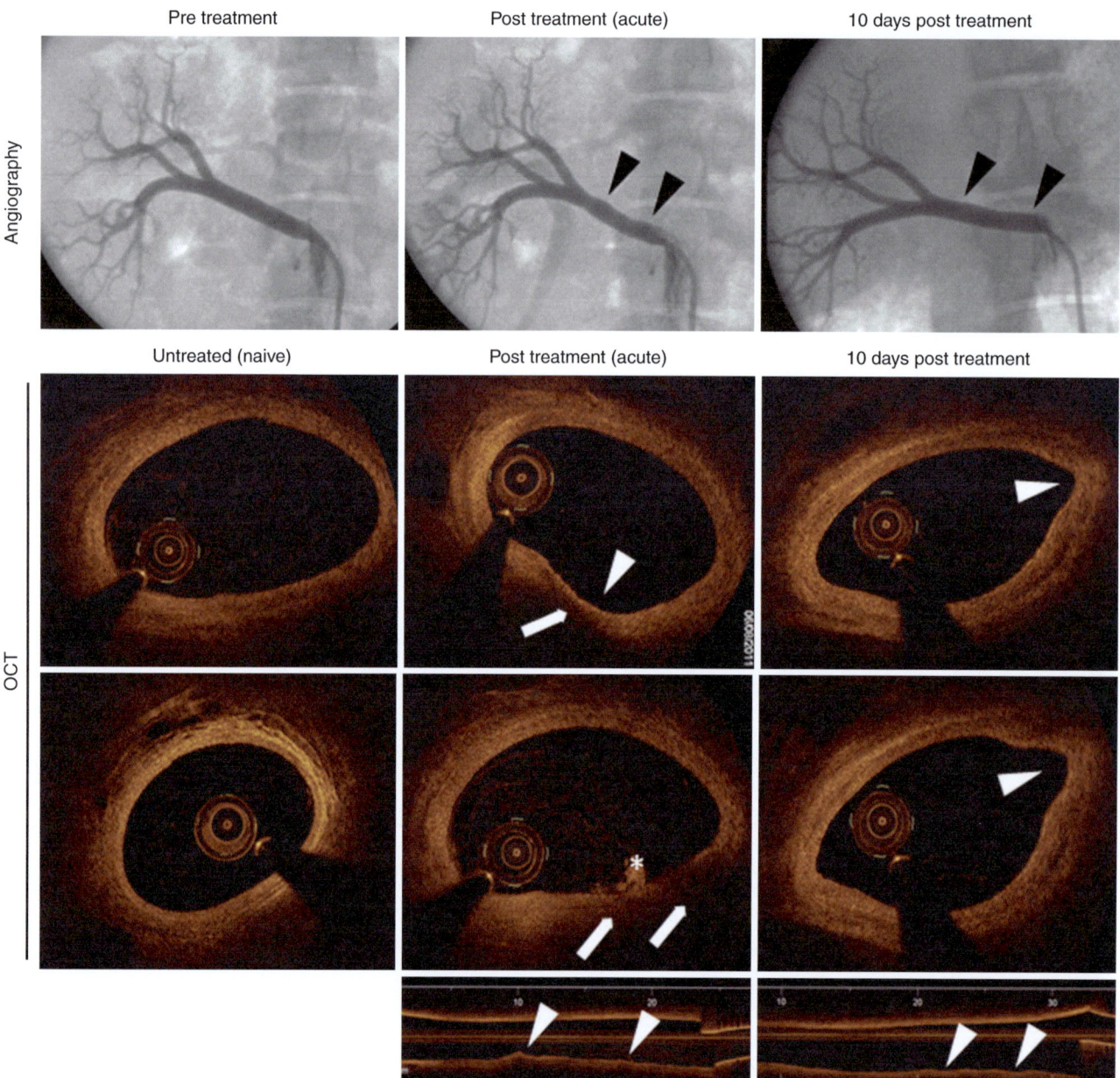

Fig. 3.2 Renal artery imaging per angiography and optical coherence tomography (OCT). *Upper panel* images: angiography images at base line (*left*), acute after radiofrequency therapy (mid) and subacute at 10 days follow-up (*right*). At the acute time point vessel notches are apparent at the lesion site (*black arrow heads*) accompanied by moderate vessel spasm. At 10 days vessel notches are still discernable. *Lower panel* images: OCT images of untreated arteries (*left*), arteries acutely after treatment (mid) and 10 days posttreatment (*right*). Lesion sites were distinguishable from naive tissue in the presence of lumen retraction (*white arrow heads*). The arteries displayed thrombotic material (*) and loss of signal intensity (*white arrows*) acutely after radiofrequency treatment (Reproduced with permission from Steigerwald et al. [33])

cellular edema, whereas thrombotic material was absent at 10-day follow-up (Fig. 3.2). Histologic findings revealed the presence of thrombus formation and depletion of endothelial cells, which were confirmed by absence of von Willebrand factor (vWF) staining (Fig. 3.3) [33]. The arterial media showed edematous cell swelling with a reduction in cellularity [33] (Fig. 3.4). Also, the adjacent adventitial layer showed coagulation necrosis of the connective tissue and cell depletion. The number of nerve fascicles around the treated arteries were significantly affected as compared to the untreated arteries. Immunostaining against neurofilament protein did not show abnormal staining pattern in the acute injured nerves (Fig. 3.5). In the sub-acute phase, re-endothelialization was evident by the presence of vWF staining (91 %) and thrombus was absent (Fig. 3.3) [33]. The recovered media showed fibrotic scar tissue comprising 11 % of the

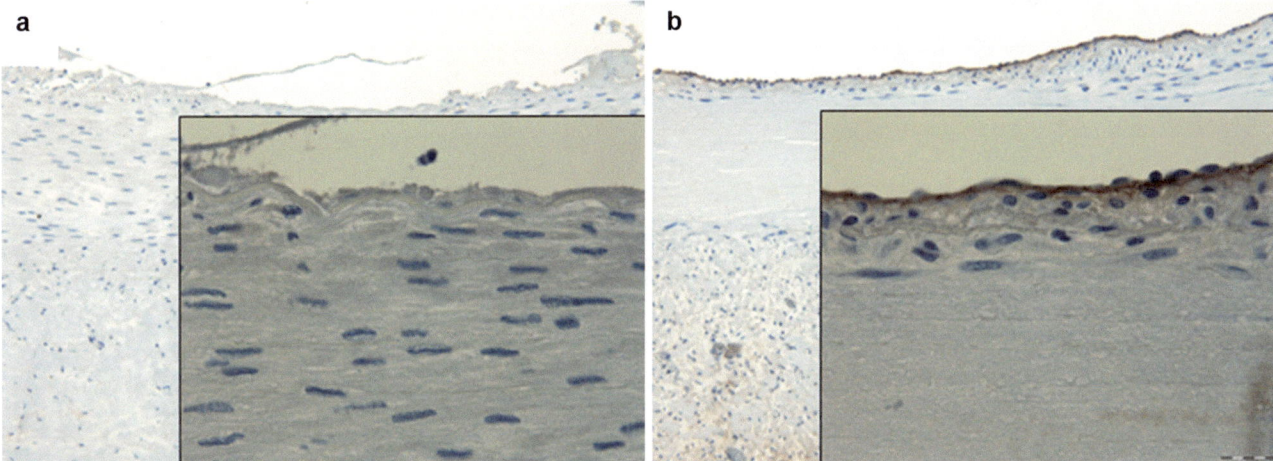

Fig. 3.3 von Willebrand factor immunohistochemical staining of arteries after radiofrequency-based renal sympathetic denervation. *Upper panel* images show the luminal surface of the renal arteries (**a**) acutely and (**b**) sub-acutely after treatment. *Inserts* represent images at higher magnification. There is absence of von Willebrand factor staining acutely following treatment, whereas there is strong staining present in the subacute phase (Reproduced with permission from Steigerwald et al. [33])

media area, however substantial variability in the degree of medial fibrosis was evident (Fig. 3.4) [33]. Nerve fascicles showed degenerative morphologic changes consisting of vacuolization and thickening of the perineurium [33]. Also, Immunostaining against neurofilament protein showed weak or loss of staining (Fig. 3.5) [33]. This study suggests the importance of difference between acute and subacute in the nerve injury and staining characteristics of pre-clinical porcine model following RF sympathetic denervation.

Rippy et al. reported on the chronic histopathologic changes of RF ablation in swine [22]. Seven swine were treated with the Symplicity Catheter System, with angiography and histopathology performed at 6-months. By angiography, there was no restenosis or other vascular complication at 6-month follow-up [22]. Histopathology of the renal arteries at 6-months showed media injury consisting of fibrotic replacement of the smooth muscle cells of the media with disruption of the IEL (10–25 %) [22]. Minimal intimal thickening was observed in treated renal arteries with complete endothelializatio [22] (Fig. 3.6). The renal nerve injury at 6 months was characterized by fibrosis of the nerve fibers and perineural thickening (Fig. 3.6) [22]. These findings show the long-term safety of RF ablation.

Histopathology of Cryoablation Induced Lesions

Cryoablation has evolved as an alternative therapy to conventional RF ablation of the conduction system since the late 1990s [34]. The catheter tip is cooled to −70 °C to −80 °C by instilling liquid NO_2 in the catheter [35]. As compared to the thermal injury caused by RF ablation, the targeted tissue is frozen, and tissue structure remains almost unchanged when used for the treatment of arrhythmia [36]. On the other hand, the limitations include a higher recurrence rate of arrhythmia following cryoablation [35].

Prochnau et al. reported the histopathologic changes of cryoablation of perirenal nerves in a sheep model [37]. A standard seven French cryocatheter, with a 6 mm tip (Freezor Xtra; Medtronic Inc., Minneapolis, MN) was used for renal denervation and the temperature was lowered to minus 81 °C for 4 min. Changes were determined at 48 h, at 1 month, and at 3 months. Histopathology of renal arteries showed focal coagulation necrosis of the intima and media at 48-h [37]. At 1 month, regeneration of endothelium, which was confirmed by immunostaining (CD31), was observed [37]. At 3 months, there was a loss of axons which was confirmed by immunohistochemistry against neurofilament protein [37].

Histopathology of Ultrasound Ablation Induced Lesions

Ultrasound energy has also been applied to achieve renal sympathetic denervation. Overall, both intravascular and extracorporeal ultrasound ablation have been used for renal denervation [14]. Mabin et al. reported the first experience with endovascular ultrasound renal denervation for the treatment of resistant hypertension [38]. They enrolled 11 consecutive patients with resistant hypertension for the treatment by transcatheter renal denervation using the CE-marked PARADISE™ technology (ReCor Medical, Ronkonkoma, NY). Clinically, 3-months results were comparable to RF renal denervation with an average reduction in office and home blood pressure of −36/−17 mmHg and −22/−12 mmHg, respectively.

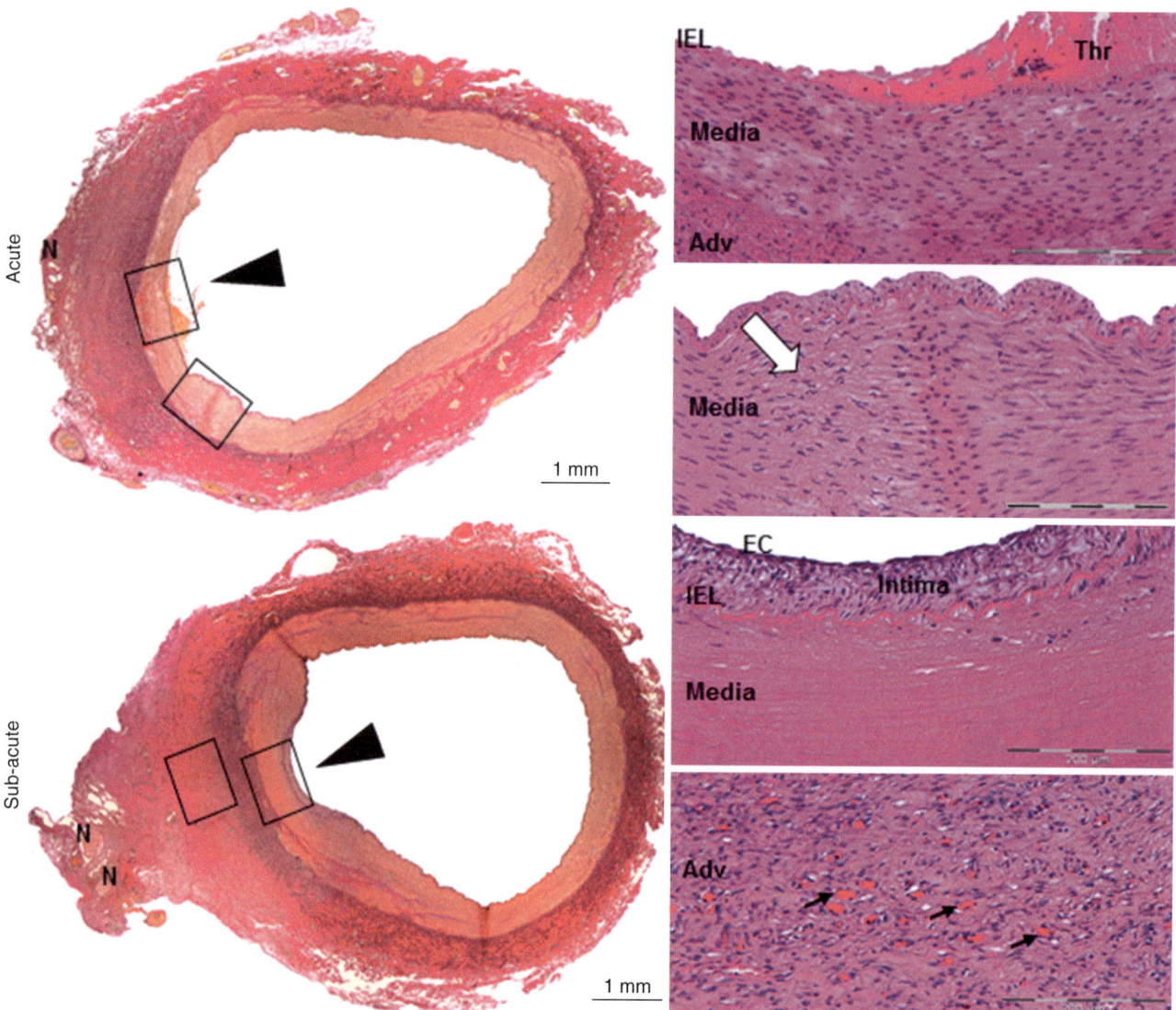

Fig. 3.4 Histological cross-sections of the treated renal arteries. Overview images represent elastica von Giesson-stained sections. Higher magnified images are stained hematoxylin and eosin (*scale bars* represent a length of 200 mm). *Black arrow* heads point to the lesion site, which engages approximately 20 % of the vessel circumference. Remnant nerve fascicles (*N*) are evident for both groups at the lesion site. *Upper panel* images: images of a renal artery cross-section acutely after radiofrequency therapy. At the lesion site the internal elastic lamina (*IEL*) shows minimal disruptions. Accumulation of thrombotic material (*Thr*) is evident at locations absent of an endothelial layer. The media is retracted and displays reduced cellular density and edema (*white arrow*). The adventitia (*Adv*) exhibits coagulation of connective tissue. *Lower panel* images: images of a renal artery cross-section subacutely (10-day follow-up) after radiofrequency therapy. Surface endothelialization (*EC*) is restored and presence of thrombus is no longer discernable. The intima is minimally thickened and the media shows presence of fibrotic scar tissue comprising full media thickness. The adventitia displays inflammatory reaction and vasculogenesis (*black arrows*) (Reproduced with permission from Steigerwald et al. [33])

On the other hand, high-intensity focused ultrasound has been developed to noninvasively ablate tissue by extracorporeal delivering of focused acoustic energy, and has been used to ablate deep solid tissue like kidney, liver, and uterine tumors [14, 39–41], and more recently brain and glaucoma [42, 43]. Wang et al. reported 6 and 28 days histopathologic findings following extracorporeal high-intensity focused ultrasound (HIFU) (36.3 ± 2.8 HIFU emission in each animal) delivered to the peri-renal tissues in the canine model

[14]. Following ablation at 28-days blood pressure and plasma noradrenaline levels were significantly decreased as compared to baseline. Gross findings at 6 day showed several hemorrhagic spots on the fatty tissue around the renal arteries also ablation lesions were observed on the renal artery adventitia following removal of the fatty tissue. At 28 days, the slightly yellow fatty tissue was adhered to the target lesion but the lesions of the fatty tissue had disappeared [14]. Histopathology at 6 day showed pyknotic nuclei and absence

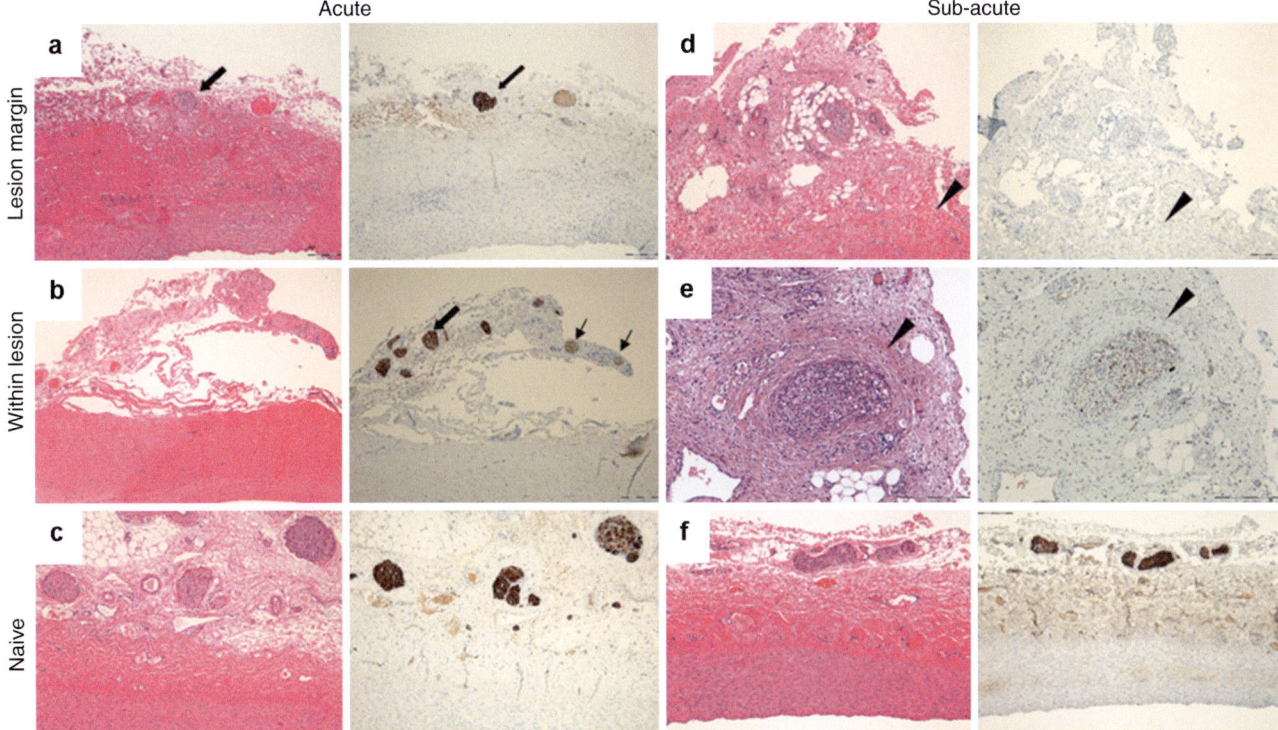

Fig. 3.5 Morphological changes of nerve fascicles after treatment. Nerve fascicles immunostained for neurofilament protein and their respective hematoxylin and eosin (H&E) stained sections are shown at high magnification (*scale bars* represent a length of 200 mm) for (**a**–**c**) acute and (**d**–**f**) subacute groups. Treatment groups are further categorized according to their location within the treated arteries with (**a**, **d**) located at the margin of the lesion, (**b**, **e**) within the lesion and (**c**, **f**) within the naive arterial segments. Nerve fascicles of the acute group show regular neurofilament protein staining intensity (*thick arrows*) as compared to the control and naive vessel segments. A loss of staining intensity (*thin arrows*) is discernable in a few number of nerve fascicles. In the subacute group, nerve fascicles within the lesion and at the lesion margin display enhanced vacuolic morphology, fibrosis and almost complete loss of neurofilament protein staining (images **e** and **f**, *arrow heads*). (**e**) Shows vacuolic degeneration and thickening of the perineurium. Here, neurofilament protein staining is reduced to evenly distributed focal areas. Remnant naive nerve fascicles remained unaffected with regards to their immunostaining profile 10 days after treatment (Reproduced with permission from Steigerwald et al. [33])

of nuclei, whereas histopathology at 28 day showed shrunken and vacuolated nerve fibers [14]. As compared to 6 days, the myxoid change of the nerve was more apparent at 28 days [14]. Also, histology of the renal vascular wall did not show any injury at 28 days. There was no inflammation, fibrosis, hyperplasia, or stenosis at 28 days [14]. By our estimation these morphologic changes of the nerves would be considered minimal or mild.

Histopathology of Beta-Radiation for Renal Nerve Denervation

Waksman et al. reported the effects of beta-radiation in the swine at 1- and 2-months [44]. Vascular brachytherapy was delivered to the renal arteries using the Beta-Cath™ 3.5 Fr delivery system at doses of 25 and 50 Gy. Follow-up angiography at 1 and 2 months showed patent renal artery without restenosis or occlusion [44]. Histopathology showed focal hypocellular nerve fascicles with degeneration, vacuolization,

and perineural inflammation with/without fibrosis [44]. Also, dose-related effect was observed at 2 months. In this study, immunohistochemistry against anti-tyrosine hydroxylase and S-100 protein was performed to confirm the functional nerve damage by beta-radiation therapy.

Histopathology of the renal artery showed focal adventitial fibrosis with myxoid change. Smaller arterioles showed varying degrees of injury, ranging from normal to perivascular inflammation, typically showing internal elastic lamina and external elastic lamina tear with medial necrosis. Overall damage of large artery and small arterioles were greater in 50-Gy as compared to 25-Gy [44].

Histopathology of Ethanol-Mediated Perivascular Renal Sympathetic Denervation

Fischell et al. reported the effects of ethanol-mediated perivascular renal sympathetic denervation in swine model at 14-days of [15]. They used a three-needle catheter delivery

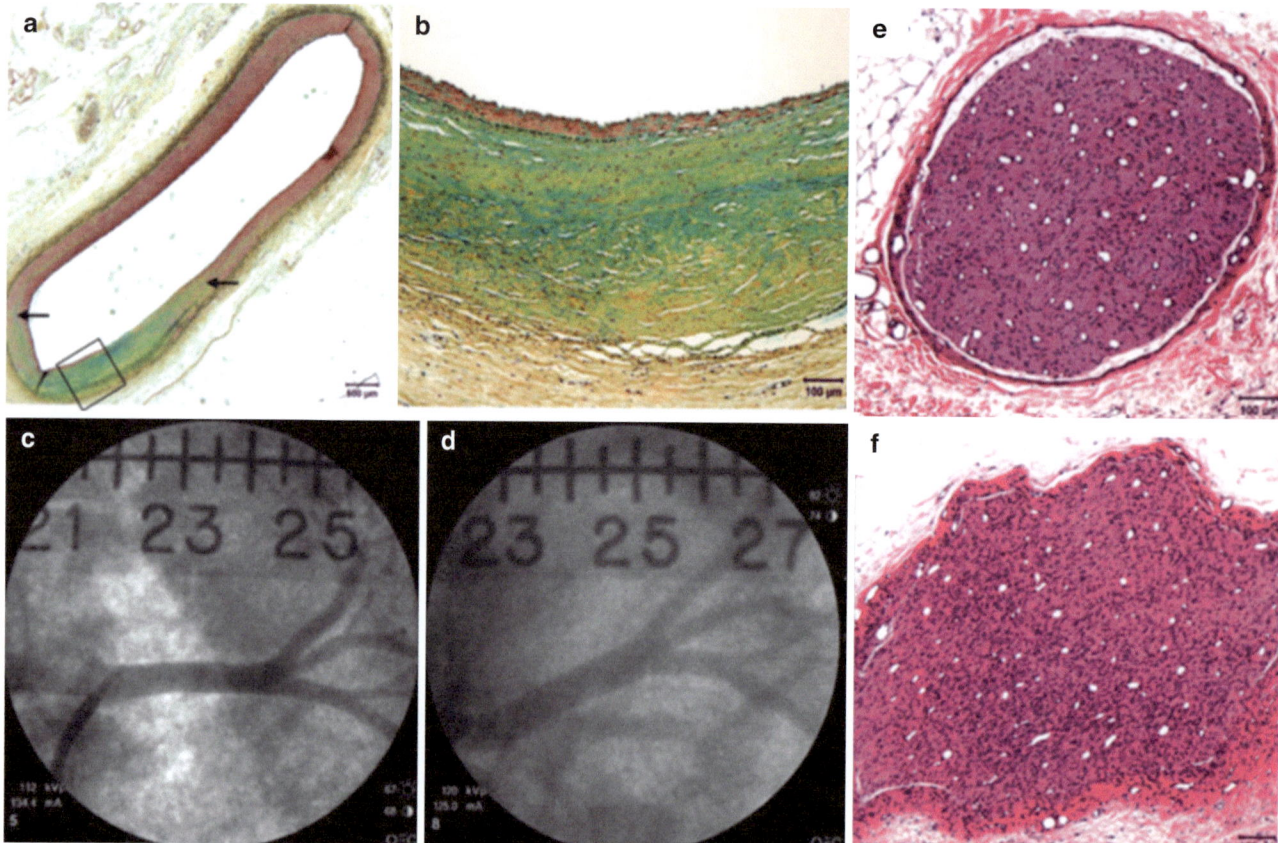

Fig. 3.6 Six-month histology results showing the most extensive medial injury (up to 25 % of the total media affected) that was noted in three sections of treated vessels. Both sections stained with Movat's pentachrome. (**a**) The area of medial injury (*yellow–green*) is located between the *arrows*. (**b**) A higher magnification of an area transmurally affected vessel wall (*rectangular area*) in (**a**). Sections show minimal intimal thickening and minimal IEL injury overlying areas of mild full thickness medial fibrosis (*yellow* [fibrosis] with *green* [proteoglycan deposition]), and adventitial fibrosis (*yellow*). No significant inflammatory cells are present suggesting that the healing process is complete.

Shown are the baseline (**c**) and 6-month (**d**) angiograms from the vessel from which the histology was taken. Angiograms at baseline and 6 months showed no findings. Six-month H&E-stained histology slides showing a nerve from an untreated (**e**) and treated vessel (**f**). Note the appearance of a periarterial nerve bundle surrounded by a thin fibrous connective tissue sheath (epineurium) in the untreated vessel. In contrast, the nerve bundle from a treated renal artery has a hypercellular appearance and the epineurium and perineurium appear thickened with prominent fibrosis and collagen deposition (Reproduced with permission from Rippy et al. [22])

system (Peregrine System™; Ablative Solutions, Inc., Kalamazoo, MI) inserted percutaneously via the femoral artery into the renal arteries of adult swine under fluoroscopic guidance [15]. Three volumes of dehydrated EtOH (98 %) were used in this study: 0.15 ml/artery (n = 3 pigs/ 6 renal arteries), 0.30 ml/artery (n = 3 pigs/6 renal arteries), and 0.60 ml/artery (n = 3 pigs/6 renal arteries). Also, saline injection was performed in the control animals as sham treatment.

Angiography at 14 days showed no abnormal findings. Histopathology of the nerve showed marked injury characterized by vacuolization, necrosis of the nerve bundles, with the development of perineural fibrosis and inflammation, while no nerve injury was observed in the sham treatment group. Histopathologic examination of the renal artery showed absence of thrombi, dissections, aneurysms, perforations, hematoma or other device-related pathologies.

However, at the higher doses (0.30 and 0.60 ml EtOH), there was occasional, focal loss of some smooth muscle cells and proteoglycan deposition in the outermost media, which typically originated at the adventitial surface and was associated with the injection sites.

Streitparth et al. investigated the Magnetic resonance image (MRI) guided spinal needle periarterial injection of ethanol for renal sympathetic denervation in pigs [45]. Unilateral renal periarterial ethanol injection was performed under general anesthesia in six pigs with the contralateral kidney serving as control [45]. All injections were performed using an open 1.0 T MRI system under real-time multiplanar guidance. Significant reduction (53 %) of norepinephrine concentration in the kidney parenchyma was observed in the treated kidney as compared to the control kidney [45]. Neural degeneration, with necrosis of the nerve fascicles peri- and endoneural fibrosis and inflammation was observed in the histology sections and calcification of the treated vessels in the adventitia was also occasionally seen [45].

Summary

Renal sympathetic denervation has emerged as a promising treatment for resistant hypertension, however, many unanswered questions regarding the efficacy of radiofrequency ablation versus placebo controlled trials remain. Nevertheless convincing preclinical results following perirenal sympathetic denervation in various animal models have shown efficacy. To date, radiofrequency ablation is the most frequently used modality in clinical as well as animal models. However, other treatment modalities including cryoablation, catheter-ultrasound, extracorporeal high-intensity focused ultrasound, and ethanol injection have been developed. Histopathology studies of peri-renal sympathetic nerves and norepinephrine levels in the kidney in preclinical models have shown both necrosis and peri-and endo-neural fibrosis correlating with norepinephrine reduction. Morphologic studies will continue to play a crucial role in the evaluation of both efficacy and safety of the new devices being developed. Standardized semi-quantitative ordinal grading systems are useful for the evaluation of the degree of changes observed in the nerve, renal artery, and peri-arterial soft tissue following renal denervation irrespective of the method utilized.

References

1. Kearney PM, Whelton M, Reynolds K, Muntner P, Whelton PK, He J. Global burden of hypertension: analysis of worldwide data. Lancet. 2005;365:217–23.
2. Chobanian AV, Bakris GL, Black HR, et al. The Seventh Report of the Joint National Committee on Prevention, Detection, Evaluation, and Treatment of High Blood Pressure: the JNC 7 report. JAMA. 2003;289:2560–72.
3. Lewington S, Clarke R, Qizilbash N, Peto R, Collins R. Age-specific relevance of usual blood pressure to vascular mortality: a meta-analysis of individual data for one million adults in 61 prospective studies. Lancet. 2002;360:1903–13.
4. Gu Q, Burt VL, Dillon CF, Yoon S. Trends in antihypertensive medication use and blood pressure control among United States adults with hypertension: the National Health and Nutrition Examination Survey, 2001 to 2010. Circulation. 2012;126:2105–14.
5. James PA, Oparil S, Carter BL, et al. 2014 evidence-based guideline for the management of high blood pressure in adults: report from the panel members appointed to the Eighth Joint National Committee (JNC 8). JAMA. 2014;311:507–20.
6. Grassi G, Mancia G. New therapeutic approaches for resistant hypertension. J Nephrol. 2012;25:276–81.
7. Sarafidis PA. Epidemiology of resistant hypertension. J Clin Hypertens (Greenwich). 2011;13:523–8.
8. Calhoun DA, Jones D, Textor S, et al. Resistant hypertension: diagnosis, evaluation, and treatment. A scientific statement from the American Heart Association Professional Education Committee of the Council for High Blood Pressure Research. Hypertension. 2008;51:1403–19.
9. Worthley SG, Tsioufis CP, Worthley MI, et al. Safety and efficacy of a multi-electrode renal sympathetic denervation system in resistant hypertension: the EnligHTN I trial. Eur Heart J. 2013;34: 2132–40.
10. Krum H, Schlaich M, Whitbourn R, et al. Catheter-based renal sympathetic denervation for resistant hypertension: a multicentre safety and proof-of-principle cohort study. Lancet. 2009;373: 1275–81.
11. Esler MD, Krum H, Sobotka PA, Schlaich MP, Schmieder RE, Bohm M. Renal sympathetic denervation in patients with treatment-resistant hypertension (The Symplicity HTN-2 Trial): a randomised controlled trial. Lancet. 2010;376:1903–9.
12. Krum H, Schlaich MP, Bohm M, et al. Percutaneous renal denervation in patients with treatment-resistant hypertension: final 3-year report of the Symplicity HTN-1 study. Lancet. 2014; 383:622–9.
13. Ahmed H, Neuzil P, Skoda J, et al. Renal sympathetic denervation using an irrigated radiofrequency ablation catheter for the management of drug-resistant hypertension. JACC Cardiovasc Interv. 2012;5:758–65.
14. Wang Q, Guo R, Rong S, et al. Noninvasive renal sympathetic denervation by extracorporeal high-intensity focused ultrasound in a preclinical canine model. J Am Coll Cardiol. 2013;61:2185–92.
15. Fischell TA, Vega F, Raju N, et al. Ethanol-mediated perivascular renal sympathetic denervation: preclinical validation of safety and efficacy in a porcine model. EuroIntervention. 2013;9:140–7.
16. Rocha-singh K. Renal artery denervation: a brave new frontier. Endovasc Today. 2012; p. 45–53.
17. Medtronic. Renal denervation. Minneapolis: RDN Press Release; 2014.
18. Kandzari DE, Bhatt DL, Sobotka PA, et al. Catheter-based renal denervation for resistant hypertension: rationale and design of the SYMPLICITY HTN-3 Trial. Clin Cardiol. 2012;35:528–35.
19. Mulder J, Hokfelt T, Knuepfer MM, Kopp UC. Renal sensory and sympathetic nerves reinnervate the kidney in a similar time-dependent fashion after renal denervation in rats. Am J Physiol Regul Integr Comp Physiol. 2013;304:R675–82.
20. Nagasu H, Satoh M, Kuwabara A, et al. Renal denervation reduces glomerular injury by suppressing NAD(P)H oxidase activity in Dahl salt-sensitive rats. Nephrol Dial Transplant. 2010;25: 2889–98.
21. Girchev R, Markova P, Vuchidolova V. Influence of renal denervation on renal effects of acute nitric oxide and ETA/ETB receptor inhibition in conscious normotensive rats. J Physiol Pharmacol. 2006;57:17–27.
22. Rippy MK, Zarins D, Barman NC, Wu A, Duncan KL, Zarins CK. Catheter-based renal sympathetic denervation: chronic preclinical evidence for renal artery safety. Clin Res Cardiol. 2011;100: 1095–101.
23. Lerman LO, Schwartz RS, Grande JP, Sheedy PF, Romero JC. Noninvasive evaluation of a novel swine model of renal artery stenosis. J Am Soc Nephrol. 1999;10:1455–65.
24. Tellez A, Rousselle S, Palmieri T, et al. Renal artery nerve distribution and density in the porcine model: biologic implications for the development of radiofrequency ablation therapies. Transl Res. 2013;162:381–9.
25. Atherton DS, Deep NL, Mendelsohn FO. Micro-anatomy of the renal sympathetic nervous system: a human postmortem histologic study. Clin Anat. 2012;25:628–33.
26. Sakakura K, Ladich E, Edelman ER et al. Methodological standardization for the preclinical evaluation of renal sympathetic denervation. JACC Cardiovasc Interv. 2014. doi:10.1016/j.jcin.2014.04.024.
27. Whitney KM, Schwartz Sterman AJ, O'Connor J, Foley GL, Garman RH. Light microscopic sciatic nerve changes in control

beagle dogs from toxicity studies. Toxicol Pathol. 2011;39: 835–40.

28. Biberthaler P, Mussack T, Wiedemann E, et al. Evaluation of S-100b as a specific marker for neuronal damage due to minor head trauma. World J Surg. 2001;25:93–7.

29. Pace V, Perentes E, Germann PG. Pheochromocytomas and ganglioneuromas in the aging rats: morphological and immunohistochemical characterization. Toxicol Pathol. 2002;30:492–500.

30. Burgi K, Cavalleri MT, Alves AS, Britto LR, Antunes VR, Michelini LC. Tyrosine hydroxylase immunoreactivity as indicator of sympathetic activity: simultaneous evaluation in different tissues of hypertensive rats. Am J Physiol Regul Integr Comp Physiol. 2011;300:R264–71.

31. Ammar S, Ladich E, Steigerwald K, Deisenhofer I, Joner M. Pathophysiology of renal denervation procedures: from renal nerve anatomy to procedural parameters. EuroIntervention. 2013;9(Suppl R):R89–95.

32. Wittkampf FH, Nakagawa H, Yamanashi WS, Imai S, Jackman WM. Thermal latency in radiofrequency ablation. Circulation. 1996;93:1083–6.

33. Steigerwald K, Titova A, Malle C, et al. Morphological assessment of renal arteries after radiofrequency catheter-based sympathetic denervation in a porcine model. J Hypertens. 2012;30:2230–9.

34. Skanes AC, Dubuc M, Klein GJ, et al. Cryothermal ablation of the slow pathway for the elimination of atrioventricular nodal reentrant tachycardia. Circulation. 2000;102:2856–60.

35. Deisenhofer I, Zrenner B, Yin YH, et al. Cryoablation versus radiofrequency energy for the ablation of atrioventricular nodal reentrant tachycardia (the CYRANO Study): results from a large multicenter prospective randomized trial. Circulation. 2010;122:2239–45.

36. Skanes AC, Klein G, Krahn A, Yee R. Cryoablation: potentials and pitfalls. J Cardiovasc Electrophysiol. 2004;15:S28–34.

37. Prochnau D, Figulla HR, Romeike BF, et al. Percutaneous catheter-based cryoablation of the renal artery is effective for sympathetic denervation in a sheep model. Int J Cardiol. 2011;152:268–70.

38. Mabin T, Sapoval M, Cabane V, Stemmett J, Iyer M. First experience with endovascular ultrasound renal denervation for the treatment of resistant hypertension. EuroIntervention. 2012;8: 57–61.

39. Ng KK, Poon RT, Chan SC, et al. High-intensity focused ultrasound for hepatocellular carcinoma: a single-center experience. Ann Surg. 2011;253:981–7.

40. Kennedy JE. High-intensity focused ultrasound in the treatment of solid tumours. Nat Rev Cancer. 2005;5:321–7.

41. Illing RO, Kennedy JE, Wu F, et al. The safety and feasibility of extracorporeal high-intensity focused ultrasound (HIFU) for the treatment of liver and kidney tumours in a Western population. Br J Cancer. 2005;93:890–5.

42. Marsac L, Chauvet D, Larrat B, et al. MR-guided adaptive focusing of therapeutic ultrasound beams in the human head. Med Phys. 2012;39:1141–9.

43. Aptel F, Charrel T, Lafon C, et al. Miniaturized high-intensity focused ultrasound device in patients with glaucoma: a clinical pilot study. Invest Ophthalmol Vis Sci. 2011;52:8747–53.

44. Waksman R, Barbash IM, Chan R, Randolph P, Makuria AT, Virmani R. Beta radiation for renal nerve denervation: initial feasibility and safety. EuroIntervention. 2013;9:738–44.

45. Streitparth F, Walter A, Stolzenburg N, et al. MR-guided periarterial ethanol injection for renal sympathetic denervation: a feasibility study in pigs. Cardiovasc Intervent Radiol. 2013;36:791–6.

The Endpoint on Measuring the Clinical Effects of Renal Denervation: What Are the Best Surrogates

Paul A. Sobotka, David G. Harrison, and Marat Fudim

Introduction

In the past several years, renal denervation has proven to be an effective treatment for resistant hypertension (HTN). Unfortunately the procedure does not always lower blood pressure and many patients continue to need drugs for HTN. While there are several potential explanations for this persistent elevation of blood pressure after renal denervation, one is that the renal nerves were not completely ablated. Another is that the HTN was not caused by increased sympathetic nerve activity (SNA) in the individual patient, and that other stimuli for HTN persists after renal denervation. In addition, accumulating evidence suggests that renal denervation also benefits other conditions including heart failure (HF), atrial fibrillation and insulin resistance. Thus in the near future this procedure might be frequently employed for several common medical problems. A major problem is that it will not be sufficient to simply measure blood pressure to ascertain successful renal denervation. Given these considerations, it is apparent that we need surrogate measures of increased sympathetic activity and procedural success. In this chapter we will discuss direct and indirect methods for assessing SNA in humans, how these can be used to screen patients for renal denervation, how they could be used to gauge technical success and how these various methods might be used in specific diseases.

P.A. Sobotka, MD (✉)
Division of Cardiology, Department of Medicine, The Ohio State University, 2015 Marywood Lane, West St. Paul, MN 55118, USA
e-mail: Sobotka@alumni.stanford.edu

D.G. Harrison, MD
Medicine and Pharmacology, Vanderbilt Medical Center,
Room 536, Robinson Research Bldg, Nashville,
TN 37232-6602, USA
e-mail: david.g.harrison@vanderbilt.edu

M. Fudim, MD
Internal Medicine, Vanderbilt Medical Center,
D-3100, Medical Center North, Nashville, TN 37232-2358, USA
e-mail: marat.fudim@vanderbilt.edu

Anatomy and Physiology or Renal Nerves

The renal sympathetic nerves arise from spinal segments T11 to L3 and enter the kidney at the hilum along with the renal artery, extending to vascular and tubular structures [1]. As is the case for most major vessels, the nerves of the renal arteries are located principally in the adventitia [2]. The kidney receives both efferent sympathetic signals and generates afferent signals [3]. There is no evidence for parasympathetic innervation of the kidney [4].

The efferent nerves densely invest numerous structures of the kidney involved in water and sodium homeostasis, including both the afferent and efferent arterioles, the proximal tubule, the loop of Henle, as well as the distal renal tubule. The efferent sympathetic nerves modulate renal function through the release of a large number of local neurotransmitters. While noradrenaline serves as primary neurotransmitter, neuropeptide Y and ATP have modulatory/stimulatory roles and are released in response to sympathetic nerve stimulation [5, 6]. Neurotransmitters released from the synapses activate postsynaptic receptors like α/β-adrenergic receptors (norepinephrine) [7, 8] and Y1 receptor (neuropeptide Y) [9] and purinergic P2 receptors (ATP) [10]. Physiological consequences of sympathetic stimulation in the kidney include modulation of tubular secretion of sodium and constriction of afferent arterioles to the glomerulus. Constriction of the efferent arteriole is less pronounced, protecting against neurogenic reductions of glomerular pressure and glomerular filtration rate (GFR). Further stimulation of efferent sympathetic nerves causes a decreased blood flow (RBF) to the renal cortex and medulla [1]. Moreover, through alteration in perfusion pressure, changes in GFR and RBF can decrease sodium and water excretion. Direct antinatriuretic effects of sympathetic stimulation appear to be independent of GFR or RBF, and are mediated by α1-adrenergic receptors [1, 11–13].

A major role of renal sympathetic nerves is modulation of renin release from the juxtaglomerular apparatus directly by norepinephrine activation of $\beta1$ adrenoreceptors, and indirectly by modulation of the afferent arteriolar tone [14, 15]. Norepinephrine causes immediate release of pre-synthesized renin and over the long term, also increases expression of renin mRNA [16].

Efferent renal sympathetic nerve activity (RSNA) is modulated by reflex mechanisms outside of the kidney. Activation of carotid and aortic baroreceptors and deactivation of carotid chemoreceptors decrease renal sympathetic efferent traffic [17–19]. On the contrary inhibition of carotid and aortic baroreceptors and activation of carotid chemoreceptors increases RSNA and renin secretion [1]. These reflex modulations of RSNA are important in maintaining volume and sodium homeostasis under normal physiological conditions, but can become maladaptive in a variety of pathological states as discussed later in this chapter and in other chapters of this textbook [20–23].

Compared to the efferent renal sympathetic nerves, the function of afferent somatic nerves is less well understood. Afferent fibers arise from a variety of receptor types throughout the kidney and project to the dorsal spinal roots to the central regions of cardiovascular control including the hypothalamus and the brainstem [24–26]. Renal vascular chemoreceptors, including osmoreceptors, monitor interstitial fluid environment, while renal mechanoreceptors sense hydrostatic pressure changes. While chemoreceptors are mainly located in the submucosal areas of renal pelvis, mechanoreceptors are present in the renal pelvis and cortex [26]. Similar to the modulatory function of reflex mechanisms on the efferent RSN, stimulation afferent RSN in animals produces heterogeneous effects on RSNA, leading to both sympathoexcitation and sympathoinhibition [26–28]. Dorsoal rhizotomy, which selectively eliminates afferent renal nerve traffic, reduces blood pressure [29, 30].

In addition to controlling body electrolyte and fluid homeostasis, afferent renal nerves also seem to play an important function in the pathophysiology of cardiovascular diseases [31]. Efferent and afferent nerves appear to function in a reflex loop where sensory signals from the kidney to the CNS stimulate the efferent sympathetic nerve output to the kidney. In return efferent sympathetic signaling to the kidney could propagate pathological positive feedback via sensory renal nerves. The sympathoexcitatory activity of the kidney, directly mediated by renal afferents or indirectly by central nervous system effects of renal angiotensin II certainly have systemic implications. For example kidney ischemia and inflammation cause a sympathoexcitatory response via renal afferent nerves [32]. While neuropeptide P and calcitonin gene-related peptide (CGRP) are the main transmitters of the afferent nerves, the transient receptor potential vanilloid type 1 (TRPV1) pathway has also been recognized to be key to the inflammatory response [33–37]. Evidence suggests that

afferent nerves not only regulate renal homoeostasis but also affect the cardiovascular system in a global fashion. Experiments in animals suggest an involvement of afferent renal nerves in the pathogenesis of cardiovascular diseases like HTN, diabetes mellitus (DM), congestion due to fluid retention or changes in venous capacitance [38–41]. Thus, effective renal afferent nerve denervation is likely associated with measurable systemic effects, such as reduction of insulin resistance, alteration of venous capacitance, and reduced heart rate and ventricular hypertrophy.

Understanding the status of renal sympathetic and afferent nerve function may provide intraprocedural and post procedural insights into treatment, optimal selection of patients, and titration of ablative therapy. Additionally, this knowledge might provide understanding of mechanisms behind lack of sustained treatment effect. Some animal and human data suggest that efferent sympathetic renal nerves can regenerate following surgical renal denervation. In rats functional reinnervation occurred 4 weeks post procedural following surgical renal denervation [42]. In a renal transplant model of the dog early histological reinnervation was observed after 3 months while complete histological reinnervation was complete at 8 months [43]. In humans there is evidence of gradual anatomical and functional efferent sympathetic reinnervation of the kidney, with partial reinnervation starting 4 weeks after renal transplantation and lasting up to the 8th month [44, 45]. There is new evidence that reinnervation of the kidney is not only restricted to the efferent arm of the sympathetic system but it also true for the afferent renal nerves. Mulder et al. demonstrated reinnervation of renal afferent nerves in a normotensive rat (up to 12 weeks) [46]. It can be assumed that anatomical and eventually also functional restoration of efferent and afferent renal nerves could also occur in humans following device based renal denervation. It should be pointed out, however that renal denervation has been associated with sustained lowering of blood pressure for up to 3 years, which suggets that nerve re-growth doesn't occur or is inconsequential.

Methods to Quantify Sympathetic Nerve Activity: Microneurography, Noradrenaline Spill-Over, Heart Rate Variability, Baroreflex and Chemoreflex Sensitivity

Sympathetic outflow does not always occur in a global fashion, but often in directed toward specific organs (Fig. 4.1). The response of any one of these therefore reflects sympathetic outflow to that specific organ, but not to other tissues [20, 47]. Increased sympathetic traffic to the heart increases chronotropic and inotropic activity. Sympathetic stimulation of vessels alters vascular tone, and generally favors vasoconstriction. As an example, splanchnic activation

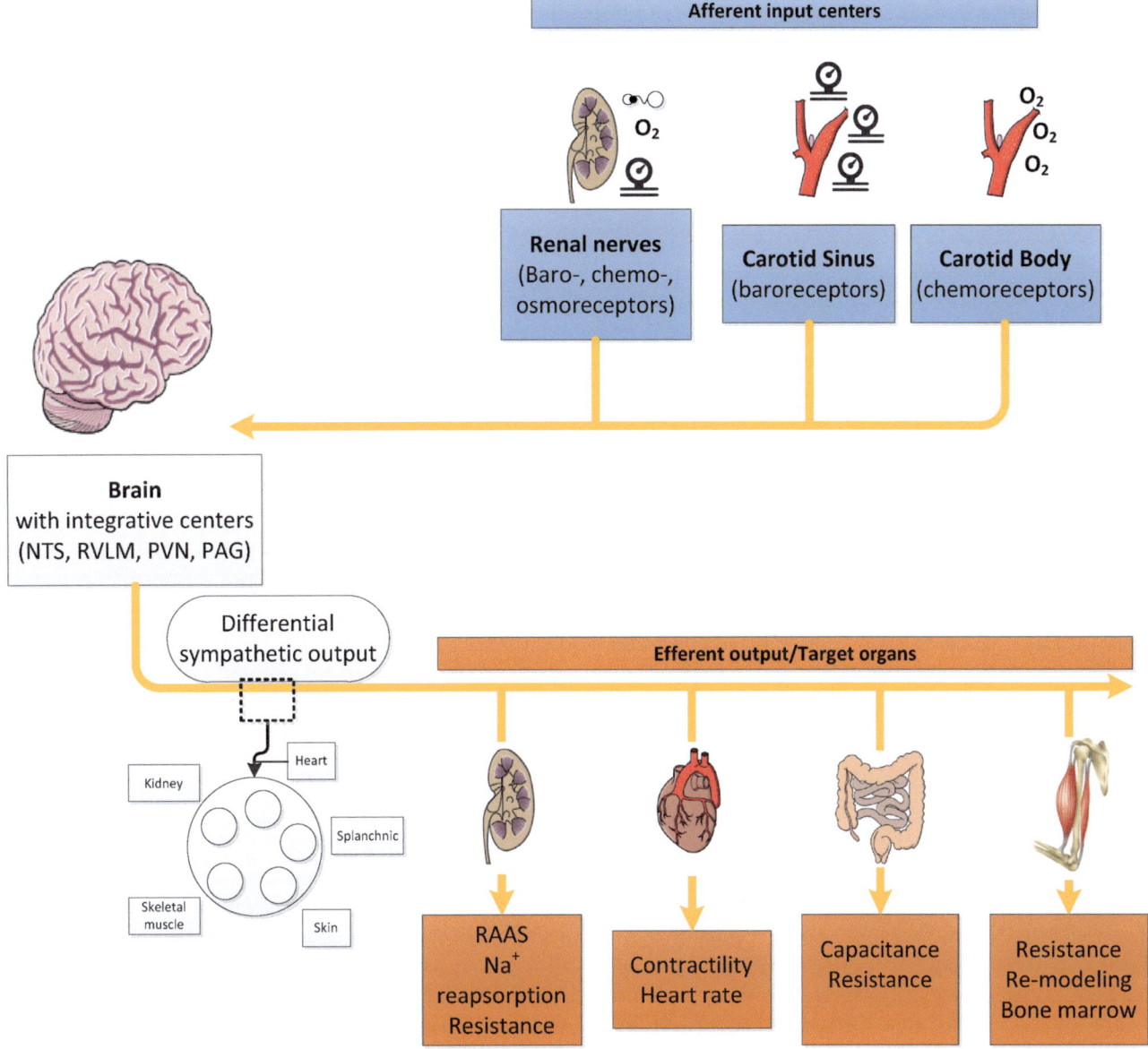

Fig. 4.1 Integration of afferent input and differential efferent sympathetic nerve output

decreases splanchnic capacitance and increases venous return [48]. Renal specific activation alters activity of the RAS, sodium reabsorption and intrarenal arterial resistance.

In animals SNA can be assessed by using electrodes to measure nerve firing or by examining the physiological responses of specific organs, including: kidneys [49], heart [50], lungs [51] and liver [52]. Such measurements are often enhanced by use of specific adrenergic antagonists or by use of genetically altered animals, which provide insight into the receptors activated. In humans quantification of SNA is more difficult. In the next section, we will discuss the currently employed approaches and discuss advantages and disadvantages of each.

Measurement of plasma or urinary noradrenaline is sometimes used as a surrogate of total sympathetic outflow but identifies only that portion of noradrenaline escaping reuptake and entering the systemic circulation. Moreover, plasma noradrenaline levels inherently fails to asses regional SNA [53, 54]. Radiotracer-based measurements of noradrenaline spill over from specific organs into the draining venous bed is accepted as a gold standard, but is complicated, requires arterial and venous cannulation and is performed in selective expert centers. Direct recording of sympathetic firing of the peroneal nerve is a elegant method to record muscle sympathetic nerve activity, but again is only performed in specific centers. These methods capture specific elements of sympathetic stimulation, when taken alone, they potentially fail to characterize differential sympathetic innervation of separate organs, the whole body sympathetic activity and contribution of peripheral sites to the whole body SNA [55].

Noradrenaline Spillover

Noradrenaline spill over uses radiotracer technology, is one of the most reliable to study whole body and regional noradrenaline kinetics in humans [56]. Radiolabelled norepinephrine (most commonly [3]) is infused intravenously and regional samples of blood are obtained from veins draining from specific organs. The variable measured is the release of noradrenaline into plasma. The difference in arteriovenous noradrenaline as measured by isotope dilution provides an estimate of regional/organ specific SNA [57, 58]. A limitation of this method is that it measures regional SNA at a single time point and does not allow continuous tracing. This method has proven very powerful, and has been used to document alterations in sympathetic innervation of the heart, the kidneys and skeletal muscle. Recent evidence suggests that at a high rate of nerve discharges there is no longer a linear correlation with the rate of noradrenaline spillover since noradrenaline released from the nerve terminals eventually reaches a plateau [59].

Microneurography

In 1968 Hagbarth and Valibo were the first to report on efficacy of microneurography to measure efferent multi-fiber sympathetic nerve activity (MSNA) [60]. Direct recordings (commonly from the peroneal nerve) reveal burst of nerve activity, synchronous with the heart beat. Observations show while repeat measurements within one subject are highly consistent, there is an up to tenfold variation of SNA from normotensive subject to the next [61–63]. This between individual variability appears to be due physiological variability, rather than variations in recording techniques. Recent refinements have led to single-fiber sympathetic nerve recording in humans [64, 65]. The results from single-fiber recording are supportive of recordings from the whole nerve [66, 67]. Similar to multi-fiber recordings, single-fiber firing is low in humans at baseline, however physiological stimuli and cardiovascular diseases increases single unit discharge rates [68, 69]. MSNA is commonly suggested to be a surrogate of global SNA. While MSNA correlates with noradrenaline spillover, it measures only the patterns of MSNA of the sampled nerve. As discussed above regional

differences in sympathetic tone do not necessarily allow conclusions from one organ region to another. There is some evidence that in patients with HF MSNA correlates with mortality [70]. MSNA recording, while a very valuable tool, requires a dedicated laboratory, specialized equipment and skilled personal. For these reasons, it is not used in the clinical setting.

Heart Rate and Blood Pressure Variability

Another commonly employed method is power spectral analysis of heart rate and blood pressure variability. This identifies oscillations in heart rate and blood pressure that are modulated by inputs from the renin-angiotensin system, sympathetic and parasympathetic neurons and by locally released vasoactive factors such as nitric oxide. Obviously, assessment of heart rate variability requires continuous ECG or pulse monitoring, and assessment of blood pressure generally requires constant measurements using arterial cannulation. Fourier analysis and similar techniques allow one to differentiate between the influence of the sympathetic and parasympathetic impact on the heart rate. The analysis is based on the fact that the SNS and parasympathetic nervous system (PNS) operate in different frequency bands. Sympathetic outflow modulates low frequency oscillations, while parasympathetic tone affects both low and high oscillations of heart rate. Thus the ratio of low to high frequency heart rate variability reflects sympathetic cardiovascular modulation. Another approach is to measure baroreflex and chemoreflex sensitivity [71–73]. Patients with HF have increased heart rate and decreased heart rate variability, both of which are associated with increased mortality [74–76]. A major limitation of this method is that no individual heart rate spectrum is selective to the SNA. Factors like age, gender, respiration and baroreflex signals interfere with use of heart rate variability [75, 77]. Similar to the heart rate variability, variability in blood pressure is increased in conditions with increased sympathetic tone and correlates with a heightened MSNA [78]. Absolute values of low frequency blood pressure oscillations provide indirect assessment of sympathetic outflow. Moreover, increased blood pressure variability is associated with higher rates of cardiovascular mortality. However high frequency fluctuations depend on mechanical impact of respiration, whereas low frequency spectral powers are largely due to the complex interaction between vasomotor tone, vascular resistance, humeral and neural factors. Similar to the heart rate variability the use of blood pressure spectral powers are limited by its dependence on various factors, lowering its specificity thus limiting its use in clinical practice [71, 79].

Baroreflex Sensitivity

SNS hyperactivity suppresses the arterial baroreceptor reflex. Consequently the carotid baroreflex is blunted in animals and humans with cardiovascular disease like HTN and HF [80, 81]. At the same time resolution of those morbidities improves the baroreflex sensitivity (BRS). BRS is defined as the change in interbeat interval (IBI) in milliseconds per unit change in BP. This is most often quantified as a slope or gain function [82]. Initially the BRS was assessed with vasoconstrictive agents that increase BP and reflexly decrease heart rate affecting the IBI. New are non-invasive methods to measure the BRS. Here the spontaneous heart rate variability and BP variability are obtained continuously using noninvasive arterial pressure monitoring devices. A major limitation of this method includes that BRS assessment requires a sinus rhythm since small amounts of noise easily disrupts the analysis.

Chemoreflex Sensitivity

Preclinical animal and surgical human studies have outlined the significance of the peripheral chemoreflex in mediating sympathetic hyperactivity, heightened RSNA, and baroreflex inhibition [18, 19, 83–85]. Peripheral chemosensitivity is clinically assessed by measuring the ventilatory response and changes in heart rate or blood pressure in response to either inhibition or stimulation of the peripheral chemoreceptor by manipulating inhaled gas mixtures or applying chemoreceptor stimulating or inhibiting drugs [86–88]. Increased sensitivity of the chemoreflex reflects dysfunction of autonomic cardiovascular control and is linked to development and/or progression of diseases like HF and HTN. Again, give some examples and discuss pluses and minuses.

Identifying Patients in Which Renal Denervation Is Likely to Be Successful

The ability to identify patients with elevated renal sympathetic efferent or afferent nerve activity may help identify optimal candidates for denervation. To guarantee success of RDN, ideal inclusion criteria are: sympathetically mediated disease with heightened sympathetic tone, originating from the renal afferent nerves. Current trials have focused on the broad spectrum of treatment resistant hypertensive patients. Present patient selection focuses to identify truly resistant hypertensive patients. Inclusion criteria for the Symplicity trials are a baseline systolic blood pressure of 160 mmHg or more ($\geq$150 mmHg for patients with type 2 diabetes), despite taking three or more antihypertensive drugs (including a diuretic). However since RDN is a rapidly evolving field newer trials started applying the novel technology in patients with moderate resistant HTN [89].

So far there are at least two screening tests that predict the outcome RDN in patients with resistant HTN. A screening tool that is currently applied by most centers includes the use of ambulatory BP monitoring (24–72 h) to identify patients with truly resistant HTN. This technique also allows to exclude patients with pseudo-resistant HTN [90]. Not surprisingly higher baseline BP predicted more pronounced BP reduction following the procedure. More interestingly impaired cardiac baroreflex sensitivity identified patients with resistant HTN who respond to RDN [91]. In a study by Zuern et al. baroreceptor sensitivity was identified to be the strongest predictor of a patient's BP response to RDN. Similarly other preprocedural measures of SNA could provide important insight into effects of RDN on patients and increase rate of procedural success. Central sympatholytic agents like clonidine could additionally be used to distinguish responders from non-responders. This is supported by the idea that RDN is more likely to be effective in patients with treatment resistant HTN with a significant component of sympathetic hyperactivation. A marked reduction in blood pressure following the use of a sympatholytic agent is more likely to result successful response to RDN [92].

More efforts are required to preselect patients for RDN in order to maximize response to the novel technology. A selection trying to quantify activity of the SNS rather than disease activity as shown by Zuern et al. opens new ways for effective and targeted screening. Further development of screening tools requires the understanding of how to measure response and how to define success of RDN. Since RDN proves itself to be successful for sympathetically mediated diseases other than HTN, novel tools need to be developed to identify responders for a broad variety of diseases including DM, HF etc..

How to Confirm Technical Success? Measuring Afferent and Efferent Denervation

In humans there are no reports of direct intraprocedural measures of technical success, neither on direct assessment of renal nerve activity during or after the intervention. A more viable and accessible option to measure activity of renal nerves may arise with the use of biomarkers of renal specific nerve activity. Since many of these biomarkers are modifiable they provide targeted measures of risk reduction following therapeutic interventions. Table 4.1 shows a list of

Table 4.1 A list of biomarkers which have been used in RDN studies or could potentially be applied to measure technical success

Outcome measurement	Biomarker
Efferent deinnervation	Renin, angiotensin and aldosteron levels
	Natriuresis, diuresis, renal vascular resistance and renal blood flow
	Renal specific noradrenaline spillover
	Systemic response to renal chemo, or mechanical sensory stimulation
Afferent deinnervation	Via interruption of neurogenic reflex loop
	Total body noradrenaline spillover
	Heart rate/heart rate variability/blood pressure variability
	Baroreflex sensitivity
	Central angiotensin levels

potential biomarkers that can be used to confirm technical success.

In today's clinical world, technical success of RDN is defined solely by a reduction in blood pressure and quantified by the extent of BP reduction. It is important to point out that a reduction in sympathetic tone does not necessarily reflect itself in a reduction of BP. This is also true for various other surrogate markers that are clearly linked to the activity of the SNA. In the case of BP as a surrogate outcome, conceivable technical success of RDN does not have to be accompanied by immediate or any BP changes at all [93]. In parts this can be attributed to the complexity of pathophysiology of HTN and the variable role that SNA can play in it. The rate of ineffective reduction in BP following RDN ranges from 10 % to 50 % [94, 95]. Additionally, blood pressure cannot be used as a technical success measure in all populations, as it is not expected to fall following renal denervation in normotensive patients undergoing the procedure in hopes of reducing the renal contribution to elevated sympathetic tone, such as patients with HF, or sympathetically mediated tachyarrhythmias. Since technical success and BP reduction do not have sufficient overlap, other biomarkers and surrogate markers or a combination of both has to be applied to define technical success. Most effective would be a combined assessment of afferent and efferent nerve activity as outlined further below in this chapter.

Unlike in animals intraprocedural and postprocedural direct nerve recordings in humans are limited by the simple fact of inaccessibility of the renal nerves and invasiveness of the procedure. Chinushi et al. first recorded renal nerve activity in animals during RDN [96]. Renal nerve stimulation prior to the ablation increased systemic BP, serum catecholamine and heart rate variability. Renal nerve ablation attenuated BP and HR responses following nerve stimulation. Thus the attenuation or elimination of the different components of the response to renal nerve stimulation following RDN could be the evidence of successful damage to renal fibers and serve as technical success of the intervention. Translated to humans this could mean that technical success eventually could require demonstration of blunted efferent and afferent response to proper stimuli (e.g. exposure to chemosensitive agent fails to trigger afferent signals).

Efferent

In the case of RDN there are various potential biomarkers which arise from direct and indirect effects of efferent deinnervation of the kidney. Renal efferent nerves regulate circulating volume and sodium as well as fluid homeostasis. Several acute and chronic renal diseases like renal ischemia, renal vascular disease, and end stage renal disease are associated with excessive renal sympathetic efferent activity. Reduction of renal sympathetic efferent signaling suppresses albuminuria, and podocyte injury in aortic insufficiency [97], preventing glomerular hyperfiltration in diabetic rats [98], prevention of angiotensin receptor over expression in HF [99], as well as in acute diseases where renal denervation prevented experimental glomerular nephritis [100] and endotoxemic associated renal injury in mice [101]. Moreover, renal sympathetic nerve traffic may mediate renal ischemic injury [102]. Thus, the renal nerves may mediate several pathologic process linked together by over activity of renal sympathetic signaling. This supports the use renal markers of disease to identify renal hyperactivity and successful therapeutic renal denervation.

Primary biomarkers of efferent deinnervation include a decreased RSNA with decreased release of noradrenaline and its co-transmitters from renal nerve endings. Since renal efferent nerves innervate all major structures of the kidney, loss of the nerves would explain a decrease in renin release from the juxtaglomerular granular cells, decrease in renal arterial vascular resistance, increase in glomerular filtration rate and increase in renal sodium excretion [103]. Changes in levels of locally secreted neurotransmitters at the terminal endings of efferent renal nerves and levels of RAS components like renin could serve as additional markers of SNA. Several small scale human studies have used noradrenaline spillover technique and renin levels to quantify the remaining renal nerve activity following RDN. In a preliminary study using radiofrequency renal nerve ablation Schlaich et al. demonstrated a reduction of renal noradrenaline spillover (left kidney −48 % and right kidney −75 %), a 50 % reduction in renin activity and increased renal blood flow at 1 month after device based denervation [104]. In a study with ten resistant hypertensive patients, device based renal denervation led to a reduction in noradrenaline spillover of 47 %, 15–30 days after the procedure [95]. In two other small scale studies RDN decreased plasma noradrenaline or catecholamine metabolites but not renin levels [105, 106]. The absent decrease in renin activity was linked to insufficient ablation of renal nerves in order to see a meaningful response. Comparable outcomes were described in patients with resistant HTN and end-stage renal disease [107]. This data shows that primary biomarkers of efferent renal denervation like renin activity and noradrenaline spillover are useful methods to document a decreased sympathetic tone following RDN. While radiotracer dependent noradrenaline spillover technique is not readily available in clinic practice nor is it practicable outside of a research environment, intra or post procedural renal venous blood sampling could be used to measure the concentration of neurotransmitters.

Secondary biomarkers of efferent denervation would include an inhibition of the renin-angiotensin system (RAS), beyond a pure decrease in renin activity. Decreased renin activity reduces angiotensin II and aldosteron levels, resulting in a number of positive effects including decreased global sympathetic tone, vasodilation, improved heart function etc. [108, 109]. Surgical renal denervation in various animal models demonstrated increased natriuresis and diuresis as well as a better response to diuretic neurohormones like ANP, which can be understood as a direct effect of efferent denervation as well as indirect effect of RAS inhibition [110–113]. Human studies on bilateral nephrectomy in renal transplant patients and device based renal denervation in treatment resistant hypertensive patients resulted in not only decreased renin but also angiotensin levels [104, 114–116].

Afferent

Unlike the effects of renal efferent nerve denervation, the effects of afferent denervation cannot be explained by a pure loss of the afferent limb of renal nerves. The renal afferent nerves are part of a neurogenic reflex which regulates the autonomic balance by alteration of the sympathetic tone. In chronic diseases states this reflex is pathologically hyperactive, resulting in over activation of sympathetic tone. These pathophysiological processes do not necessary have to involve the kidney. However CKD serves as a good example to explain the relevance of the renal afferents for this reflex. In CKD, local ischemic and inflammatory changes could increase discharge of local chemoreceptors [32, 100, 117]. As a consequence sensory output from the kidney to the brain is elevated resulting in an increased discharge and potentially also new set point for SNA. Further, successful renal transplantation restores renal function however SNA does not decrease as long as native kidneys remain in place. Removal of bilateral native kidneys restores central sympathetic outflow represented by a decrease in whole body noradrenaline spillover [30, 118]. This speaks most

likely for the persistent activity of sensory fibers if native kidneys remain in situ.

Apart from direct nerve traffic recordings, biomarkers of successful renal afferent nerve denervation are related to the interruption of the reflex arc. This includes assessments of the sympathetic nervous system with methods like MSNA, noradrenaline spillover (regional and whole body), baroreflex sensitivity and heart rate variability. There are multiple studies showing a reduction of MSNA in patients who underwent a device based renal denervation when compared with controls. In a study with 20 patients there was a significant reduction in MSNA 3 months following renal denervation procedure [119]. Schlaich et al. measured a reduced whole body noradrenaline spillover and MSNA in patients with CKD undergoing renal denervation [107].

Apart from multi-unit MSNA there is emerging evidence for the use of single-unit MSNA to measure technical success following RDN. Single-unit MSNA recording is technically more challenging, however appears to be more specific and quantitative in patients with cardiovascular disease including essential HTN than multi-unit MSNA [66, 120]. Hering et al. were able to show a reduction in single- unit and multi-unit MSNA in 25 patients 3 months following RDN [65].

While the responder rate to RDN (defined as a reduction in systolic BP of at least 10 mmHg) was up to 100 % in the first landmark trial (Symplicity HTN-1) within the first 12 months following the procedure, the magnitude of blood pressure reduction was more distinct in the time from 6 to 12 months. This finding could potentially be explained by the delayed integration of afferent renal nerve input to the CNS.

Several clinical trials have studied the effects of RDN on the SNA with methods other than MSNA and noradrenaline spillover. Animal studies RDN resulted in an improvement in cardiac and sympathetic baroreflex sensitivity [94, 121, 122]. Interestingly even unilateral RDN was beneficial on the baroreflex function [123]. So far only few studies have studied the effects of RDN on baroreflex sensitivity in humans. Comparable to animal experiments Hart et al. demonstrated improvements in the cardiac and sympathetic baroreflex sensitivity in resistant hypertensive patients [94]. Interestingly these changes were also observed in patients who had no BP response to RDN. Beyond its use as a potential biomarker of successful denervation, impaired baroreflex sensitivity was also able to predict response to therapy [91]. In contrast Brinkman et al. demonstrated no changes in baroreflex function [124]. Notably RDN did not result in any blood pressure changes in this study population.

With an increasing number of clinical trials studying the effects of RDN on the SNA, some studies have not show a reduction in SNA in patients with resistant hypertensive patients following RDN. In a study by Brinkmann et al. RDN did not alter the MSNA, heart rate, blood pressure variability or baroreceptor activity 3–6 months following RDN. Interestingly only 3/10 patients had a reduction in their office blood pressure without any relation to MSNA changes [124]. Similar results on blood pressure and MSNA in humans were demonstrated by Hart et al. 1 and 6 months following RDN. Unlike spontaneously hypertensive rats in a sample size of eight patients only four human subjects had a response in blood pressure to RDN (10 % reduction) which did not necessarily correlate with MSNA [94]. It is possible that response of MSNA to RDN is dependent on baseline MSNA which was lower in these two studies when compared to previously presented studies showing improvement in MSNA [104, 119].

Further biomarkers of successful RDN could be found in the CNS. Today we know that central RAS plays a significant role in controlling systemic sympathetic activity and central integration of the afferent limb of the neurogenic reflex loop originating from the kidney [125]. Central angiotensin II has been implicated to promote development and maintenance of HTN [126] while central infusion of angiotensin II inhibitors attenuated the increases in RSNA and BP in response to renal afferent nerve stimulation [125]. This data suggest central RAS to be a key mechanism for several effects of RDN in humans. Measuring the physiologic response to administration of central angiotensin or measuring central levels of angiotensin are all potential methods to assess the effects of RDN in animals [127]. So far there are no comparable studies in humans advocating the use of new biomarkers or surrogate outcomes.

Despite the limited number of published data a majority of studies point towards a beneficial effect of RDN on SNA. A number of biomarkers provide evidence for a successful reduction in local and general sympathetic tone in animal disease models as well as humans with resistant HTN. As expected for a new technology in its early clinical phase the effects on biomarkers are heterogeneous. Discrepancies between animal and human data can potentially be explained by the difference in pathophysiology of HTN, renal disease as well as the role of SNS for disease development and progression between animal models and humans. An explanation for varying results in humans could be based in the inconsistent selection criteria of resistant hypertensive patients.

Role of Surrogate Markers in Renal Denervation

The initial safety and durability experience for therapeutic RDN document infrequent serious adverse events and durable treatment benefits in patients with elevated blood pressure and drug resistant HTN [128]. Besides a reduction in ambulatory and office blood pressure, animal and human studies provide evidence for a variety of other beneficial effects on cardiovascular physiology and concomitant diseases. Some of the effects are an improvement in reduced heart rate [129, 130], insulin resistance [131, 132], improved exercise tolerance [133] and renal function [134, 135], with attenuation of HF [136–138] as well as improved sleep apnea and cardiac arrhythmia [139–142]. Developing a vision of endpoints and surrogates of treatment efficacy becomes a critical next step in the development and application of RDN. Measuring the success of RDN requires careful differentiation of the technical success (biomarker) from the two measures of successful clinical outcome; surrogate endpoint and clinical endpoint.

Selection and validation of a biomarker and successive advancement to a surrogate endpoint are key processes in the development of new drug and device therapies as shown in Fig. 4.2. Streamlining the use of biomarkers over surrogate outcomes to clinical outcomes requires deep understanding of the pathophysiology of the underlying disease. Thoughtful selection, validation, and application of surrogate endpoints of clinical outcomes offers the potential to bring valuable interventions to clinical care expeditiously. Reduction in sample size and trial duration are important motivations for the use of surrogate endpoints that replace rare or distal endpoints by more frequent or proximate ones.

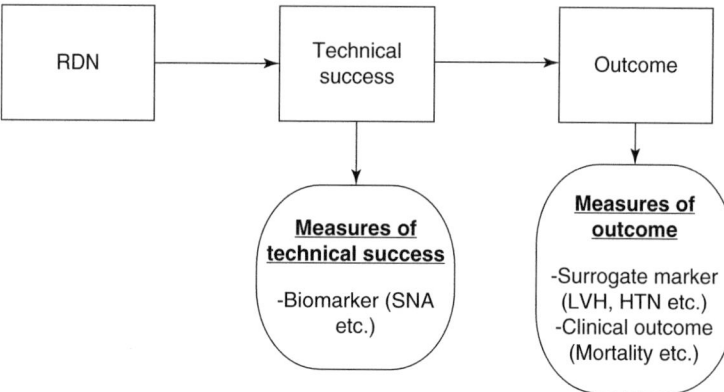

Fig. 4.2 Effective denervation by the RDN procedure can be evaluated intra- or postprocedural (technical success/ biomarkers). The clinical effects on outcome can be evaluated with surrogate outcomes or clinical outcomes

Table 4.2 A list of surrogate outcomes and clinical outcomes which have been used in RDN studies or could potentially be applied

Outcome measurement	Surrogate outcome	Clinical outcome
Efferent deinnervation	Blood pressure (ambulatory, office, blood pressure variability)	All cause mortality, cardiovascular mortality, stroke, MI, angina
	Renal function (GFR, proteinuria, albuminuria etc.)	
Afferent deinnervation	Via interruption of neurogenic reflex loop	Via interruption of neurogenic reflex loop
	Blood pressure (ambulatory, office, blood pressure variability)	All cause mortality, cardiovascular mortality, stroke, MI, angina
	Endothelial dysfunction	
	Heart rate	
	Insulin resistance	
	Renal function (GFR, albuminuria, proteinuria etc.)	
	Left ventricular mass by ECHO or MRI	
	EKG LVH with repolarization abnormalities	
	Tachycardic arrhythmias	
	Endothelial dysfunction	

It is obvious that long term endpoints such as mortality are the ultimately desired endpoints of every clinical study. However no study has studied the effects of RDN on hard clinical outcomes. Prudent consideration of clinical surrogate standards and biomarkers of desired outcomes may accelerate appropriate applications of therapeutic RDN. It is unrealistic to demand mortality endpoints for all new promising therapies especially if the procedure like RDN continues to show low serious adverse events. Moreover, some clinical endpoints, such as blood pressure, as a surrogate for mortality and morbidity in HTN, have attained an indisputable status, and several biomarkers convey confidence about prognosis. Table 4.2 summarizes surrogate and clinical outcomes that have been used or can be used for past and future RDN studies.

Disease Specific Outcomes

In the following part of this chapter we would like to identify disease specific measures which can be used to assess the effect of RDN on a particular disease. We will focus on surrogate outcomes as well as biomarkers which could be used to describe qualitative and quantitative result of RDN. A variety of measures can be used to characterize disease activity however not all of them can necessarily be used to capture the immediate or short-term effects of RDN on a particular organ or organ system.

Cardiovascular

Blood Pressure
Surrogate Outcomes: Ambulatory BP, Office BP, BP Variability, Night Time BP
BP reduction is the most commonly studied surrogate outcome in clinical trials and clinical practice. The first major RDN trials used changes in BP as a surrogate of successful

RDN. According to the Symplicity trials patients with an office systolic BP drop of more than 10 mmHg were considered to be responders to the intervention [143]. The positive effect of RDN on arterial BP are most likely a combined result of efferent renal denervation and decreased SNA following afferent kidney denervation. There are several reasons why BP is primarily chosen as surrogate outcome. Control of arterial HTN is a well-accepted risk reduction intervention for primary and secondary prevention of cardiovascular events. There is a well-established continuous and independent relationship between (office and ambulatory) BP and cardiovascular risk. Interventions leading to a reduction of BP have consistently been demonstrated to improve clinical outcome [144]. Based on this relationship it is assumed that successful reduction in BP following RDN will eventually also result in better clinical outcomes. Additional benefit of BP as a surrogate outcome is its universal availability and comparability of results. Ambulatory blood pressure monitoring (ABPM) is more sensitive and specific for cardiovascular risk stratification than office BP measurements [145, 146]. Also, 24 h ABPM correlates better with hypertensive and diabetic end-organ damage than office BP measurements do [147, 148]. Night time BP is related to sympathetic hyperactivation and more indicative of cardiovascular morbidity and mortally [149, 150]. The Dublin Outcome Study studied over 5,000 hypertensive patients and showed that an increase of 10 mmHg in mean night time systolic ABPM increased the cardiovascular mortality by 21 % [151]. Further ABPM is recommended in resistant hypertensive patients to rule out pseudoresistance [152]. Today we know that reduction in BP does not equally affect the outcome, rather the mode of BP control seems to play an important role [153, 154]. It is important to keep in mind that BP alteration and changes in SNA (e.g. MSNA) are not mutually inclusive. While HTN is clearly linked to the activity of the SNA, technical success of RDN does not have to be accompanied by BP changes [93].

RDN trials have investigated both the ambulatory and office blood pressure. While RDN significantly reduced ambulatory and office blood pressure, office BP reductions were more distinct than reductions in ABPM [90, 143]. The landmark trial Symplicity HTN-2 demonstrated a reduction in office BP of 32/12 mm Hg and 11/7 mm Hg in ambulatory 24-h BP [143]. The relative lower change in ABPM may be explained in part by selection criteria for the HTN 1 and 2 trials that did not exclude white coat HTN, thus inherently limiting the opportunity to realize reductions in the post procedure ABPM. Just as entry blood pressure predicts the outcome of renal denervation, entry ABPM is likely a major determinate in its response to the therapy. This relationship is consistent with results from drug treatment trials [155]. Office blood pressure lowering effects have been observed for a period of at least 2 years [128]. Beyond changes in mean arterial pressure RDN also reduces 24-h BP variability [156]. The clinical relevance of standard deviation of systolic BP has been demonstrated by Parati et al. in 109 hypertensive patients, where higher BP variability led to more end organ damage independent from the mean systolic BP [157]. Moreover it appears that visit to visit or day to day BP variability is a similar negative prognostic factor for cardiovascular mortality, stroke and overall mortality [158–160]. Taken together parameters like office and ambulatory BP, as well as its characteristics like BP variability and the pattern/time-dependence of BP reduction are all well suited surrogate outcomes for RDN. Further, risk factors like endothelial dysfunction are clearly linked to increased cardiovascular disease like essential HTN and could be used as accessory markers to measure effects of RDN [161]. Whilst HTN control is the current gold standard in the assessment of technical success in RDN, hard clinical outcomes like mortality may be impacted without BP changes. This urges for additional clinical surrogates in future clinical trials.

Left Ventricular Mass
Surrogate Outcomes: LV Mass by Echocardiogram, ECG or MRI, LV Diastolic and Systolic Heart Function

Left ventricular hypertrophy (LVH) documented by ECHO, ECG and MRI is a common finding in patients with HTN and HF with preserved and reduced ejection fraction. LVH, diastolic and systolic dysfunction are associated with an increased cardiovascular morbidity and mortality [162, 163]. Reduction in LVH by any metric reduces cardiovascular risk, improve mortality in interventional pharmaceutical trials which qualifies it as a surrogate outcome [164–166]. Perhaps of most interest are the well documented associations of ECG repolarization changes and both all-cause and cardiovascular mortality, and the improvements in the mortality following HTN therapy associated with improvements in ECG findings [167, 168]. Herein rests a surrogate, LVH with repolarization abnormalities that might

more closely link the therapy with morbidity and mortality changes, however it fails to have utility in predicting response to intervention or guiding intraprocedural therapy. There is also evidence suggesting that LVH regression influences cardiovascular outcomes in HTN independent of blood pressure changes and more strongly than any other risk factor except age [169]. Multiple retrospective and observational ECG and echocardiography studies shown that cardiovascular outcome is better in individuals in whom LVH regresses rather than progresses. This is indicative of the fact that reversal of LVH improves outcome beyond pure blood pressure treatment and reduction [170]. Using this information left ventricular mass can serve as a surrogate of disease progression and its control. This is supported by ECG trial data from the HOPE [168] and the LIFE [171, 172]. Further echocardiographic left ventricular mass predicts independently complications in the general population [173, 174] and patients with coronary artery disease (CAD) [175–177].

Brandt et al. studied the effect of RDN on left ventricular hypertrophy, systolic and diastolic function. In a group of 46 patients with resistant HTN, RDN significantly reduced left ventricular mass and improved systolic as well as diastolic heart function when compared to control [137]. Notably LV mass reduction was also observed in patients who did not respond to RDN with BP reduction, suggesting multiple pathways like fibrosis in which the SNA might contribute to LVH.

Exercise Capacity
Surrogate Outcomes: Exercise Capacity, Chronotropic Competence, Peak Exercise BP and HR

Decreased exercise capacity as well as excessive increases in systolic BP and heart rate during exercise are associated with increased cardiovascular morbidity and mortality [178, 179]. Meanwhile improvement in exercise tolerance is associated with an improved outcome. RDN improves exercise capacity with attenuated blood pressure at peak exercise (21 mmHg) without compromising chronotropic competence [133]. So far there is only one study targeting the HF population directly. In the REACH pilot study seven patients with HF with reduced ejection fraction underwent RDN. This resulted in a trend toward improved 6 min walk test and reduced diuretic therapy over a 6 months follow up period [138]. Unfortunately, the association of exercise endpoints and mortality in HTN is limited, and hardly serves as a convenient surrogate for diseases other than HF.

Arterial Stiffness
Surrogate Outcomes: Arterial Stiffness, Arterial Wall Inflammation?

Arterial stiffness is an established risk factor and independent predictor of cardiovascular morbidity and mortality

[180–182]. Decreased aortic distensibility has been linked to worse cardiovascular outcome especially in the hypertensive population [183]. Arterial stiffness can be assessed with the so called augmentation index which shows good correlation with coronary artery disease, all-cause and cardiovascular mortality [184, 185]. Hering et al. measured the arterial stiffness using finger tonometry-derived augmentation index in 40 patients who underwent catheter based RDN which resulted in a significant and rapid reduction of augmentation index [65]. Effects on arterial stiffness were independent from BP and MSNA changes. Interestingly drug studies with RAS blockade reduced arterial stiffness independent from BP changes which could speak for the fact that arterial stiffness is due to structural changes in the vessel wall rather than hemodynamic changes only [186–188]. Similar to EKG and repolarization abnormalities, the several metrics of arterial stiffness may closely associate to reductions of mortality and end organ disability, but will fail to provide guidance in screening patients or making intraprocedural therapy.

Heart Rate
Surrogate Outcomes: Resting HR
Elevated resting heart rate is considered a risk factor for arterial HTN [189], CAD [190], HF [191] and is a well established surrogate outcome of cardiovascular mortality [192, 193]. Pharmacological suppression of heart rate with ivabradine decreased composite outcome of cardiovascular death and hospitalization in a HF population [194]. In a sub population of patients with a resting heart rate >75 ivabradine reduced cardiovascular and all-cause mortality [195]. These data make heart rate a potential surrogate outcome and target for RDN. Repeatedly RDN trials were able to demonstrate a reduction in heart rate [89, 129]. The effect was more pronounced with higher baseline heart rate at baseline. Theoretical candidates, such as changes in heart rate and alterations of heart rate variability are complicated by the concurrent requirements for analgesia and anxiolytics during the procedure. Unfortunately, while reducing heart rate may associate with long term benefits of therapeutic renal denervation, it cannot be valuable in guiding patient selection or intraprocedural therapy.

Electrophysiology
Surrogate Outcomes: Freedom of Atrial Fibrillation and Ventricular Tachycardia and Fibrillation, Proarrhythmia, Ventricular Rate, Premature Ventricular Complex, ST-T Abnormalities

The SNA affects important electrophysiological properties of the heart including chronotropy and dromotropy. Consequently SNA plays a significant role in the development and persistence of atrial and ventricular tachyarrhythmias [196, 197]. An increased sympathetic tone becomes particularly relevant in context of existing co-morbidities like HTN, HF, DM, CAD and SDB. Atrial and ventricular tachyarrhythmias are clearly linked to an increased risk of mortality, making tachyarrhythmias a potential surrogate outcome for RDN [198, 199]. In animal models of tachyarrhythmias RDN resulted in negative chronotropic and dromotropic effects on the heart, leading to an improved rate control during induced atrial fibrillation (AF) and decreased AF susceptibility [140, 141]. In humans RDN improved ventricular rate in AF and decreased inducibility of AF in patients undergoing pulmonary vein isolation (PVI) vs. PVI alone [142]. Potential benefit of RDN on tachyarrhythmias in humans might also be explained by the effects of RDN on comorbidities which are associated with an increased SNA and tachyarrhythmias. Guidelines for clinical trials on atrial fibrillation suggest a variety of outcome measures to validate therapy effects of new drugs and technologies. Suggested clinical outcomes include mortality, stroke, AF related life quality as well as ECG based outcomes like freedom from AF, change in AF pattern, proarrhythmia (ventricular tachycardia, torsades de pointes, atrial flutter, bradycardia, AV nodal block), ventricular rate during AF at rest and during exercise [200].

Comparable to supraventricular arrhythmias RDN was studied in ventricular arrhythmias. In an animal model of myocardial ischemia induced ventricular arrhythmias/fibrillation RDN reduced the occurrence of ventricular arrhythmias/fibrillation [201]. First human studies on RDN and ventricular arrhythmias are restricted to a case series of two patients with HF and electrical storm. The off-label use of RDN decreased incidence of ventricular arrhythmias [202]. Likewise to guidelines for atrial fibrillation the use of hard clinical outcomes and ECG based outcomes can be used to investigate the effect of RDN on ventricular arrhythmias.

Lastly electrocardiographical ST-T wave changes could be used as a surrogate outcome. While a clear relationship with the SNA has not been established, ST-T patterns represented by ST-T wave abnormalities are clearly linked to a higher cardiovascular mortality in patient with underlying cardiovascular disease like HTN, coronary disease etc. [203].

Atherosclerosis and Cardiovascular Events
Surrogate Outcomes: Intima Media Thickness, Inflammatory Markers
Reduction in sympathetic tone could also benefit atherosclerosis and future cardiovascular events. There is an established link between sympathetic hyperactivation and cardiac events like myocardial infarction and angina. Although RDN trials have not yet looked into potential benefits, future trials could use established surrogate outcomes of CAD like carotid intima media thickness and inflammatory markers like CRP [204, 205].

Renal

Surrogate Outcomes: GFR, Proteinuria, Albuminuria, Renal Noradrenaline Levels, Renal Vascular Resistance and Renal Arterial Flow

Increased SNA correlates with worsening renal function [30, 118, 206]. Levels of noradrenaline predict mortality and cardiovascular events in patients with chronic kidney disease (CKD). CKD is an established independent risk factor for cardiovascular and all-cause mortality in the general population [207–209]. Besides the traditional estimate of renal function with the glomerular filtration function (GFR), albuminuria and proteinuria have been established as independent risk factors for all-cause mortality [209, 210]. Thus GFR, albuminuria and proteinuria can potentially serve as surrogate outcomes for RDN. Surgical RDN has favourable effects on acute kidney injury and CKD in a number of different animal models [211]. RDN resulted in improvement of renal hemodynamic and filtration dysfunction caused by chemical toxic or ischemic damage to the kidney. In humans there are currently only several small scale studies looking into potential effects of RDN on renal function. Human trials have studied the effects of RDN on normal and deceased kidneys in resistant hypertensives. Initial landmark studies have used decreased GFR as an exclusion criterion for RDN. Effects of RDN on the kidney function include biomarkers of successful renal denervation like decreased renin secretion and increased RBF [104]. Further Krum et al. demonstrated in a single-arm study an improved GFR in 24 % of patients with resistant HTN and a normal renal function over a 12 months period. In a comparable study with a control group RDN reduced the incidence of microalbuminuria while GFR remained unchanged [134]. Denervation resulted in a decreased proportion of patients with detectable urinary albumin excretion 6 months after the procedure. Other renal vascular hemodynamics could be additional biomarkers of efferent and afferent denervation. Renal vascular resistance and renal blood flow could reflect a reduction in SNA of renal nerves. However despite improved central and peripheral blood pressure, decreased renal vascular resistance, the renal function (GFR) and renal perfusion remain unchanged after the procedure [95, 212].

Subsequent studies investigated the safety and potential benefit of RDN in CKD. Hering et al. studied the short term effects of RDN in CKD three to four patients. RDN reduced the BP however did not result in significant changes of GFR, proteinuria or albuminuria [213]. Three additional studies investigated the effects of RDN in end stage renal disease (ESRD) for up to 12 months [107, 116, 214]. These studies confirm the anti-hypertensive effect of RDN in ESRD without a change in GFR which could suggest a protective effect of this intervention on renal function. Since most studies lack a control group the potentially beneficial effect and its role as a surrogate outcome need to be further investigated in randomized controlled trials.

Metabolic

Diabetes
Surrogate Outcomes: Insulin Level, Insulin Resistance, Fasting Glucose and Glucose Tolerance Test

There is a clear link between activation of the SNS, hyperinsulinemia and development of diabetes mellitus type 2 (DM) [215–217]. Moreover SNA is associated with pathophysiology of metabolic syndrome, obesity and resistant HTN [217]. At the same time the metabolic syndrome and DM are clearly linked to an increased cardiovascular morbidity and mortality [218]. Increased fasting glucose, impaired glucose tolerance and increased insulin levels have been established as surrogate outcomes for the metabolic syndrome and DM.

In animals models of insulin induced HTN, renal denervation improved BP [131]. Mahfoud et al. studied the effects of RDN in humans with resistant HTN [132]. In a population of patients with resistant HTN and metabolic syndrome, 40 % of whom had a confirmed diagnosis of DM2, RDN decreased fasting glucose from 118 to 108 mg/dL, insulin levels from 20.8 to 9.3 µIU/mL and C-peptide levels from 5.3 to 3.0 ng/mL. Further the insulin resistance index as well as a postprandial glucose tolerance test improved by 30–40 % following 3 months after the procedure. Moreover oral glucose tolerance tests improved in the studied population resulting in decreased number of patients with impaired fasting hyperglycemia and impaired glucose tolerance test.

While the association between renal sympathetic denervation in resistant HTN has been documented, neither insulin resistance by HOMA or reduction of insulin levels themselves have been documented as mortality surrogates.

Conclusion

1. There is no current intraprocedural test of technical success to assist in titration of therapy that both is sensitive and specific as well as provide immediate results to the interventional clinician. The low complication rates and cost of therapeutic renal denervation for treatment resistant HTN render the value for these tools low. However, if more aggressive or potentially toxic interventions or the titration of ablation therapy is associated with renal or vascular toxicity the need for measures of technical success will be more obvious.

2. Screening tests for identification of optimal candidates for renal denervation could reduce futile therapy. For the population of drug resistant HTN, where the cost and morbidity of the procedure are apparently low while the underlying morbidity of excessive blood pressure is high, a screening test has to overcome high burdens to prove themselves useful. In populations, other than HTN, where the benefit: risk of therapy is lower, a screening test with excellent positive predictive value of benefit could be necessary and may require organ system specific metrics.

3. Beyond the reduction of office blood pressure, a well vetted surrogate of cardiovascular morbidity and mortality are improvements in left ventricular electrocardiographic findings, such left ventricular voltage and strain patterns represented by ST-T wave abnormalities. A less sensitive and more specific surrogate for mortality may be the reduction of LV mass documented by either ECHO or MRI. The reporting of these changes in renal denervation trails for the treatment of HTN could empower clinicians and patients considering therapeutic options.

4. Various measures of sympathetic activity remain scientifically interesting and perhaps valuable in comparing the method of action between denervation tools, but these measures are themselves poorly linked to mortality rates and the sensitivity of these measures to changes in mortality rates remains untested.

References

1. Johns EJ, Kopp UC, Dibona GF. Neural control of renal function. Compr Physiol. 2011;1:731–67.
2. Atherton DS, Deep NL, Mendelsohn FO. Micro-anatomy of the renal sympathetic nervous system: a human postmortem histologic study. Clin Anat. 2012;25:628–33.
3. Campese VM. Neurogenic factors and hypertension in renal disease. Kidney Int Suppl. 2000;75:S2–6.
4. Kopp UC. Neural control of renal function. San Rafael: Morgan & Claypool Life Sciences; 2011.
5. Pernow J, Schwieler J, Kahan T, Hjemdahl P, Oberle J, Wallin BG, Lundberg JM. Influence of sympathetic discharge pattern on norepinephrine and neuropeptide y release. Am J Physiol. 1989;257:H866–72.
6. Schwartz DD, Malik KU. Renal periarterial nerve stimulation-induced vasoconstriction at low frequencies is primarily due to release of a purinergic transmitter in the rat. J Pharmacol Exp Ther. 1989;250:764–71.
7. Williams NG, Zhong H, Minneman KP. Differential coupling of alpha1-, alpha2-, and beta-adrenergic receptors to mitogen-activated protein kinase pathways and differentiation in transfected pc12 cells. J Biol Chem. 1998;273:24624–32.
8. Azroyan A, Morla L, Crambert G, Laghmani K, Ramakrishnan S, Edwards A, Doucet A. Regulation of pendrin by camp: possible involvement in beta-adrenergic-dependent nacl retention. Am J Physiol Renal Physiol. 2012;302:F1180–7.
9. Pernow J, Lundberg JM. Modulation of noradrenaline and neuropeptide y (npy) release in the pig kidney in vivo: involvement of alpha 2, npy and angiotensin ii receptors. Naunyn Schmiedebergs Arch Pharmacol. 1989;340:379–85.
10. Unwin RJ, Bailey MA, Burnstock G. Purinergic signaling along the renal tubule: the current state of play. News Physiol Sci Int J Physiol Produced Jointly Int Union Physiol Sci Am Physiol Soc. 2003;18:237–41.
11. Barajas L, Powers K, Wang P. Innervation of the renal cortical tubules: a quantitative study. Am J Physiol. 1984;247:F50–60.
12. Barajas L, Powers K. Innervation of the renal proximal convoluted tubule of the rat. Am J Anat. 1989;186:378–88.
13. Barajas L, Powers K. Monoaminergic innervation of the rat kidney: a quantitative study. Am J Physiol. 1990;259:F503–11.
14. Zanchetti AS. Neural regulation of renin release: experimental evidence and clinical implications in arterial hypertension. Circulation. 1977;56:691–8.
15. Osborn JL, DiBona GF, Thames MD. Beta-1 receptor mediation of renin secretion elicited by low-frequency renal nerve stimulation. J Pharmacol Exp Ther. 1981;216:265–9.
16. Holmer S, Rinne B, Eckardt KU, Le Hir M, Schricker K, Kaissling B, Riegger G, Kurtz A. Role of renal nerves for the expression of renin in adult rat kidney. Am J Physiol. 1994;266:F738–45.
17. Barrett CJ, Navakatikyan MA, Malpas SC. Long-term control of renal blood flow: what is the role of the renal nerves? Am J Physiol Regul Integr Comp Physiol. 2001;280:R1534–45.
18. Abdala AP, McBryde FD, Marina N, Hendy EB, Engelman Z, Fudim M, Sobotka PA, Gourine A, Paton J. Hypertension is critically dependent on the carotid body input in the spontaneously hypertensive rat. J Physiol. 2012;590(Pt 17):4269–77.
19. Paton JF, Sobotka PA, Fudim M, Engleman ZJ, Hart EC, McBryde FD, Abdala AP, Marina N, Gourine AV, Lobo M, Patel N, Burchell A, Ratcliffe L, Nightingale A. The carotid body as a therapeutic target for the treatment of sympathetically mediated diseases. Hypertension. 2013;61(1):5–13.
20. Esler M, Jennings G, Korner P, Willett I, Dudley F, Hasking G, Anderson W, Lambert G. Assessment of human sympathetic nervous system activity from measurements of norepinephrine turnover. Hypertension. 1988;11:3–20.
21. Lundin S, Ricksten SE, Thoren P. Interaction between "mental stress" and baroreceptor reflexes concerning effects on heart rate, mean arterial pressure and renal sympathetic activity in conscious spontaneously hypertensive rats. Acta Physiol Scand. 1984;120: 273–81.
22. Hasking GJ, Esler MD, Jennings GL, Burton D, Johns JA, Korner PI. Norepinephrine spillover to plasma in patients with congestive heart failure: evidence of increased overall and cardiorenal sympathetic nervous activity. Circulation. 1986;73:615–21.
23. Ramchandra R, Hood SG, Denton DA, Woods RL, McKinley MJ, McAllen RM, May CN. Basis for the preferential activation of cardiac sympathetic nerve activity in heart failure. Proc Natl Acad Sci U S A. 2009;106:924–8.
24. Solano-Flores LP, Rosas-Arellano MP, Ciriello J. Fos induction in central structures after afferent renal nerve stimulation. Brain Res. 1997;753:102–19.
25. Ciriello J, de Oliveira CV. Renal afferents and hypertension. Curr Hypertens Rep. 2002;4:136–42.
26. Stella A, Zanchetti A. Functional role of renal afferents. Physiol Rev. 1991;71:659–82.
27. Smits JF, Brody MJ. Activation of afferent renal nerves by intrarenal bradykinin in conscious rats. Am J Physiol. 1984;247:R1003–8.
28. Katholi RE, Whitlow PL, Hageman GR, Woods WT. Intrarenal adenosine produces hypertension by activating the sympathetic nervous system via the renal nerves in the dog. J Hypertens. 1984;2:349–59.

29. Campese VM, Kogosov E. Renal afferent denervation prevents hypertension in rats with chronic renal failure. Hypertension. 1995;25:878–82.

30. Hausberg M, Kosch M, Harmelink P, Barenbrock M, Hohage H, Kisters K, Dietl KH, Rahn KH. Sympathetic nerve activity in end-stage renal disease. Circulation. 2002;106:1974–9.

31. Kopp UC, Cicha MZ, Smith LA. Endogenous angiotensin modulates pge(2)-mediated release of substance p from renal mechanosensory nerve fibers. Am J Physiol Regul Integr Comp Physiol. 2002;282:R19–30.

32. Siddiqi L, Joles JA, Grassi G, Blankestijn PJ. Is kidney ischemia the central mechanism in parallel activation of the renin and sympathetic system? J Hypertens. 2009;27:1341–9.

33. Gontijo JA, Kopp UC. Activation of renal pelvic chemoreceptors in rats: role of calcitonin gene-related peptide receptors. Acta Physiol Scand. 1999;166:159–65.

34. Kopp UC, Cicha MZ, Farley DM, Smith LA, Dixon BS. Renal substance p-containing neurons and substance p receptors impaired in hypertension. Hypertension. 1998;31:815–22.

35. Zhu Y, Xie C, Wang DH. Trpv1-mediated diuresis and natriuresis induced by hypertonic saline perfusion of the renal pelvis. Am J Nephrol. 2007;27:530–7.

36. Ditting T, Freisinger W, Siegel K, Fiedler C, Small L, Neuhuber W, Heinlein S, Reeh PW, Schmieder RE, Veelken R. Tonic postganglionic sympathetic inhibition induced by afferent renal nerves? Hypertension. 2012;59:467–76.

37. Feng NH, Lee HH, Shiang JC, Ma MC. Transient receptor potential vanilloid type 1 channels act as mechanoreceptors and cause substance p release and sensory activation in rat kidneys. Am J Physiol Renal Physiol. 2008;294:F316–25.

38. Fallick C, Sobotka PA, Dunlap ME. Sympathetically mediated changes in capacitance: redistribution of the venous reservoir as a cause of decompensation. Circ Heart Fail. 2011;4:669–75.

39. Bencsath P, Szenasi G, Takacs L. Water and electrolyte transport in henle's loop and distal tubule after renal sympathectomy in the rat. Am J Physiol. 1985;249:F308–14.

40. Bachmann S, Bosse HM, Mundel P. Topography of nitric oxide synthesis by localizing constitutive no synthases in mammalian kidney. Am J Physiol. 1995;268:F885–98.

41. Kopp UC, Cicha MZ, Smith LA. Impaired responsiveness of renal mechanosensory nerves in heart failure: role of endogenous angiotensin. Am J Physiol Regul Integr Comp Physiol. 2003;284:R116–24.

42. Kline RL, Mercer PF. Functional reinnervation and development of supersensitivity to NE after renal denervation in rats. Am J Physiol. 1980;238:R353–8.

43. Couch NP, Mc BR, Dammin GJ, Murray JE. Observations on the nature of the enlargement, the regeneration of the nerves, and the function of the canine renal autograft. Br J Exp Pathol. 1961;42:106–13.

44. Gazdar AF, Dammin GJ. Neural degeneration and regeneration in human renal transplants. N Engl J Med. 1970;283:222–4.

45. Hansen JM, Abildgaard U, Fogh-Andersen N, Kanstrup IL, Bratholm P, Plum I, Strandgaard S. The transplanted human kidney does not achieve functional reinnervation. Clin Sci (Lond). 1994;87:13–20.

46. Mulder J, Hokfelt T, Knuepfer MM, Kopp UC. Renal sensory and sympathetic nerves reinnervate the kidney in a similar time-dependent fashion after renal denervation in rats. Am J Physiol Regul Integr Comp Physiol. 2013;304:R675–82.

47. Friberg P, Meredith I, Jennings G, Lambert G, Fazio V, Esler M. Evidence for increased renal norepinephrine overflow during sodium restriction in humans. Hypertension. 1990;16:121–30.

48. Dunlap ME, Sobotka PA. Fluid re-distribution rather than accumulation causes most cases of decompensated heart failure. J Am Coll Cardiol. 2013;62:165–6.

49. Ma MC, Huang HS, Chen CF. Impaired renal sensory responses after unilateral ureteral obstruction in the rat. J Am Soc Nephrol: JASN. 2002;13:1008–16.

50. Pan HL, Longhurst JC, Eisenach JC, Chen SR. Role of protons in activation of cardiac sympathetic c-fibre afferents during ischaemia in cats. J Physiol. 1999;518(Pt 3):857–66.

51. Kostreva DR, Zuperku EJ, Hess GL, Coon RL, Kampine JP. Pulmonary afferent activity recorded from sympathetic nerves. J Appl Physiol. 1975;39:37–40.

52. Kostreva DR, Castaner A, Kampine JP. Reflex effects of hepatic baroreceptors on renal and cardiac sympathetic nerve activity. Am J Physiol. 1980;238:R390–4.

53. Vaz M, Jennings G, Turner A, Cox H, Lambert G, Esler M. Regional sympathetic nervous activity and oxygen consumption in obese normotensive human subjects. Circulation. 1997;96:3423–9.

54. Malpas SC. Sympathetic nervous system overactivity and its role in the development of cardiovascular disease. Physiol Rev. 2010;90:513–57.

55. Iriki M, Simon E. Differential control of efferent sympathetic activity revisited. J Physiol Sci J Physiol Sci. 2012;62:275–98.

56. Esler M, Jennings G, Korner P, Blombery P, Sacharias N, Leonard P. Measurement of total and organ-specific norepinephrine kinetics in humans. Am J Physiol. 1984;247:E21–8.

57. Esler M, Jennings G, Korner P, Blombery P, Burke F, Willett I, Leonard P. Total, and organ-specific, noradrenaline plasma kinetics in essential hypertension. Clin Exp Hypertens A Theory Pract. 1984;6:507–21.

58. Esler M, Willett I, Leonard P, Hasking G, Johns J, Little P, Jennings G. Plasma noradrenaline kinetics in humans. J Auton Nerv Syst. 1984;11:125–44.

59. Bradley T, Hjemdahl P. Further studies on renal nerve stimulation induced release of noradrenaline and dopamine from the canine kidney in situ. Acta Physiol Scand. 1984;122:369–79.

60. Hagbarth KE, Vallbo AB. Pulse and respiratory grouping of sympathetic impulses in human muscle-nerves. Acta Physiol Scand. 1968;74:96–108.

61. Charkoudian N, Joyner MJ, Johnson CP, Eisenach JH, Dietz NM, Wallin BG. Balance between cardiac output and sympathetic nerve activity in resting humans: role in arterial pressure regulation. J Physiol. 2005;568:315–21.

62. Wallin BG, Charkoudian N. Sympathetic neural control of integrated cardiovascular function: insights from measurement of human sympathetic nerve activity. Muscle Nerve. 2007;36:595–614.

63. Fagius J, Wallin BG. Long-term variability and reproducibility of resting human muscle nerve sympathetic activity at rest, as reassessed after a decade. Clin Auton Res. 1993;3:201–5.

64. Macefield VG, Wallin BG, Vallbo AB. The discharge behaviour of single vasoconstrictor motoneurones in human muscle nerves. J Physiol. 1994;481(Pt 3):799–809.

65. Hering D, Lambert EA, Marusic P, Walton AS, Krum H, Lambert GW, Esler MD, Schlaich MP. Substantial reduction in single sympathetic nerve firing after renal denervation in patients with resistant hypertension. Hypertension. 2013;61:457–64.

66. Lambert E, Dawood T, Schlaich M, Straznicky N, Esler M, Lambert G. Single-unit sympathetic discharge pattern in pathological conditions associated with elevated cardiovascular risk. Clin Exp Pharmacol Physiol. 2008;35:503–7.

67. Macefield VG, Wallin BG. Respiratory and cardiac modulation of single sympathetic vasoconstrictor and sudomotor neurones to human skin. J Physiol. 1999;516(Pt 1):303–14.

68. Murai H, Takata S, Maruyama M, Nakano M, Kobayashi D, Otowa K, Takamura M, Yuasa T, Sakagami S, Kaneko S. The activity of a single muscle sympathetic vasoconstrictor nerve unit is affected by physiological stress in humans. Am J Physiol Heart Circ Physiol. 2006;290:H853–60.

69. Macefield VG, Rundqvist B, Sverrisdottir YB, Wallin BG, Elam M. Firing properties of single muscle vasoconstrictor neurons in the sympathoexcitation associated with congestive heart failure. Circulation. 1999;100:1708–13.

70. Barretto AC, Santos AC, Munhoz R, Rondon MU, Franco FG, Trombetta IC, Roveda F, de Matos LN, Braga AM, Middlekauff HR, Negrao CE. Increased muscle sympathetic nerve activity predicts mortality in heart failure patients. Int J Cardiol. 2009;135:302–7.

71. Parati G, Saul JP, Di Rienzo M, Mancia G. Spectral analysis of blood pressure and heart rate variability in evaluating cardiovascular regulation. A critical appraisal. Hypertension. 1995;25:1276–86.

72. Task force of the European Society of Cardiology and the North American Society of Pacing and Electrophysiology. Heart rate variability. Standards of measurement, physiological interpretation, and clinical use. Eur Heart J. 1996;17:354–81.

73. Gilder M, Ramsbottom R. Measures of cardiac autonomic control in women with differing volumes of physical activity. J Sports Sci. 2008;26:781–6.

74. La Rovere MT, Bigger Jr JT, Marcus FI, Mortara A, Schwartz PJ. Baroreflex sensitivity and heart-rate variability in prediction of total cardiac mortality after myocardial infarction. Atrami (autonomic tone and reflexes after myocardial infarction) investigators. Lancet. 1998;351:478–84.

75. Malpas SC. Neural influences on cardiovascular variability: possibilities and pitfalls. Am J Physiol Heart Circ Physiol. 2002;282:H6–20.

76. Fox K, Borer JS, Camm AJ, Danchin N, Ferrari R, Lopez Sendon JL, Steg PG, Tardif JC, Tavazzi L, Tendera M. Resting heart rate in cardiovascular disease. J Am Coll Cardiol. 2007;50:823–30.

77. Julien C, Chapuis B, Cheng Y, Barres C. Dynamic interactions between arterial pressure and sympathetic nerve activity: role of arterial baroreceptors. Am J Physiol Regul Integr Comp Physiol. 2003;285:R834–41.

78. Narkiewicz K, Winnicki M, Schroeder K, Phillips BG, Kato M, Cwalina E, Somers VK. Relationship between muscle sympathetic nerve activity and diurnal blood pressure profile. Hypertension. 2002;39:168–72.

79. Parati G, Esler M. The human sympathetic nervous system: its relevance in hypertension and heart failure. Eur Heart J. 2012;33:1058–66.

80. Bristow JD, Honour AJ, Pickering GW, Sleight P, Smyth HS. Diminished baroreflex sensitivity in high blood pressure. Circulation. 1969;39:48–54.

81. Ellenbogen KA, Mohanty PK, Szentpetery S, Thames MD. Arterial baroreflex abnormalities in heart failure. Reversal after orthotopic cardiac transplantation. Circulation. 1989;79:51–8.

82. Parati G, Di Rienzo M, Mancia G. How to measure baroreflex sensitivity: from the cardiovascular laboratory to daily life. J Hypertens. 2000;18:7–19.

83. Despas F, Lambert E, Vaccaro A, Labrunee M, Franchitto N, Lebrin M, Galinier M, Senard JM, Lambert G, Esler M, Pathak A. Peripheral chemoreflex activation contributes to sympathetic baroreflex impairment in chronic heart failure. J Hypertens. 2012;30:753–60.

84. Ponikowski P, Chua TP, Anker SD, Francis DP, Doehner W, Banasiak W, Poole-Wilson PA, Piepoli MF, Coats AJ. Peripheral chemoreceptor hypersensitivity: an ominous sign in patients with chronic heart failure. Circulation. 2001;104:544–9.

85. McBryde FD, Abdala AP, Hendy EB, Pijacka W, Marvar P, Moraes DJ, Sobotka PA, Paton JF. The carotid body as a putative therapeutic target for the treatment of neurogenic hypertension. Nat Commun. 2013;4:2395.

86. Niewinski P, Engelman ZJ, Fudim M, Tubek S, Paleczny B, Jankowska EA, Banasiak W, Sobotka PA, Ponikowski P. Clinical predictors and hemodynamic consequences of elevated peripheral chemosensitivity in optimally treated men with chronic systolic heart failure. J Card Fail. 2013;19:408–15.

87. Biaggioni I, Olafsson B, Robertson RM, Hollister AS, Robertson D. Cardiovascular and respiratory effects of adenosine in conscious man. Evidence for chemoreceptor activation. Circ Res. 1987;61:779–86.

88. Stickland MK, Fuhr DP, Haykowsky MJ, Jones KE, Paterson DI, Ezekowitz JA, McMurtry MS. Carotid chemoreceptor modulation of blood flow during exercise in healthy humans. J Physiol. 2011;589:6219–30.

89. Ott C, Mahfoud F, Schmid A, Ditting T, Sobotka PA, Veelken R, Spies A, Ukena C, Laufs U, Uder M, Bohm M, Schmieder RE. Renal denervation in moderate treatment-resistant hypertension. J Am Coll Cardiol. 2013;62:1880–6.

90. Mahfoud F, Ukena C, Schmieder RE, Cremers B, Rump LC, Vonend O, Weil J, Schmidt M, Hoppe UC, Zeller T, Bauer A, Ott C, Blessing E, Sobotka PA, Krum H, Schlaich M, Esler M, Bohm M. Ambulatory blood pressure changes after renal sympathetic denervation in patients with resistant hypertension. Circulation. 2013;128:132–40.

91. Zuern CS, Eick C, Rizas KD, Bauer S, Langer H, Gawaz M, Bauer A. Impaired cardiac baroreflex sensitivity predicts response to renal sympathetic denervation in patients with resistant hypertension. J Am Coll Cardiol. 2013;62(22):2124–30.

92. Rocha-Singh KJ, Katholi RE. Renal sympathetic denervation for treatment-resistant hypertension…in moderation. J Am Coll Cardiol. 2013;62:1887–9.

93. Morlin C, Wallin BG, Eriksson BM. Muscle sympathetic activity and plasma noradrenaline in normotensive and hypertensive man. Acta Physiol Scand. 1983;119:117–21.

94. Hart EC, McBryde FD, Burchell AE, Ratcliffe LE, Stewart LQ, Baumbach A, Nightingale A, Paton JF. Translational examination of changes in baroreflex function after renal denervation in hypertensive rats and humans. Hypertension. 2013;62(3):533–41.

95. Krum H, Schlaich M, Whitbourn R, Sobotka PA, Sadowski J, Bartus K, Kapelak B, Walton A, Sievert H, Thambar S, Abraham WT, Esler M. Catheter-based renal sympathetic denervation for resistant hypertension: a multicentre safety and proof-of-principle cohort study. Lancet. 2009;373:1275–81.

96. Chinushi M, Izumi D, Iijima K, Suzuki K, Furushima H, Saitoh O, Furuta Y, Aizawa Y, Iwafuchi M. Blood pressure and autonomic responses to electrical stimulation of the renal arterial nerves before and after ablation of the renal artery. Hypertension. 2013;61:450–6.

97. Rafiq K, Noma T, Fujisawa Y, Ishihara Y, Arai Y, Nabi AH, Suzuki F, Nagai Y, Nakano D, Hitomi H, Kitada K, Urushihara M, Kobori H, Kohno M, Nishiyama A. Renal sympathetic denervation suppresses de novo podocyte injury and albuminuria in rats with aortic regurgitation. Circulation. 2012;125:1402–13.

98. Luippold G, Beilharz M, Muhlbauer B. Chronic renal denervation prevents glomerular hyperfiltration in diabetic rats. Nephrol Dial Transplant. 2004;19:342–7.

99. Clayton SC, Haack KK, Zucker IH. Renal denervation modulates angiotensin receptor expression in the renal cortex of rabbits with chronic heart failure. Am J Physiol Renal Physiol. 2011;300:F31–9.

100. Veelken R, Vogel EM, Hilgers K, Amann K, Hartner A, Sass G, Neuhuber W, Tiegs G. Autonomic renal denervation ameliorates experimental glomerulonephritis. J Am Soc Nephrol: JASN. 2008;19:1371–8.

101. Wang W, Falk SA, Jittikanont S, Gengaro PE, Edelstein CL, Schrier RW. Protective effect of renal denervation on normotensive endotoxemia-induced acute renal failure in mice. Am J Physiol Renal Physiol. 2002;283:F583–7.

102. Salman IM, Ameer OZ, Sattar MA, Abdullah NA, Yam MF, Najim HS, Khan AH, Johns EJ. Role of the renal sympathetic

nervous system in mediating renal ischaemic injury-induced reductions in renal haemodynamic and excretory functions. Pathology. 2010;42:259–66.

103. van de Borne P. The kidney and the sympathetic system: a short review. Curr Clin Pharmacol. 2013;8(3):175–81.

104. Schlaich MP, Sobotka PA, Krum H, Lambert E, Esler MD. Renal sympathetic-nerve ablation for uncontrolled hypertension. N Engl J Med. 2009;361:932–4.

105. Ezzahti M, Moelker A, Friesema EC, van der Linde NA, Krestin GP, van den Meiracker AH. Blood pressure and neurohormonal responses to renal nerve ablation in treatment-resistant hypertension. J Hypertens. 2014;32(1):135–41.

106. Ahmed H, Neuzil P, Skoda J, Petru J, Sediva L, Schejbalova M, Reddy VY. Renal sympathetic denervation using an irrigated radiofrequency ablation catheter for the management of drug-resistant hypertension. JACC Cardiovasc Interv. 2012;5:758–65.

107. Schlaich MP, Bart B, Hering D, Walton A, Marusic P, Mahfoud F, Bohm M, Lambert EA, Krum H, Sobotka PA, Schmieder RE, Ika-Sari C, Eikelis N, Straznicky N, Lambert GW, Esler MD. Feasibility of catheter-based renal nerve ablation and effects on sympathetic nerve activity and blood pressure in patients with end-stage renal disease. Int J Cardiol. 2013;168(3):2214–20.

108. Seva Pessoa B, van der Lubbe N, Verdonk K, Roks AJ, Hoorn EJ, Danser AH. Key developments in renin-angiotensin-aldosterone system inhibition. Nat Rev Nephrol. 2013;9:26–36.

109. Wagman G, Fudim M, Kosmas CE, Panni RE, Vittorio TJ. The neurohormonal network in the raas can bend before breaking. Curr Heart Fail Rep. 2012;9:81–91.

110. Kowalski R, Kreft E, Kasztan M, Jankowski M, Szczepanska-Konkel M. Chronic renal denervation increases renal tubular response to p2x receptor agonists in rats: implication for renal sympathetic nerve ablation. Nephrol Dial Transplant. 2012;27:3443–8.

111. Christy IJ, Denton KM, Anderson WP. Renal denervation potentiates the natriuretic and diuretic effects of atrial natriuretic peptide in anaesthetized rabbits. Clin Exp Pharmacol Physiol. 1994;21:41–8.

112. Kompanowska-Jezierska E, Walkowska A, Johns EJ, Sadowski J. Early effects of renal denervation in the anaesthetised rat: natriuresis and increased cortical blood flow. J Physiol. 2001;531:527–34.

113. Pettersson A, Hedner J, Hedner T. Renal interaction between sympathetic activity and anp in rats with chronic ischaemic heart failure. Acta Physiol Scand. 1989;135:487–92.

114. Wenting GJ, Blankestijn PJ, Poldermans D, van Geelen J, Derkx FH, Man in't Veld AJ, Schalekamp MA. Blood pressure response of nephrectomized subjects and patients with essential hypertension to ramipril: indirect evidence that inhibition of tissue angiotensin converting enzyme is important. Am J Cardiol. 1987;59:92D–7.

115. Wang L, Lu CZ, Zhang X, Luo D, Zhao B, Yu X, Xia DS, Chen X, Zhao XD. The effect of catheter based renal synthetic denervation on renin-angiotensin-aldosterone system in patients with resistant hypertension. Zhonghua Xin Xue Guan Bing Za Zhi. 2013;41:3–7.

116. Di Daniele N, De Francesco M, Violo L, Spinelli A, Simonetti G. Renal sympathetic nerve ablation for the treatment of difficult-to-control or refractory hypertension in a haemodialysis patient. Nephrol Dial Transplant. 2012;27:1689–90.

117. Masuo K, Lambert GW, Esler MD, Rakugi H, Ogihara T, Schlaich MP. The role of sympathetic nervous activity in renal injury and end-stage renal disease. Hypertens Res. 2010;33:521–8.

118. Converse Jr RL, Jacobsen TN, Toto RD, Jost CM, Cosentino F, Fouad-Tarazi F, Victor RG. Sympathetic overactivity in patients with chronic renal failure. N Engl J Med. 1992;327:1912–8.

119. Hering D, Lambert EA, Marusic P, Ika-Sari C, Walton AS, Krum H, Sobotka PA, Mahfoud F, Bohm M, Lambert GW, Esler MD, Schlaich

MP. Renal nerve ablation reduces augmentation index in patients with resistant hypertension. J Hypertens. 2013;31(9):1893–900.

120. Greenwood JP, Stoker JB, Mary DA. Single-unit sympathetic discharge: quantitative assessment in human hypertensive disease. Circulation. 1999;100:1305–10.

121. Oliveira VL, Irigoyen MC, Moreira ED, Strunz C, Krieger EM. Renal denervation normalizes pressure and baroreceptor reflex in high renin hypertension in conscious rats. Hypertension. 1992;19:II17–21.

122. Janssen BJ, van Essen H, Vervoort-Peters LH, Struyker-Boudier HA, Smits JF. Role of afferent renal nerves in spontaneous hypertension in rats. Hypertension. 1989;13:327–33.

123. Schiller ACP, Haack K, Zucker I. Unilateral renal denervation enhances baroreflex function in concious rabbits with chronic heart failure. Physiologist. 2012;55:A13.19.43.

124. Brinkmann J, Heusser K, Schmidt BM, Menne J, Klein G, Bauersachs J, Haller H, Sweep FC, Diedrich A, Jordan J, Tank J. Catheter-based renal nerve ablation and centrally generated sympathetic activity in difficult-to-control hypertensive patients: prospective case series. Hypertension. 2012;60:1485–90.

125. Fujisawa Y, Nagai Y, Lei B, Nakano D, Fukui T, Hitomi H, Mori H, Masaki T, Nishiyama A. Roles of central renin-angiotensin system and afferent renal nerve in the control of systemic hemodynamics in rats. Hypertens Res. 2011;34:1228–32.

126. Ito S, Komatsu K, Tsukamoto K, Kanmatsuse K, Sved AF. Ventrolateral medulla at1 receptors support blood pressure in hypertensive rats. Hypertension. 2002;40:552–9.

127. Weyhenmeyer JA, Phillips MI. Angiotensin-like immunoreactivity in the brain of the spontaneously hypertensive rat. Hypertension. 1982;4:514–23.

128. Krum H, Barman N, Schlaich M, Sobotka P, Esler M, Mahfoud F, Bohm M, Dunlap M, Sadowski J, Bartus K, Kapelak B, Rocha-Singh KJ, Katholi RE, Witkowski A, Kadziela J, Januszewicz A, Prejbisz A, Walton AS, Sievert H, Id D, Wunderlich N, Whitbourn R, Rump LC, Vonend O, Saleh A, Thambar S, Nanra R, Zeller T, Erglis A, Sagic D, Boskovic S, Brachmann J, Schmidt M, Wenzel UO, Bart BA, Schmieder RE, Scheinert D, Börgel J, Straley C. Catheter-based renal sympathetic denervation for resistant hypertension: durability of blood pressure reduction out to 24 months. Hypertension. 2011;57:911–7.

129. Ukena C, Mahfoud F, Spies A, Kindermann I, Linz D, Cremers B, Laufs U, Neuberger HR, Bohm M. Effects of renal sympathetic denervation on heart rate and atrioventricular conduction in patients with resistant hypertension. Int J Cardiol. 2013; 167(6):2846–51.

130. Brandt MC, Reda S, Mahfoud F, Lenski M, Bohm M, Hoppe UC. Effects of renal sympathetic denervation on arterial stiffness and central hemodynamics in patients with resistant hypertension. J Am Coll Cardiol. 2012;60:1956–65.

131. Huang WC, Fang TC, Cheng JT. Renal denervation prevents and reverses hyperinsulinemia-induced hypertension in rats. Hypertension. 1998;32:249–54.

132. Mahfoud F, Schlaich M, Kindermann I, Ukena C, Cremers B, Brandt MC, Hoppe UC, Vonend O, Rump LC, Sobotka PA, Krum H, Esler M, Bohm M. Effect of renal sympathetic denervation on glucose metabolism in patients with resistant hypertension: a pilot study. Circulation. 2011;123:1940–6.

133. Ukena C, Mahfoud F, Kindermann I, Barth C, Lenski M, Kindermann M, Brandt MC, Hoppe UC, Krum H, Esler M, Sobotka PA, Bohm M. Cardiorespiratory response to exercise after renal sympathetic denervation in patients with resistant hypertension. J Am Coll Cardiol. 2011;58:1176–82.

134. Mahfoud F, Cremers B, Janker J, Link B, Vonend O, Ukena C, Linz D, Schmieder R, Rump LC, Kindermann I, Sobotka PA, Krum H, Scheller B, Schlaich M, Laufs U, Bohm M. Renal hemodynamics and renal function after catheter-based renal

sympathetic denervation in patients with resistant hypertension. Hypertension. 2012;60:419–24.

135. Schmieder RE, Mann JF, Schumacher H, Gao P, Mancia G, Weber MA, McQueen M, Koon T, Yusuf S. Changes in albuminuria predict mortality and morbidity in patients with vascular disease. J Am Soc Nephrol: JASN. 2011;22:1353–64.

136. Villarreal D, Freeman RH, Johnson RA, Simmons JC. Effects of renal denervation on postprandial sodium excretion in experimental heart failure. Am J Physiol. 1994;266:R1599–604.

137. Brandt MC, Mahfoud F, Reda S, Schirmer SH, Erdmann E, Bohm M, Hoppe UC. Renal sympathetic denervation reduces left ventricular hypertrophy and improves cardiac function in patients with resistant hypertension. J Am Coll Cardiol. 2012;59:901–9.

138. Davies JE, Manisty CH, Petraco R, Barron AJ, Unsworth B, Mayet J, Hamady M, Hughes AD, Sever PS, Sobotka PA, Francis DP. First-in-man safety evaluation of renal denervation for chronic systolic heart failure: primary outcome from reach-pilot study. Int J Cardiol. 2013;162:189–92.

139. Linz D, Schotten U, Neuberger HR, Bohm M, Wirth K. Negative tracheal pressure during obstructive respiratory events promotes atrial fibrillation by vagal activation. Heart Rhythm. 2011;8: 1436–43.

140. Linz D, Mahfoud F, Schotten U, Ukena C, Neuberger HR, Wirth K, Bohm M. Renal sympathetic denervation suppresses postapneic blood pressure rises and atrial fibrillation in a model for sleep apnea. Hypertension. 2012;60:172–8.

141. Linz D, Mahfoud F, Schotten U, Ukena C, Hohl M, Neuberger HR, Wirth K, Bohm M. Renal sympathetic denervation provides ventricular rate control but does not prevent atrial electrical remodeling during atrial fibrillation. Hypertension. 2013;61:225–31.

142. Pokushalov E, Romanov A, Corbucci G, Artyomenko S, Baranova V, Turov A, Shirokova N, Karaskov A, Mittal S, Steinberg JS. A randomized comparison of pulmonary vein isolation with versus without concomitant renal artery denervation in patients with refractory symptomatic atrial fibrillation and resistant hypertension. J Am Coll Cardiol. 2012;60:1163–70.

143. Esler MD, Krum H, Sobotka PA, Schlaich MP, Schmieder RE, Bohm M. Renal sympathetic denervation in patients with treatment-resistant hypertension (the symplicity HTN-2 trial): a randomised controlled trial. Lancet. 2010;376:1903–9.

144. Law MR, Morris JK, Wald NJ. Use of blood pressure lowering drugs in the prevention of cardiovascular disease: meta-analysis of 147 randomised trials in the context of expectations from prospective epidemiological studies. BMJ. 2009;338:b1665.

145. Ohkubo T, Imai Y, Tsuji I, Nagai K, Watanabe N, Minami N, Itoh O, Bando T, Sakuma M, Fukao A, Satoh H, Hisamichi S, Abe K. Prediction of mortality by ambulatory blood pressure monitoring versus screening blood pressure measurements: a pilot study in ohasama. J Hypertens. 1997;15:357–64.

146. Pickering TG, Shimbo D, Haas D. Ambulatory blood-pressure monitoring. N Engl J Med. 2006;354:2368–74.

147. Mancia G, Zanchetti A, Agabiti-Rosei E, Benemio G, De Cesaris R, Fogari R, Pessina A, Porcellati C, Rappelli A, Salvetti A, Trimarco B. Ambulatory blood pressure is superior to clinic blood pressure in predicting treatment-induced regression of left ventricular hypertrophy. Sample study group. Study on ambulatory monitoring of blood pressure and lisinopril evaluation. Circulation. 1997;95:1464–70.

148. Mancia G, Parati G. Ambulatory blood pressure monitoring and organ damage. Hypertension. 2000;36:894–900.

149. Fagard RH, Celis H, Thijs L, Staessen JA, Clement DL, De Buyzere ML, De Bacquer DA. Daytime and nighttime blood pressure as predictors of death and cause-specific cardiovascular events in hypertension. Hypertension. 2008;51:55–61.

150. Metoki H, Ohkubo T, Kikuya M, Asayama K, Obara T, Hashimoto J, Totsune K, Hoshi H, Satoh H, Imai Y. Prognostic significance for stroke of a morning pressor surge and a nocturnal blood pressure decline: the Ohasama study. Hypertension. 2006;47:149–54.

151. Dolan E, Stanton A, Thijs L, Hinedi K, Atkins N, McClory S, Den Hond E, McCormack P, Staessen JA, O'Brien E. Superiority of ambulatory over clinic blood pressure measurement in predicting mortality: the Dublin outcome study. Hypertension. 2005;46: 156–61.

152. Mancia G, De Backer G, Dominiczak A, Cifkova R, Fagard R, Germano G, Grassi G, Heagerty AM, Kjeldsen SE, Laurent S, Narkiewicz K, Ruilope L, Rynkiewicz A, Schmieder RE, Struijker Boudier HA, Zanchetti A, Vahanian A, Camm J, De Caterina R, Dean V, Dickstein K, Filippatos G, Funck-Brentano C, Hellemans I, Kristensen SD, McGregor K, Sechtem U, Silber S, Tendera M, Widimsky P, Zamorano JL, Erdine S, Kiowski W, Agabiti-Rosei E, Ambrosioni E, Lindholm LH, Manolis A, Nilsson PM, Redon J, Struijker-Boudier HA, Viigimaa M, Adamopoulos S, Bertomeu V, Clement D, Farsang C, Gaita D, Lip G, Mallion JM, Manolis AJ, O'Brien E, Ponikowski P, Ruschitzka F, Tamargo J, van Zwieten P, Waeber B, Williams B, The task force for the management of arterial hypertension of the European Society of H, The task force for the management of arterial hypertension of the European Society of C. 2007 guidelines for the management of arterial hypertension: the task force for the management of arterial hypertension of the European Society of Hypertension (esh) and of the European Society of Cardiology (esc). Eur Heart J. 2007;28:1462–536.

153. Williams B, Lacy PS, Thom SM, Cruickshank K, Stanton A, Collier D, Hughes AD, Thurston H, O'Rourke M. Differential impact of blood pressure-lowering drugs on central aortic pressure and clinical outcomes: principal results of the conduit artery function evaluation (cafe) study. Circulation. 2006;113:1213–25.

154. Lindholm LH, Carlberg B, Samuelsson O. Should beta blockers remain first choice in the treatment of primary hypertension? A meta-analysis. Lancet. 2005;366:1545–53.

155. Mancia G, Parati G. Office compared with ambulatory blood pressure in assessing response to antihypertensive treatment: a meta-analysis. J Hypertens. 2004;22:435–45.

156. Zuern CS, Rizas KD, Eick C, Stoleriu C, Bunk L, Barthel P, Balletshofer B, Gawaz M, Bauer A. Effects of renal sympathetic denervation on 24-hour blood pressure variability. Front Physiol. 2012;3:134.

157. Parati G, Pomidossi G, Albini F, Malaspina D, Mancia G. Relationship of 24-hour blood pressure mean and variability to severity of target-organ damage in hypertension. J Hypertens. 1987;5:93–8.

158. Kikuya M, Hozawa A, Ohokubo T, Tsuji I, Michimata M, Matsubara M, Ota M, Nagai K, Araki T, Satoh H, Ito S, Hisamichi S, Imai Y. Prognostic significance of blood pressure and heart rate variabilities: the Ohasama study. Hypertension. 2000;36:901–6.

159. Muntner P, Shimbo D, Tonelli M, Reynolds K, Arnett DK, Oparil S. The relationship between visit-to-visit variability in systolic blood pressure and all-cause mortality in the general population: findings from nhanes iii, 1988 to 1994. Hypertension. 2011;57:160–6.

160. Hsieh YT, Tu ST, Cho TJ, Chang SJ, Chen JF, Hsieh MC. Visit-to-visit variability in blood pressure strongly predicts all-cause mortality in patients with type 2 diabetes: a 5.5-year prospective analysis. Eur J Clin Invest. 2012;42:245–53.

161. Perticone F, Ceravolo R, Pujia A, Ventura G, Iacopino S, Scozzafava A, Ferraro A, Chello M, Mastroroberto P, Verdecchia P, Schillaci G. Prognostic significance of endothelial dysfunction in hypertensive patients. Circulation. 2001;104:191–6.

162. Redfield MM, Jacobsen SJ, Burnett Jr JC, Mahoney DW, Bailey KR, Rodeheffer RJ. Burden of systolic and diastolic ventricular dysfunction in the community: appreciating the scope of the heart failure epidemic. JAMA: J Am Med Assoc. 2003;289:194–202.

163. Bombelli M, Facchetti R, Carugo S, Madotto F, Arenare F, Quarti-Trevano F, Capra A, Giannattasio C, Dell'Oro R, Grassi G, Sega R, Mancia G. Left ventricular hypertrophy increases cardiovascular risk independently of in-office and out-of-office blood pressure values. J Hypertens. 2009;27:2458–64.

164. Koren MJ, Devereux RB, Casale PN, Savage DD, Laragh JH. Relation of left ventricular mass and geometry to morbidity and mortality in uncomplicated essential hypertension. Ann Intern Med. 1991;114:345–52.

165. Okin PM, Devereux RB, Jern S, Kjeldsen SE, Julius S, Nieminen MS, Snapinn S, Harris KE, Aurup P, Edelman JM, Wedel H, Lindholm LH, Dahlof B. Regression of electrocardiographic left ventricular hypertrophy during antihypertensive treatment and the prediction of major cardiovascular events. JAMA: J Am Med Assoc. 2004;292:2343–9.

166. Pierdomenico SD, Cuccurullo F. Risk reduction after regression of echocardiographic left ventricular hypertrophy in hypertension: a meta-analysis. Am J Hypertens. 2010;23:876–81.

167. Vakili BA, Okin PM, Devereux RB. Prognostic implications of left ventricular hypertrophy. Am Heart J. 2001;141:334–41.

168. Mathew J, Sleight P, Lonn E, Johnstone D, Pogue J, Yi Q, Bosch J, Sussex B, Probstfield J, Yusuf S, Heart Outcomes Prevention Evaluation I. Reduction of cardiovascular risk by regression of electrocardiographic markers of left ventricular hypertrophy by the angiotensin-converting enzyme inhibitor ramipril. Circulation. 2001;104:1615–21.

169. Mancini GB, Dahlof B, Diez J. Surrogate markers for cardiovascular disease: structural markers. Circulation. 2004;109: IV22–30.

170. Devereux RB, Agabiti-Rosei E, Dahlof B, Gosse P, Hahn RT, Okin PM, Roman MJ. Regression of left ventricular hypertrophy as a surrogate end-point for morbid events in hypertension treatment trials. J Hypertens Suppl. 1996;14:S95–101; discussion S101–2.

171. Dahlof B, Devereux R, de Faire U, Fyhrquist F, Hedner T, Ibsen H, Julius S, Kjeldsen S, Kristianson K, Lederballe-Pedersen O, Lindholm LH, Nieminen MS, Omvik P, Oparil S, Wedel H. The losartan intervention for endpoint reduction (life) in hypertension study: rationale, design, and methods. The life study group. Am J Hypertens. 1997;10:705–13.

172. Okin PM, Devereux RB, Jern S, Kjeldsen SE, Julius S, Nieminen MS, Snapinn S, Harris KE, Aurup P, Edelman JM, Wedel H, Lindholm LH, Dahlof B, Investigators LS. Regression of electrocardiographic left ventricular hypertrophy during antihypertensive treatment and the prediction of major cardiovascular events. JAMA: J Am Med Assoc. 2004;292:2343–9.

173. Levy D, Garrison RJ, Savage DD, Kannel WB, Castelli WP. Prognostic implications of echocardiographically determined left ventricular mass in the Framingham Heart Study. N Engl J Med. 1990;322:1561–6.

174. Bikkina M, Levy D, Evans JC, Larson MG, Benjamin EJ, Wolf PA, Castelli WP. Left ventricular mass and risk of stroke in an elderly cohort. The Framingham Heart Study. JAMA: J Am Med Assoc. 1994;272:33–6.

175. Liao Y, Cooper RS, McGee DL, Mensah GA, Ghali JK. The relative effects of left ventricular hypertrophy, coronary artery disease, and ventricular dysfunction on survival among black adults. JAMA: J Am Med Assoc. 1995;273:1592–7.

176. Ghali JK, Liao Y, Simmons B, Castaner A, Cao G, Cooper RS. The prognostic role of left ventricular hypertrophy in patients with or without coronary artery disease. Ann Intern Med. 1992;117:831–6.

177. Bolognese L, Dellavesa P, Rossi L, Sarasso G, Bongo AS, Scianaro MC. Prognostic value of left ventricular mass in uncomplicated acute myocardial infarction and one-vessel coronary artery disease. Am J Cardiol. 1994;73:1–5.

178. Fagard RH, Pardaens K, Staessen JA, Thijs L. Prognostic value of invasive hemodynamic measurements at rest and during exercise in hypertensive men. Hypertension. 1996;28:31–6.

179. Kokkinos P, Myers J, Faselis C, Panagiotakos DB, Doumas M, Pittaras A, Manolis A, Kokkinos JP, Karasik P, Greenberg M, Papademetriou V, Fletcher R. Exercise capacity and mortality in older men: a 20-year follow-up study. Circulation. 2010; 122:790–7.

180. Blacher J, Guerin AP, Pannier B, Marchais SJ, Safar ME, London GM. Impact of aortic stiffness on survival in end-stage renal disease. Circulation. 1999;99:2434–9.

181. Laurent S, Boutouyrie P, Asmar R, Gautier I, Laloux B, Guize L, Ducimetiere P, Benetos A. Aortic stiffness is an independent predictor of all-cause and cardiovascular mortality in hypertensive patients. Hypertension. 2001;37:1236–41.

182. Willum-Hansen T, Staessen JA, Torp-Pedersen C, Rasmussen S, Thijs L, Ibsen H, Jeppesen J. Prognostic value of aortic pulse wave velocity as index of arterial stiffness in the general population. Circulation. 2006;113:664–70.

183. Laurent S, Cockcroft J, Van Bortel L, Boutouyrie P, Giannattasio C, Hayoz D, Pannier B, Vlachopoulos C, Wilkinson I, Struijker-Boudier H. Expert consensus document on arterial stiffness: methodological issues and clinical applications. Eur Heart J. 2006;27:2588–605.

184. London GM, Blacher J, Pannier B, Guerin AP, Marchais SJ, Safar ME. Arterial wave reflections and survival in end-stage renal failure. Hypertension. 2001;38:434–8.

185. Weber T, Auer J, O'Rourke MF, Kvas E, Lassnig E, Berent R, Eber B. Arterial stiffness, wave reflections, and the risk of coronary artery disease. Circulation. 2004;109:184–9.

186. Tropeano AI, Boutouyrie P, Pannier B, Joannides R, Balkestein E, Katsahian S, Laloux B, Thuillez C, Struijker-Boudier H, Laurent S. Brachial pressure-independent reduction in carotid stiffness after long-term angiotensin-converting enzyme inhibition in diabetic hypertensives. Hypertension. 2006;48:80–6.

187. Karalliedde J, Smith A, DeAngelis L, Mirenda V, Kandra A, Botha J, Ferber P, Viberti G. Valsartan improves arterial stiffness in type 2 diabetes independently of blood pressure lowering. Hypertension. 2008;51:1617–23.

188. Stewart AD, Jiang B, Millasseau SC, Ritter JM, Chowienczyk PJ. Acute reduction of blood pressure by nitroglycerin does not normalize large artery stiffness in essential hypertension. Hypertension. 2006;48:404–10.

189. Gillman MW, Kannel WB, Belanger A, D'Agostino RB. Influence of heart rate on mortality among persons with hypertension: the Framingham Study. Am Heart J. 1993;125:1148–54.

190. Wannamethee G, Shaper AG, Macfarlane PW. Heart rate, physical activity, and mortality from cancer and other noncardiovascular diseases. Am J Epidemiol. 1993;137:735–48.

191. Bohm M, Swedberg K, Komajda M, Borer JS, Ford I, Dubost-Brama A, Lerebours G, Tavazzi L. Heart rate as a risk factor in chronic heart failure (shift): the association between heart rate and outcomes in a randomised placebo-controlled trial. Lancet. 2010;376:886–94.

192. Reil JC, Custodis F, Swedberg K, Komajda M, Borer JS, Ford I, Tavazzi L, Laufs U, Bohm M. Heart rate reduction in cardiovascular disease and therapy. Clin Res Cardiol. 2011;100:11–9.

193. Kannel WB, Kannel C, Paffenbarger Jr RS, Cupples LA. Heart rate and cardiovascular mortality: the Framingham study. Am Heart J. 1987;113:1489–94.

194. Swedberg K, Komajda M, Bohm M, Borer JS, Ford I, Dubost-Brama A, Lerebours G, Tavazzi L. Ivabradine and outcomes in chronic heart failure (shift): a randomised placebo-controlled study. Lancet. 2010;376:875–85.

195. Bohm M, Borer J, Ford I, Gonzalez-Juanatey JR, Komajda M, Lopez-Sendon J, Reil JC, Swedberg K, Tavazzi L. Heart rate at

baseline influences the effect of ivabradine on cardiovascular outcomes in chronic heart failure: analysis from the shift study. Clin Res Cardiol. 2013;102:11–22.

196. He B, Scherlag BJ, Nakagawa H, Lazzara R, Po SS. The intrinsic autonomic nervous system in atrial fibrillation: a review. ISRN Cardiol. 2012;2012:490674.

197. Podrid PJ, Fuchs T, Candinas R. Role of the sympathetic nervous system in the genesis of ventricular arrhythmia. Circulation. 1990;82:I103–13.

198. Knecht S, O'Neill MD, Verbeet T. Rhythm control versus rate control for atrial fibrillation. N Engl J Med. 2008;359:1522; author reply 1522.

199. Benjamin EJ, Wolf PA, D'Agostino RB, Silbershatz H, Kannel WB, Levy D. Impact of atrial fibrillation on the risk of death: the Framingham heart study. Circulation. 1998;98:946–52.

200. Kirchhof P, Auricchio A, Bax J, Crijns H, Camm J, Diener HC, Goette A, Hindricks G, Hohnloser S, Kappenberger L, Kuck KH, Lip GY, Olsson B, Meinertz T, Priori S, Ravens U, Steinbeck G, Svernhage E, Tijssen J, Vincent A, Breithardt G. Outcome parameters for trials in atrial fibrillation: executive summary. Eur Heart J. 2007;28:2803–17.

201. Linz D, Wirth K, Ukena C, Mahfoud F, Poss J, Linz B, Bohm M, Neuberger HR. Renal denervation suppresses ventricular arrhythmias during acute ventricular ischemia in pigs. Heart Rhythm. 2013;10(10):1525–30.

202. Ukena C, Bauer A, Mahfoud F, Schreieck J, Neuberger HR, Eick C, Sobotka PA, Gawaz M, Bohm M. Renal sympathetic denervation for treatment of electrical storm: first-in-man experience. Clin Res Cardiol. 2012;101:63–7.

203. Daviglus ML, Liao Y, Greenland P, Dyer AR, Liu K, Xie X, Huang CF, Prineas RJ, Stamler J. Association of nonspecific minor st-t abnormalities with cardiovascular mortality: the Chicago Western Electric Study. JAMA: J Am Med Assoc. 1999;281:530–6.

204. de Groot E, Hovingh GK, Wiegman A, Duriez P, Smit AJ, Fruchart JC, Kastelein JJ. Measurement of arterial wall thickness as a surrogate marker for atherosclerosis. Circulation. 2004;109: III33–8.

205. Danesh J, Wheeler JG, Hirschfield GM, Eda S, Eiriksdottir G, Rumley A, Lowe GD, Pepys MB, Gudnason V. C-reactive protein and other circulating markers of inflammation in the prediction of coronary heart disease. N Engl J Med. 2004;350:1387–97.

206. Klein IH, Ligtenberg G, Neumann J, Oey PL, Koomans HA, Blankestijn PJ. Sympathetic nerve activity is inappropriately increased in chronic renal disease. J Am Soc Nephrol: JASN. 2003;14:3239–44.

207. Wen CP, Cheng TY, Tsai MK, Chang YC, Chan HT, Tsai SP, Chiang PH, Hsu CC, Sung PK, Hsu YH, Wen SF. All-cause mortality attributable to chronic kidney disease: a prospective cohort study based on 462 293 adults in Taiwan. Lancet. 2008;371: 2173–82.

208. Weiner DE, Tabatabai S, Tighiouart H, Elsayed E, Bansal N, Griffith J, Salem DN, Levey AS, Sarnak MJ. Cardiovascular outcomes and all-cause mortality: exploring the interaction between ckd and cardiovascular disease. Am J Kidney Dis. 2006;48: 392–401.

209. Go AS, Chertow GM, Fan D, McCulloch CE, Hsu CY. Chronic kidney disease and the risks of death, cardiovascular events, and hospitalization. N Engl J Med. 2004;351:1296–305.

210. Matsushita K, van der Velde M, Astor BC, Woodward M, Levey AS, de Jong PE, Coresh J, Gansevoort RT. Association of estimated glomerular filtration rate and albuminuria with all-cause and cardiovascular mortality in general population cohorts: a collaborative meta-analysis. Lancet. 2010;375:2073–81.

211. Wang Y, Seto SW, Golledge J. Therapeutic effects of renal denervation on renal failure. Curr Neurovasc Res. 2013;10:172–84.

212. Ott C, Janka R, Schmid A, Titze S, Ditting T, Sobotka PA, Veelken R, Uder M, Schmieder RE. Vascular and renal hemodynamic changes after renal denervation. Clin J Am Soc Nephrol: CJASN. 2013;8:1195–201.

213. Hering D, Mahfoud F, Walton AS, Krum H, Lambert GW, Lambert EA, Sobotka PA, Bohm M, Cremers B, Esler MD, Schlaich MP. Renal denervation in moderate to severe ckd. J Am Soc Nephrol: JASN. 2012;23:1250–7.

214. Ott C, Schmid A, Ditting T, Sobotka PA, Veelken R, Uder M, Schmieder RE. Renal denervation in a hypertensive patient with end-stage renal disease and small arteries: a direction for future research. J Clin Hypertens (Greenwich). 2012;14:799–801.

215. Mancia G, Bousquet P, Elghozi JL, Esler M, Grassi G, Julius S, Reid J, Van Zwieten PA. The sympathetic nervous system and the metabolic syndrome. J Hypertens. 2007;25:909–20.

216. Huggett RJ, Scott EM, Gilbey SG, Stoker JB, Mackintosh AF, Mary DA. Impact of type 2 diabetes mellitus on sympathetic neural mechanisms in hypertension. Circulation. 2003;108:3097–101.

217. Esler M, Rumantir M, Wiesner G, Kaye D, Hastings J, Lambert G. Sympathetic nervous system and insulin resistance: from obesity to diabetes. Am J Hypertens. 2001;14:304S–9.

218. Isomaa B, Almgren P, Tuomi T, Forsen B, Lahti K, Nissen M, Taskinen MR, Groop L. Cardiovascular morbidity and mortality associated with the metabolic syndrome. Diabetes Care. 2001;24:683–9.

Appraisal of the Clinical Trial Data on Renal Denervation for the Management of Resistant Hypertension

5

Aung Myat and Deepak L. Bhatt

Key Points

- Treatment-resistant systemic HTN can be described as a blood pressure that remains uncontrolled (i.e., seated office BP >140/90 mmHg) despite adherence to treatment with at least three complementary antihypertensive agents (one of which is a diuretic) already taken at optimal or best-tolerated doses.
- Apparent or pseudo-resistant hypertension, defined as inadequate blood pressure control in a patient who does not have true resistant hypertension but is receiving appropriate treatment, must first be excluded before a diagnosis of resistant hypertension can be confirmed.
- Pseudo-resistant hypertension most commonly arises from: incorrect office blood pressure measurement technique, the 'white coat' effect, poor patient adherence with prescribed therapy, and/or a suboptimal antihypertensive treatment regimen.
- Current expert consensus documents on catheter-based renal denervation all advocate ruling out pseudo-resistant hypertension and thereafter confirming the validity of persistently high office blood pressure recordings with the use of ambulatory blood pressure monitoring.

- The prevalence of secondary hypertension is greater in the resistant hypertension cohort than in the general hypertensive population, with studies indicating 5–10 % of those patients have an identifiable cause. As such it is fundamentally important for a trial of renal denervation to incorporate a selection protocol through which those patients with a secondary cause are excluded prior to randomization.
- The Global SYMPLICITY Registry reiterates yet again the significant heterogeneity in pharmacotherapy used to treat poorly controlled hypertension and the continued need to establish an evidence-based drug combination that should first be exhausted before even considering invasive measures.
- The open-label designs of both SYMPLICITY HTN-1 and HTN-2 make them susceptible to expectation, performance, and evaluation biases, particularly when the primary outcome measure in HTN-2 – seated office blood pressure – was not recorded by assessors blinded to treatment assignment.
- The SYMPLICITY HTN-3 trial did not meet either its primary or secondary efficacy outcomes at 6 months. This follow-up time point may however be too short to establish a significant dichotomy in blood pressure reduction when compared to the sham control arm of the trial.
- Preliminary feasibility data from studies of alternative renal denervation catheters and devices are all encouraging in terms of safety and efficacy but all suffer to some extent from those same limitations that have hampered the SYMPLICITY HTN-1 and HTN-2 trials.
- The holy grail of renal denervation must be to identify a reliable, reproducible, and easily attainable imaging test or biomarker of successful denervation.

A. Myat, BSc (Hons), MBBS, MRCP
The Rayne Institute, British Heart Foundation Center of Research Excellence, St Thomas' Hospital, King's College London, 4th Floor, Lambeth Wing, Westminster Bridge Road, London SE1 7EH, UK
e-mail: aungmyat25@hotmail.com

D.L. Bhatt, MD, MPH, FACC, FAHA, FSCAI, FESC (✉)
Interventional Cardiovascular Programs, Brigham and Women's Hospital Heart and Vascular Center, Harvard Medical School, 75 Francis Street, Boston, MA 02115, USA
e-mail: DLBHATTMD@post.harvard.edu

What Is Resistant Hypertension?

Over the past decade several national and international societies/regulatory bodies have proposed definitions of resistant hypertension (RHTN) (Table 5.1). There are subtle differences between these definitions, but treatment-resistant systemic HTN can be described as a blood pressure (BP) that remains uncontrolled (i.e., seated office BP >140/90 mmHg) despite adherence to treatment with at least three complementary antihypertensive agents (one of which is a diuretic) already taken at optimal or best-tolerated doses [1, 3, 11, 12]. In the UK, the National Institute for Health and Care Excellence (NICE) Clinical Guideline 127 [4] (Table 5.1) has been more proscriptive with their definition by suggesting that the three antihypertensives would usually be a regimen of an angiotensin converting enzyme (ACE) inhibitor or

angiotensin receptor blocker (ARB) plus a calcium channel blocker plus a thiazide-type diuretic (i.e., A+C+D regimen), in accordance with the NICE treatment algorithm (http://guidance.nice.org.uk/CG127). The NICE guidance has also suggested that RHTN should only be diagnosed after confirming inadequate BP control by use of ambulatory blood pressure monitoring (ABPM – i.e., mean daytime BP >135/85), thereby excluding so-called "white coat" hypertension. The optimal target BP in patients treated for RHTN is widely accepted to be <140/90 mmHg, although lower targets might be appropriate in those with diabetes and/or chronic kidney disease (CKD) (Table 5.1) [11]. Furthermore, it should be remembered that an individual whose BP is controlled by the incorporation of a 4th line agent continues to be labelled as having RHTN. Likewise, RHTN should not be confused with uncontrolled HTN, the latter being an umbrella

Table 5.1 The evolution of treatment-resistant hypertension definitions

National or international society	Date published	Definition of resistant hypertension
Seventh Report of the JNC on Prevention, Detection, Evaluation, and Treatment of High Blood Pressure [1]	2003	The failure to achieve goal BP (<140/90 mmHg) in patients who are adhering to full doses of an appropriate 3-drug regimen that includes a diuretic
ESH and ESC Guidelines for the Management of Arterial Hypertension [2]	2007	When a therapeutic plan that has included attention to lifestyle measures and the prescription of at least three drugs (including a diuretic) in adequate doses has failed to lower systolic and diastolic BP to goal (<140/90 mmHg)
AHA Professional Education Committee of the Council for High Blood Pressure Research [3]	2008	BP that remains above goal (<140/90 mmHg) in spite of the concurrent use of 3 antihypertensive agents of different classes. Ideally, one of the 3 agents should be a diuretic and all agents should be prescribed at optimal dose amounts
NICE Clinical Guideline 127. Hypertension – The Clinical Management of Primary Hypertension in Adults [4]	2011	BP not controlled to <140/90 mmHg despite optimal or best tolerated doses of third line treatment. Third line treatment comprises angiotensin-converting enzyme inhibitor or angiotensin receptor blocker plus a calcium channel blocker plus a diuretic
Joint UK Societies' Consensus Summary Statement on Renal Denervation for Resistant Hypertension [5]	2011	Sustained clinic BP ≥160 mmHg (≥150 mmHg in type 2 diabetes mellitus) in patients on 3 or more antihypertensive medications. Confirmation of sustained raised BP using ambulatory BP monitoring is essential
ESH Position Paper on Renal Denervation [6]	2012	BP levels above goal in spite of the concurrent use of three antihypertensive agents in adequate doses from different classes including a diuretic
ASH and ISH Clinical Practice Guidelines for the Management of Hypertension in the Community [7]	2013	BP not controlled to target (<140/90 mmHg in most patients) by using either 1, 2, or 3 drugs (angiotensin-converting enzyme inhibitor or angiotensin receptor blocker/calcium channel blocker/diuretic) in full or maximally tolerated doses
ESC Consensus Document on Catheter-Based Renal Denervation [8]	2013	BP >140/90 mmHg, >130–139/80–85 mmHg in diabetes mellitus or >130/80 mmHg in chronic kidney disease in the presence of three or more antihypertensives of different classes, including a diuretic, at maximal or the highest tolerated dose
International Expert Consensus Statement [9]	2013	BP higher than target levels despite the use of 3 antihypertensive agents in adequate doses from different classes, including a diuretic agent
ESH Working Group on the Interventional Treatment of Hypertension [10]	2014	Office systolic BP ≥160 mmHg (≥150 mmHg in type 2 diabetes) despite treatment with ≥3 antihypertensive drugs of different types in adequate doses, including one diuretic

Key: *BP* blood pressure, *JNC* Joint National Committee, *ESH* European Society of Hypertension, *ESC* European Society of Cardiology, *AHA* American Heart Association, *NICE* National Institute of Health and Care Excellence, *ASH* American Society of Hypertension, *ISH* International Society of Hypertension

term to include all those individuals unable to achieve adequate BP targets, including that due to non-adherence, despite therapeutic intervention.

Interest regarding the assessment, diagnosis, and subsequent management of RHTN has been noticeably accelerated in recent times for several reasons: recognition that patients with true RHTN appear to lie at the extreme end of an already high-risk cardiovascular (CV) morbidity and mortality continuum [11, 13, 14]; acceptance that estimates of the incidence and prevalence of RHTN remain largely anecdotal [14–17]; the need to establish robust prognostic associations to benchmark the degree of benefit gained from timely and consistent management of RHTN; the need to define the optimal pharmacotherapeutic regimen for RHTN; evidence that RHTN may, at least in part, be mediated by chronic activation of the sympathetic nervous system (SNS) [18]; and the subsequent emergence of percutaneous sympathetic denervation of the renal arteries – an intervention that could possibly stimulate a paradigm shift in the way we manage treatment-resistant systemic HTN [11, 12, 19].

The predominant focus of this chapter is a critical appraisal of the data emanating from trials involving the use of all renal denervation (RDN) devices currently available in the market place. To fully appreciate whether each trial has recruited an appropriate treatment-resistant HTN population we also concentrate on how best to isolate true RHTN individuals from those actually describing apparent or "pseudo" RHTN and highlight how crucial medical optimization pre-procedure, exclusion of secondary causes of systemic HTN, adequate compliance with pharmacotherapy and instigation of lifestyle modification is – before RDN should be considered.

Assessment of True Resistant Hypertension

Physician inertia has an important role to play in the suboptimal management of HTN, particularly when patients require multiple medications. Poor knowledge of clinical guidelines, a misguided acceptance of elevated BP levels, potentially spurious reasons to avoid intensification of existing therapy, and an underestimation of CV disease risk can all lead to suboptimal BP control and thereafter a misdiagnosis of RHTN [20].

Exclusion of Apparent or Pseudo-Resistant Hypertension

Apparent or pseudo-RHTN, defined as inadequate BP control in a patient who does not have true RTHN but is receiving appropriate treatment, must first be excluded before consigning a an individual to a diagnosis of true RHTN [12].

Pseudo-RHTN most commonly arises from: poor office BP measurement technique, the 'white coat' effect, poor patient adherence with prescribed therapy, and/or a suboptimal antihypertensive treatment regimen. Complicated dosing regimens, inadequate patient education, and the rising cost of medication (within some healthcare systems) must also be borne in mind. It is of prime importance to conduct a thorough exploration of these patient and physician barriers to sustained BP control and eliminate them first, before establishing a definitive diagnosis of RHTN. Trials of RDN should ideally stipulate this process has been performed thoroughly before a patient is recruited.

Office BP Versus Home BP Versus Ambulatory BP Monitoring

Up to a third of patients, defined as having RHTN according to office BP recordings, are later found to manifest a white coat effect (i.e., a persistently elevated office BP but a normal home or ambulatory daytime average BP of <135/85 mmHg) [16, 21]. This serves to emphasize the importance of using ABPM to confirm a true RHTN diagnosis [3, 4, 5, 22]. The long-term prognostic implications of the white-coat effect appear to be intermediate between sustained hypertension and normotension, and there is evidence to suggest that these individuals do have an increased risk of developing a sustained hypertensive state [23]. A white coat effect should be suspected in any individual with persistently elevated office BP readings but no signs of target organ damage or signs/symptoms of over-treatment such as postural hypotension, dizziness, or syncope [24].

Office BP measurements could be deemed more reliable if taken using an automated device with the patient alone in a quiet room [25]. There is little doubt, however, that out-of-office BP measurements are more reproducible, reflect diurnal variation, reduce observer bias if automated devices are used, and provide multiple recordings from which to base a firm diagnosis or monitor response to therapy [26]. Furthermore two recent meta-analyses have confirmed a more accurate estimation of treatment response with out-of-office (home BP monitoring – HBPM and 24-h ABPM) recordings, ABPM also giving rise to an attenuated reduction in BP, when compared to clinic BP measurements [27, 28].

The landmark PAMELA study drew attention to the significant disparity between clinic and out-of-office BP measurements and established normal values for HBPM and ABPM [29]. It is now widely accepted that CV risk is more tightly correlated to out-of-office BP than to clinic BP [30, 31]. Furthermore, elevated ambulatory BP can predict CV morbidity and mortality in patients with RHTN, whereas clinic BP has less prognostic value [32]. These data provide compelling evidence for the routine use of out-of-office BP monitoring when assessing patients for presumed RHTN and should be a prerequisite inclusion criterion in trials of RDN. Indeed, an International Expert Consensus Statement for the performance of percutaneous RDN recommends confirmation of persistently elevated BP above target by using 24-h ABPM [9]. Similarly, expert consensus documents issued by the European Society of Cardiology (ESC) and the European Society of Hypertension (ESH) on catheter-based RDN also advocate ruling out pseudo-RHTN and thereafter confirming the validity of persistently high office BP recordings with the use of ABPM [6, 8, 10].

Management After Confirmation of Resistant Hypertension

Once out-of-office BP monitoring has confirmed a diagnosis of RHTN, the clinician must instigate conservative therapeutic measures, and possibly further investigations, before an individual can be considered for enrolment in a RDN trial [6, 8–10].

Lifestyle Modifications

Once a diagnosis of RHTN has been reliably established, individuals should be evaluated for potentially remediable lifestyle factors such as obesity, alcohol, and caffeine consumption, and excess dietary sodium, which all contribute to the hypertensive state [11]. Thereafter, a survey for the potential use or abuse of exogenous substances that raise BP should be performed (Table 5.2). Once identified, the offending agents should be discontinued, minimized or substituted as required. Intuitive interventions such as weight loss, regular exercise and a high-fiber, low-salt diet must be attempted.

Exclusion of Secondary Causes of Resistant Hypertension

The next recommended step in the diagnostic pathway is to exclude a potentially remediable secondary cause [6, 8–10]. The prevalence of secondary hypertension is greater in the RHTN cohort than in the general hypertensive population, with studies indicating 5–10 % of RHTN patients with an identifiable cause [33, 34]. The most common causes are hyperaldosteronism, CKD (either the cause or result of chronic, poorly controlled HTN), renal artery stenosis (RAS), and obstructive sleep apnea [11, 35]. Less common causes include renal parenchymal disease, pheochromocytoma, thyroid diseases, Cushing's syndrome, coarctation of the aorta, and intracranial tumours. It is

Table 5.2 Drug-related causes of resistant hypertension [11]

Non-steroidal anti-inflammatory drugs
Contraceptive hormones – combined oral contraceptives are more often associated with elevated BP
Adrenal steroid hormones
Sympathomimetic agents (nasal decongestants, diet pills)
Erythropoietin, cyclosporine and tacrolimus
Liquorice – suppresses the metabolism of cortisol
Herbal supplements (ephedra, ma huang, bitter orange, etc.)
Use of cocaine and/or amphetamines

fundamentally important for an RDN trial to incorporate a selection protocol through which those RHTN patients with a secondary cause are excluded prior to randomization. As such, the trial screening should include a focused history, thorough physical examination, biochemical evaluation, non-invasive imaging, and subsequent onward referral to a specialist clinic if deemed necessary prior to potential enrolment [9, 36].

Assessment of Adherence to Therapy

Adherence to prescribed therapy is of particular relevance in this scenario since RHTN is largely an asymptomatic condition treated with multiple medications, each with their own array of potentially troublesome side effects. Measures to improve drug adherence such as improving patient education, motivation, and ownership of their management program along with setting realistic goals in achieving BP targets warrant careful attention.

Existing antihypertensive drug treatment requires optimization. Recent medication changes or dose adjustments should be given time to work – this can take up to a month to take effect [12]. If the standard A+C+D treatment algorithm is pursued, as recommended by NICE [4], the optimal fourth line agent for the pharmacologic treatment of RHTN remains open to debate. Although mineralocorticoid receptor antagonists appear to be the obvious contender, their long-term safety, particularly in patients with impaired renal function, is still unknown. As such, an individualized approach to tailor the best antihypertensive regimen for the patient is currently advocated with the addition of aldosterone antagonists if they are considered safe in the circumstances [6, 8–10]. At present there is currently no robust evidence available to define with absolute confidence the most clinically effective 4th or 5th line agent to attain target BP in RHTN [12]. It is little wonder, therefore, that RDN has been seen as a potential game-changer. It is imperative that trials of RDN should ensure potential recruits have had their current medications optimized and that their treatment regimen is in alignment with international consensus standards.

Clinical Trial Data in Renal Denervation for Resistant Hypertension

Excitement about RDN was kindled by a case report published in the *New England Journal of Medicine* in 2009 [37]. A 59-year-old patient with poorly controlled essential hypertension resistant to treatment with seven antihypertensive medications was administered radiofrequency ablation (RFA) to both renal arteries. Secondary hypertension had been excluded but there was no record of ABPM utilization to confirm a RHTN diagnosis. The case report did of course pre-date the current crop of consensus guidelines on the procedure [4, 6, 8–10, 22]. Renal norepinephrine spillover along with whole body norepinephrine spillover and muscle sympathetic nerve activity, surrogates of renal sympathetic efferent and afferent nerve activity respectively, were both reduced suggesting adequate penetration of the RF energy emitted from the catheter to ablate the renal nerves. Systemic BP was reduced from an office BP of 161/107 mmHg at baseline to 141/90 mmHg at 30 days and 127/81 mmHg at 12 months. There were no apparent procedural or vascular complications and renal function remained unaltered.

The SYMPLICITY HTN-1 Trial

This was the original proof-of-concept non-randomized cohort study designed to show that RDN was feasible, safe and effective [38]. Krum and colleagues treated 45 patients from five centers in Australia and Europe, including the patient described in the case report above [37], using the Symplicity™ Renal Denervation system (Medtronic, Santa Rosa, CA, USA). An office systolic BP ≥160 mmHg (or ≥150 mmHg in Type 2 diabetics) based on an average of three readings was required for trial entry. Mean baseline office systolic and diastolic blood pressures were 177 ± 20 and 101 ± 15 mmHg respectively. Patients were taking an average of 4.7 medications, although diuretic therapy was not taken by all trial participants (95 %). Given the predominance of volume and sodium overload in these patients, attempts at achieving sustained BP control with diuretic medication is now regarded as a prerequisite therapeutic intervention before a RHTN diagnosis can be made [4, 22]. Secondary causes of RHTN had to be excluded prior to inclusion into the study. The trial required preserved renal function (estimated glomerular filtration rate – eGFR >45 mL/min/1.73 m²) to be eligible for RDN.

Office systolic and diastolic blood pressures after the procedure (while maintaining patients on their usual antihypertensive medication therapy) were reduced by 14/10, 21/10, 22/11, 24/11, and 27/17 mmHg at 1, 3, 6, 9, and 12 months, respectively. At the 12-month follow-up stage RDN appeared to be safe with successful completion of the procedure in 43 out of 45 patients. A single intraprocedural renal artery dissection was recorded. This had occurred prior to the application of RF energy without further sequelae. There were no other renovascular complications (such as vessel spasm or RAS) [38]. One patient developed a pseudoaneurysm at the femoral access site.

By 3 years, HTN-1 had recruited 153 patients, 88 of whom had complete data for the entire follow-up period [39]. The premise was to determine the durability of the BP lowering effect seen after RDN in light of concerns that renal afferent and efferent re-innervation may occur in the medium term post procedure. Again, the intervention was shown to be safe with a total of four complications out of the entire patient cohort (one renal artery dissection previously noted in the first 12-month report of HTN-1 [38] and three access-related groin complications). A single patient developed a significant right RAS 24 months after RDN which required angioplasty [39]. At 36 months, significant reductions in office systolic (−32.0 mmHg, 95 % confidence interval [CI] −35.7 to −28.2) and diastolic BP (−14.4 mmHg, CI−16.9 to −11.9) were noted in the 88 patients in whom data were available. In terms of response rate, 55/80 (69 %) had reductions in systolic BP ≥10 mmHg at 1 month. This rose to 82/88 (93 %) at 36 months, which some interpreted as a delayed response phenomenon, although the pathophysiological basis of this remains unclear. Of note, the need for antihypertensive medications actually rose over the 36-month period from a mean of 5.1 at baseline to 5.2 at study termination despite the purported gains in BP control [39]. Further analysis of medication dose or drug changes is precluded, however, by lack of medication data after 12 months – a major limitation of the study.

The SYMPLICITY HTN-2 Trial

Whereas HTN-1 was a single-arm proof-of-principle study, and therefore exposed to confounding issues such as regression to the mean, placebo, and Hawthorne effects, HTN-2 was a prospective, multicenter trial in which 106 patients were randomly allocated to RDN (n=52) or control (n=54) [40]. A 2-week 'Baseline Evaluation Period' was used to analyze BP patterns in potential recruits with twice-daily home BP monitoring and a daily medication log to monitor compliance prior to formal randomization. Despite the opportunity to use these out-of-office BP recordings, the investigators restricted their RHTN diagnosis to the mean of office BP measurements. This potentially limits the generalizability of the trial's results [12]. Much like HTN-1, therefore, patients with a systolic BP ≥160 mmHg (≥150 mmHg in Type 2 diabetics) despite adherence to ≥3 antihypertensive agents were eligible for recruitment. Furthermore, inclusion criteria stipulated a 'stable' treatment regimen of ≥3 antihypertensives, which prevented any change in drug or dose 2 weeks prior to randomization and maintenance of the same baseline combination for at least 6 months post RDN to avoid adjustments confounding the results [12, 40]. In HTN-1, 22 % of patients were taking an aldosterone antagonist at baseline [38] and only 17 % in HTN-2 [40], perhaps reflecting the relative lack of conclusive data on what constitutes best practice in terms of pharmacotherapy in RHTN patients. Exclusion of patients with a known secondary cause of HTN is routine at present and was actively performed in HTN-1 [38, 41]. The protocol for HTN-2 excluded Type I diabetics but did not explicitly exclude those with a known secondary cause – the reasoning behind the shift in recruitment protocols is unclear [40].

At the 6-month time point, office BP fell by $32/12 \pm 23/11$ mmHg from 178/96 mmHg $\pm 18/16$ mmHg at baseline in those receiving RDN compared to a change of only $1/0 \pm 21/10$ mmHg from $178/97 \pm 17/16$ mmHg at baseline in the control arm. Note, however, the wide standard deviation in the latter cohort. When ABPM measurements were analysed, the reductions were less impressive. In the RDN group, there was a mean reduction of $11/7 \pm 15/11$ mmHg (n=20) at 6 months using out-of-office recordings. Much like in HTN-1, RDN was shown to be safe with no serious complications related to the device or the procedure [40]. Renal function remained the same overall in both groups at 6 months.

Results from HTN-2 at 1 year included the original RDN group at baseline (n=47) and control subjects who crossed over to the RDN arm and had the procedure performed per protocol at 6 months (n=35) [42]. An overall fall in BP in the original RDN group of 28/10 mmHg remained durable at 12 months. The crossover group also demonstrated a fall in BP of 24/8 mmHg at 6 months. A crossover patient suffered renal artery dissection during guide catheter insertion for angiography. Aside from this, there were no other renovascular complications reported thereby reaffirming the safety of this procedure. No significant changes in estimated glomerular filtration rate (eGFR) were noted in either group at this time point. At 36-month follow up, the data had been locked and was only available in the RDN group (n=40). The BP lowering effect remained durable with a reduction of 33/14 mmHg [43].

Limitations of the SYMPLICITY HTN-1 and HTN-2 Trials

Both HTN-1 and HTN-2 were trials that introduced a seemingly safe and effective procedure to the interventional world at large. There were, however, a number of limitations to the studies, which prevent the widespread generalizability of the data:

- Less than 250 patients combined received RDN in the HTN-1 and HTN-2 trials. These relatively small trial numbers tend to overestimate treatment effect and underestimate adverse effects.

- 36-month results from both HTN-1 and HTN-2 provide some reassurance that re-innervation of efferent and afferent nerve fibers following RDN does not occur or if re-innervation does occur, the nerves no longer contribute to the positive feedback loop that causes the hypertensive state [39, 43–45]. However, the distance of peri-renal nerves from the lumen of the renal artery follows a normal distribution ranging from 0.5 mm through to >10 mm (mean 2.0–4.0 mm). As such, there is no guarantee that the energy from each ablation will successfully reach a nerve bundle and that the treated renal nerve fully extends to the kidney [44] – this could in part explain the early non-responsiveness to RDN therapy and underlines the need to seek alternative reproducible predictors of procedural success other than high baseline BP, which is not specific enough to enhance patient selection [46].

- Renal norepinephrine spillover (measure of renal efferent activity), total body norepinephrine spillover (measure of central sympathetic drive via the renal afferent pathway) and microneurography (measure of muscle sympathetic nerve activity) are accessible metrics that can be used to evaluate the durability of effect post RDN, and therefore the effectiveness of the RF energy to ablate renal afferent and efferent nerves. They were not reported in all patients exposed to the intervention [19, 37].

- It remains uncertain what effect, if any, a renewed motivation for lifestyle modification and medication adherence could have contributed to this sustained BP reduction in patients, not only enthused by the encouraging results from their RDN procedure but also monitored more closely in an artificial trial environment.

- Importantly, follow-up was incomplete in both HTN-1 and HTN-2 and changes to antihypertensive regimens were not monitored after the 12-month post procedure visit. Indeed enthusiasm has been tempered by the more modest reduction of approximately −10 mmHg of systolic BP when ambulatory recordings were available [47].

- A small sample size precludes a direct association between any compromise in eGFR post RDN with the deleterious consequences of the underlying hypertensive state, exposure to contrast media, diuretic sensitivity heightened by RDN rendering the kidney less able to autoregulate against falls in perfusion pressure, an adverse effect on renal hemodynamics, or damage to the renal artery during the procedure, e.g., prolonged spasm or dissection, or delayed development of RAS [48–50].

- The open-label designs of both HTN-1 and HTN-2 make them susceptible to expectation, performance, and evaluation biases, particularly when the primary outcome measure in HTN-2 – seated office BP – was not recorded by assessors blinded to treatment assignment. Patients were also predominantly Caucasian (>95 % for both trials) and obese, making it difficult to generalize the findings to a wider hypertensive population [40, 41].

- There was no systematic imaging in place to identify RAS in the short to medium term. Furthermore choice of imaging modality was not standardized either at baseline or follow-up. Magnetic resonance angiography and computerized tomographic resonance angiography were used in only a minority of patients in HTN-1 and HTN-2. As such, the occurrence of adverse renovascular sequelae remains a legitimate concern, particularly beyond 6 months follow-up.

The Global SYMPLICITY Registry

The Global SYMPLICITY Registry (GSR) (ClinicalTrials. gov Identifier: NCT01534299) is consecutively enrolling up to 5,000 patients from over 200 sites worldwide to determine the real-world durability of effect and safety of the Symplicity RDN catheter. It also incorporates the GREAT SYMPLICITY registry initiated in Germany [51]. The registry aims to establish procedural benchmarking and practice patterns, assess the effect of geographical variation and procedural characteristics on outcome, and to collect quality of life data post procedure and in relation to patient comorbidity [51].

Data from the first 1,000 patients consecutively enrolled to the registry and followed up for 6 months were presented at the American College of Cardiology Scientific Sessions in March 2014 [52]. Safety solely related to the procedure appeared to be maintained with vascular complications occurring in only 0.4 % (n=4) of the cohort (n=913) at 6 months. There were no new cases of RAS. Both new onset end stage renal disease and a doubling of the serum creatinine were also rare (0.2 % each).

Perhaps most striking were those patients with a baseline office systolic BP ≥160 mmHg (i.e., the RHTN cut-off used in HTN-1 and HTN-2) or an ambulatory systolic BP ≥135 mmHg on ≥3 antihypertensive medications, which represented only a third (n=327) of the 1,000-patient cohort studied for this preliminary analysis. This cohort achieved the greatest reduction in office BP post procedure, whereas those patients with a relatively "normal" baseline BP actually saw an increase over time (Table 5.3). It is not clear whether this latter cohort corresponded to those patients in whom the primary indication for RDN therapy was to treat a

disease state characterized by SNS hyperactivation outside of the standard uncontrolled HTN parameter (i.e., heart failure, sleep apnea, insulin resistance, chronic kidney disease, or atrial fibrillation). Overall, the average reduction in office systolic BP from baseline to 6 months was a modest 11.9 mmHg for all patients. Among the subset of patients who met the BP criteria used in HTN-1 and HTN-2 and who were taking maximally tolerated doses of ≥3 antihypertensive agents the fall in mean BP was 17.3 mmHg.

On the upside, the GSR proved once again the procedure is safe. As it continues to accumulate patients, the GSR may also help to identify specific patient populations that will gain the most post RDN from a real world perspective. Conversely, the GSR reiterates yet again the significant heterogeneity in pharmacotherapy used to treat poorly controlled HTN and the continued need to establish an evidence-based drug combination that should first be exhausted before considering invasive measures. Ultimately, the real crux lies in elucidating a robust biometric parameter of successful RF ablation that will allow the interventionalist some degree of confidence that true denervation has actually occurred following the procedure. Until such a biomarker is used in clinical practice, we cannot be entirely sure the results gleaned from the GSR thus far, or from any trial of a denervation device for that matter, truly reflect renal nerve ablation, are merely a placebo effect, or indicate regression to the mean.

A French registry of 35 consecutive patients with RHTN, as defined by a home BP >160 mmHg despite the use of ≥3 antihypertensive drugs (100 % of patients were taking a diuretic, only 11.4 % were taking an aldosterone antagonist), used ABPM and home BP monitoring (HBPM) in all patients for initial assessment and follow up post percutaneous RDN using the Symplicity catheter [53]. Unlike the SYMPLICITY trials, 11.4 % of the cohort had renal impairment (eGFR <45 mL/min). Baseline out-of-office BP was 179/100±21/20 mmHg. Successful bilateral RDN was performed in 33/35 patients (one RAS on renal arteriography – not ablated and one renal artery spasm – unilateral denervation only). At 6 months, mean out-of-office BP had fallen to 152/88±22/14 mmHg. By 2 years this had fallen to 144/83±15/13 mmHg suggesting both durability of antihypertensive effect and safety given the fact no adverse events were noted during follow-up and renal function remained stable in all patients. As this was a small single-center study, it needs to be interpreted cautiously [53].

Table 5.3 Changes in office systolic blood pressure seen in the global SYMPLICITY Registry [53]

Patient group	3 months	6 months	P value
All patients	−10.0 mmHg	−11.9 mmHg	<0.0001 (at 3 and 6 months)
<140 mmHg	+12.9 mmHg	+14.2 mmHg	<0.0001 (at 3 and 6 months)
140–159 mmHg	−2.0 mmHg	−4.6 mmHg	0.14 (3 months) 0.0006 (6 months)
≥160 mmHg	−18.9 mmHg	−21.4 mmHg	<0.0001 (at 3 and 6 months)

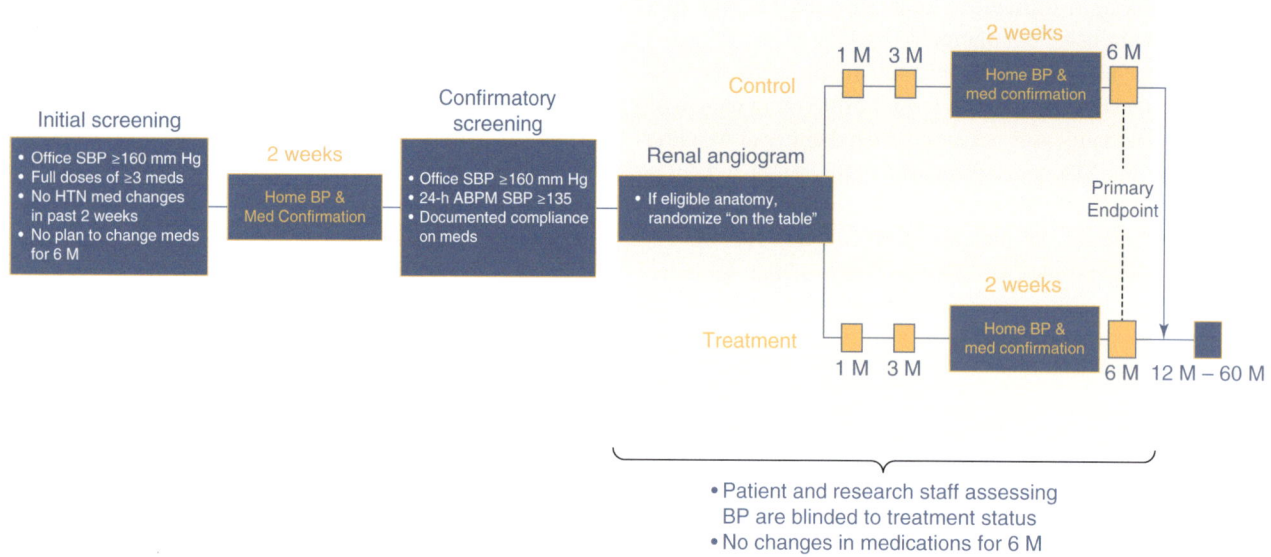

Fig. 5.1 SYMPLICITY HTN-3 Trial Flow. *ABPM* ambulatory blood pressure monitoring, *HTN* hypertension (Reproduced and adapted from Kandzari et al. [57] with permission from John Wiley and Sons)

The SYMPLICITY HTN-3 Trial

SYMPLICITY HTN-3 (ClinicalTrials.gov Identifier NCT01418261) was designed to overcome several of the methodological limitations of HTN-1 and HTN-2 [54, 55]. It was a prospective, randomized, masked procedure, single-blind trial that enrolled patients in a 2 (treatment):1 (control) design at 88 sites within the United States between October 2011 and May 2013 [56, 57]. Patients were blinded to the extent possible (through conscious sedation, sensory isolation, and lack of familiarity with the RDN procedure and its duration) by means of a sham control procedure. Pre-designated BP assessors were also blinded to treatment allocation, thereby providing the first truly controlled assessment of this intervention and minimizing confounding from expectation and evaluation bias respectively. The sham control was a renal angiogram, which the patient would have required anyway prior to randomization. A crossover from the control arm to RDN at 6 months was allowed if the patient continued to meet the inclusion criteria, and hence all randomized patients had the opportunity to be treated, circumventing any potential ethical concerns (Fig. 5.1).

There was a rigorous screening process that comprised a patient home diary to confirm compliance with pharmacotherapy and ambulatory recordings prior to the second trial visit during which time an office systolic BP of ≥160 mmHg was also reconfirmed. An ambulatory average systolic BP <135 mmHg was used to exclude patients with white coat HTN. Additionally, patients had to be treated with three or more optimally dosed antihypertensive medications from different, complementary classes, one of which had to be an appropriately dosed diuretic. There was, however, no mandated

use of an aldosterone antagonist as a 4th line agent. Changes in therapeutic regimen were not permitted prior to randomization. Routine assessment for RAS at 6 months was performed. There was also a concerted effort to exclude patients with a secondary cause of RHTN [56, 57]. All patients were maintained on their baseline antihypertensive regimen for the 6-month follow-up period unless clinical circumstances justified an alteration in pharmacotherapy. All patients, irrespective of treatment arm, are to be followed for 5 years post randomization.

A total of 535 patients (RDN group n=364 vs. sham procedure group n=171) were enrolled into the trial. Patients were taking on average 5 antihypertensive medications and almost all at maximally tolerated doses. Again, RDN was shown to be a safe procedure. There were no significant differences between the treatment arms in kidney function at any time point. New onset end stage renal disease did not occur post procedure. A single RAS occurred in the RDN arm (0.3 %).

The trial however did not meet either its primary or secondary efficacy outcomes at 6 months [57]. For the former, there was no significant between-group difference in office systolic BP (RDN -14.13 ± 23.93 mmHg vs. sham -11.74 ± 25.94 mmHg for a difference of -2.39 mmHg, 95 % CI -6.89 to 2.12, P=0.26). For the latter again there was no significant between-group difference in ambulatory BP (RDN -6.75 ± 15.11 mmHg vs. sham -4.79 ± 17.25 mmHg, for a difference of -1.96 mmHg, 95 % CI -4.97 to 1.06, P=0.98). The absolute magnitude of reduction in either office or ambulatory BP was also much lower than those observed in the HTN-1 and HTN-2 trials.

So what went wrong? In terms of trial design rigor, HTN-3 cannot be faulted. Admittedly, absolute compliance with adjunctive medical therapy cannot be guaranteed in trial participants, but this is true of all randomized trials not incorporating directly observed therapy systems or measuring drug metabolite levels. As such, we can feel confident that the individuals exposed to RDN were indeed those suffering treatment-resistant HTN and not pseudo RHTN. Moreover, HTN-3 compared the intervention with a sham-control, whereas previous trials and the existing literature are replete with studies comparing treatment results with corresponding baseline measurements taken, perhaps in triplicate, but on a single day.

Perhaps the 6-month follow up period was too short. All those participating in HTN-3 will be followed up for 5 years. We may indeed see a further divergence in BP reductions as the placebo effect diminishes over time, but this is merely supposition. Typical of all RDN devices and procedures is again the lack of a biometric signal that assures the operator that actual denervation has taken place. The search for an easily applied and measured neurophysiological biomarker to indicate adequate denervation continues. Nevertheless, the Symplicity catheter used in HTN-3 was similar to that used in part of HTN-2 [58].

Symplicity Spyral™ Multi-Electrode Catheter Study Data

In October 2012, Medtronic reported successful completion of the first phase of their feasibility study into a next-generation RDN system featuring a simultaneously firing four-electrode catheter designed to significantly reduce ablation time. Nine patients were treated with a 100 % successful procedure completion rate [59]. The new catheter was designed for ease of deliverability and consistency of RF energy application. Since then, the Symplicity Spyral catheter and G3™ RF generator have received their CE mark in Europe and Therapeutic Goods Administration (TGA) listing in Australia in December 2013. Preliminary results from a prospective, non-randomized, open label, first-in-man feasibility study (n=29) to determine the efficacy and safety of the new Spyral catheter revealed a fall in office BP of 16/7±21/12 mmHg at 1 month [60]. Aside from two femoral artery aneurysms there were no other renovascular or hemodynamic complications. Further procedural details and 3-month follow up of the entire planned cohort of 50 patients will be presented in due course.

Preliminary Data for Alternative Renal Denervation Devices

By 2012 five RDN catheters had already received their CE mark – Medtronic's Symplicity, St. Jude Medical's EnligHTN™ (St Paul, Minnesota, USA), Vessix V2™ (Boston Scientific Corp, Natick, Massachusetts, USA), Covidien's OneShot™ (Mansfield, Massachusetts, USA) and Recor Medical's Paradise™ (Menlo Park, California, USA). Most of these systems use RF energy to target renal sympathetic nerves, apart from the Paradise system, which uses ultrasound energy delivered uniformly in every treatment site.

The EnligHTN I Trial

This was a first-in-human, multicenter, single arm, non-randomized study designed to evaluate the safety and efficacy of the EnligHTN catheter [61]. The single-electrode Symplicity catheter requires the operator to navigate the catheter to achieve four to six discrete ablations separated longitudinally and rotationally along the length of each renal artery. Clearly, this can be a relatively time consuming process and exposes the patient to a heightened risk of renovascular injury. Conversely, the EnligHTN catheter is a multi-electrode RF system with electrodes arranged geometrically in pre-specified positions. As such a single burst of RF energy will simultaneously ablate at several predefined areas along the renal artery thereby moderating the need for catheter manipulation and theoretically attenuating the risk of procedure-related endothelial injury.

Patients were eligible for the study if they had an office systolic BP persistently ≥160 mmHg (≥150 mmHg in Type 2 diabetic patients) despite the concurrent use of ≥3 antihypertensive agents (one of which had to be a diuretic) at maximally tolerated doses. The drug regimen was to remain stable for at least 2 weeks prior to enrolment and through the initial 6-month follow-up. A known secondary cause of HTN meant exclusion from the trial but a specific protocol was not in place to make a *de novo* diagnosis. Akin to the limitations of HTN-1 and HTN-2 [38, 40], out-of-office BP measurements were not formally utilized in making the RHTN diagnosis despite patients having to take home BP recordings every day during the 2-week screening period in addition to having an ABPM assessment. No emphasis was made towards optimization of lifestyle modifications.

Post procedure, patients were followed up at 1, 3, and 6-month intervals continuing to 12, 18, and 24 months. Importantly, and unlike HTN-1 and HTN-2, renal artery imaging by computed tomography (CT) and duplex ultrasound was completed for all patients at the 6-month follow up visit.

Of the 62 patients who gave their consent, 46 ultimately went on to receive RDN. Minor peri-procedural side effects intrinsic to the procedure (i.e., vasospasm, access site hematoma, bradycardia, vasovagal responses, and flank pain) were reasonably common but did not give rise to permanent sequelae. Three patients (6.5 %) suffered a serious adverse event including hypotension, progression of hypertensive renal disease, and progression of a pre-existing RAS lesion. Aside from these, no patient developed a new hemodynamically significant RAS lesion at the 6-month imaging assessment. No patient experienced a reduction in eGFR >50 %, a twofold increase in serum creatinine, or progressed to end-stage renal disease.

The mean office BP at baseline was 176/96 mmHg. Post RDN this fell by 28/10 mmHg at 1 month, 27/10 mmHg at 3 months, and 26/10 mmHg at 6 months. As expected, ABPM figures were less impressive but did remain consistent throughout the 6-month period. At baseline mean ambulatory BP was 150/83 mmHg. By 1 month this had fallen by 10/5 mmHg, by 3 months 10/5 mmHg, and 10/6 mmHg at 6 months. The investigators deserve praise for ensuring follow-up was virtually complete in the study. Unlike HTN-1, this would suggest a more uniform and rapid response to RF ablation from the entire cohort when compared with results achieved by the Symplicity catheter. Here the investigators propose the multielectrode array of the EnligHTN catheter may have given rise to a more complete denervation compared with the single electrode format of the Symplicity catheter. This assumption would not, however, explain the eventual response of those patients in the HTN-1 and HTN-2 cohorts over time. Moreover the reductions in BP did not stimulate a widespread streamlining of pharmacotherapy in the EnligHTN I study group. Longer-term follow up results are awaited.

The REDUCE-HTN Trial

The REDUCE-HTN Post-Market Study (n = 128), including the first-in-man cohort (n = 18), is a prospective, non-randomized, single arm, open label multicenter study designed to evaluate the safety and efficacy of the Vessix V2 multi-electrode RDN catheter [62]. Patients were enrolled based on an office systolic BP ≥160 mmHg despite maximally tolerated doses of ≥3 antihypertensives (including a diuretic unless there was a documented intolerance). The final results of the trial have not yet been formally published and as such specific selection criteria are not available. At 1 (n = 142), 3 (n = 144), 6 (n = 139), and 12 (n = 41) months, there were reductions of 23/10, 21/8, 25/10 and 30/14 mmHg in office BP respectively [62]. Procedure-related adverse events occurred in 5.5 % of the 146-patient cohort (including hematoma, bilateral flank pain, vomiting, access site pseudoaneurysm, access site thrombus, infection, and a single RAS requiring intervention). At 6 months 222/224 renal arteries treated remained patent according to core lab duplex ultrasound analysis [62]. Boston Scientific ultimately plans to enroll 1,200 RHTN patients worldwide in the REDUCE HTN clinical series.

The REDUCE Trial

The purpose of the REDUCE study was to determine the technical feasibility along with the safety and efficacy of the CE-marked Paradise catheter, which incorporates a cylindrical transducer that emits ultrasound energy circumferentially [63]. A fluid-filled low-pressure balloon cools the endothelium during energy delivery and as such minimizes potential damage to surrounding tissues. RHTN was defined according to European Society of Hypertension (ESH) and European Society of Cardiology (ESC) guidelines: i.e., a minimum BP of 140/90 mmHg (office), 135/85 mmHg (home), and 130/80 mmHg (ambulatory) despite treatment with ≥3 antihypertensive drugs including a diuretic [63]. Bilateral denervation was achieved by delivering ultrasound energy in up to three locations within each renal artery.

The average office BP was 180/109 ± 20/13 mmHg, home BP 169/101 ± 14/13 mmHg, and ambulatory BP 168/98 ± 16/15 mmHg in 11 consecutive patients taking a mean of 4.5 antihypertensive medications with 100 % diuretic uptake. There was however no medication stabilization period, compliance monitoring, exhaustion of lifestyle modifications, or active exclusion of secondary causes of HTN. Overall, the procedure was safe although one patient suffered a renal artery dissection upon placement of the guiding catheter.

Office BP at 1, 2, and 3 months fell by 30/15, 32/14, and 36/17 mmHg respectively. Home BP measurements followed suit with reductions in BP of 20/11, 19/10, and 22/12 mmHg at the same time intervals respectively. The investigators should be commended for their use of out-of-office BP measurements in all trial participants. This gives the results notable credence and proves for now that ultrasound denervation is safe. Clearly, long-term follow-up is required to demonstrate durability of effect and imaging of the renal arteries should continue beyond the original 6-month protocol.

The WAVE I and WAVE II Trials

The Surround Sound® RDN system developed by Kona Medical (Bellevue, Washington, USA) externally delivers ultrasound energy to a target tissue obviating the need to expose patients to the dangers of radiation. In theory, directed ultrasound energy creates an ablative field around the vessel, which ablates the renal nerves without the risk of endothelial injury or access site issues.

The WAVE I first-in-man study (n = 24) demonstrated BP reductions of 22/9 mmHg at 3 months and 29/12 mmHg at 6 months [64]. The WAVE I protocol involved making 18 focused lesions over 12.6 min bilaterally. In WAVE II (n = 17), an optimized protocol involving 14 focused lesions bilaterally, created in under 3 min, was assessed [65]. An average fall in BP of 19/7 mmHg was achieved. There were no device-related serious adverse events in either study. The WAVE III study is currently enrolling.

The SOUND-ITV Study

This was a first-in-man feasibility trial used to evaluate the Sound 360™ ultrasonic RDN system (Sound Interventions Inc., Stony Brook, New York, USA) [66]. The catheter incorporates a cylindrical transducer encased within a non-cylindrical, non-occlusive balloon. An average of 1.8 applications were delivered bilaterally to the renal arteries of 17 RHTN patients resulting in an average reduction of 31/10 mmHg at 1 month. Acutely and through follow up there were no device or procedure-related complications. Longer term follow up and clearly more patients are required to confirm these results.

Discussion

Prior to HTN-3, all looked very positive in the field of RDN [57]. A systematic review and meta-analysis of two randomized controlled trials, one observational study with a control group and nine observational studies without a control group had confirmed a substantial reduction in average BP at 6 months in patients with reported RHTN encompassing the use of five different catheters [67]. RDN was also shown to be safe in this analysis. There were, however, legitimate criticisms of the data. Howard and colleagues examined the suspected office versus ambulatory BP discrepancy yet further through a meta-analysis of 31 antihypertensive drug trials (n=4,121 patients) and 23 RDN trials (n=720 patients) [68]. Their findings served to confirm what hypertension and clinical trial experts had suspected: without randomization or masking in drug trials, reductions in office BP were being over-estimated when compared with ambulatory BP recordings [69]. With randomization or masking in place, office and ambulatory BP figures were virtually identical. The investigators therefore predicted that once randomization and masking were in place, vis-à-vis the HTN-3 trial [57], trials of RDN would reveal a convergence of office and ambulatory BP reductions [68]. The results from HTN-3 would later confirm their predictions.

So how is the interventional community to move forward? If we are to pursue RDN as a viable therapy for the treatment of RHTN then the following points must be borne in mind:

- Absolute due diligence must be taken to identify patients with true RHTN and every effort must be made to rule out pseudo RHTN [11]. On the ground, this means optimization of lifestyle modifications, complete adherence to a pharmacotherapeutic regimen of ≥3 antihypertensive

agents including a diuretic, and the use of ABPM to irrefutably include those suffering from treatment-resistant systemic HTN.

- We must take a step back from the interventional forum and concentrate our efforts on establishing a standardized, stepwise, evidence-based pharmacotherapeutic regimen that must first be attempted prior to consideration for percutaneous RDN. This means efforts to determine whether aldosterone antagonists are indeed the best 4th line agent in this particular patient cohort [70–75] and if not, what agent is. Is there indeed just one specific combination to utilize or should we accept that individual tailoring of therapy is inevitable given the multitude of adverse effects that can lead to intolerance of different drugs?

- If device companies maintain interest in the RDN field, the holy grail of RDN must be to identify a reliable, reproducible, and easily attainable imaging test or biomarker of successful denervation.

Percutaneous RDN remains a safe procedure supported by sound physiological principles, and further study in clinical trials is warranted. Is it better suited to managing conditions bearing the hallmarks of SNS hyperactivation other than RHTN? Is it best reserved for patients who are non-adherent to their antihypertensive regimen? Further studies will be necessary to address these important questions. Longer-term follow up of HTN-3 will also be intriguing, as one might expect the placebo effect to decrease over time, for any true effect of RDN to persist. Future rigorously designed clinical trials with various devices should be pursued to see if the lack of efficacy in SYMPLICITY HTN-3 was due to that particular device or the way that device was used. Importantly, these future trials will need to incorporate many of the trial design elements from SYMPLICITY HTN-3.

References

1. Chobanian A, Bakris G, Black H, Cushman WC, Green LA, Izzo Jr JL, et al. The Seventh Report of the Joint National Committee on Prevention, Detection, Evaluation, and Treatment of High Blood Pressure. The JNC 7 report. JAMA. 2003;289:2560–72.
2. Mancia G, De Backer G, Dominiczak A, Cifkova R, Fagard R, Germano G, et al. Guidelines for the management of arterial hypertension: the task force for the management of arterial hypertension of the European Society of Hypertension (ESH) and of the European Society of Cardiology (ESC). Eur Heart J. 2007;28: 1462–536.
3. Calhoun DA, Jones D, Textor S, Goff DC, Murphy TP, Toto RD, et al. Resistant hypertension: diagnosis, evaluation, and treatment. A scientific statement from the American Heart Association Professional Education Committee of the Council for High Blood Pressure Research. Hypertension. 2008;51:1403–19.
4. National Clinical Guideline Centre. CG127 Hypertension: the clinical management of primary hypertension in adults. 2011. p. 1–328.

5. Caulfield M, Belder M De, Cleveland T, Collier D, Gray H, Knight C, et al. Joint UK Societies' consensus summary statement on renal denervation for resistant hypertension. 2011. p. 1–2.

6. Schmieder RE, Redon J, Grassi G, Kjeldsen SE, Mancia G, Narkiewicz K, et al. ESH position paper: renal denervation – an interventional therapy of resistant hypertension. J Hypertens. 2012;30:837–41.

7. Weber MA, Schiffrin EL, White WB, Mann S, Lindholm LH, Kenerson JG, et al. Clinical practice guidelines for the management of hypertension in the community: a statement by the American Society of Hypertension and the International Society of Hypertension. J Clin Hypertens. 2014;16:14–26.

8. Mahfoud F, Lüscher TF, Andersson B, Baumgartner I, Cifkova R, Dimario C, et al. Expert consensus document from the European Society of Cardiology on catheter-based renal denervation. Eur Heart J. 2013;34:2149–57.

9. Schlaich MP, Schmieder RE, Bakris G, Blankestijn PJ, Böhm M, Campese VM, et al. International expert consensus statement: percutaneous transluminal renal denervation for the treatment of resistant hypertension. J Am Coll Cardiol. 2013;62:2031–45.

10. Tsioufis C, Mahfoud F, Mancia G, Redon J, Damascelli B, Zeller T, et al. What the interventionalist should know about renal denervation in hypertensive patients: a position paper by the ESH WG on the interventional treatment of hypertension. EuroIntervention. 2014;9:1027–35.

11. Myat A, Redwood SR, Qureshi AC, Spertus JA, Williams B. Resistant hypertension. BMJ. 2012;345:e7473.

12. Myat A, Redwood SR, Qureshi AC, Thackray S, Cleland JGF, Bhatt DL, et al. Renal sympathetic denervation therapy for resistant hypertension: a contemporary synopsis and future implications. Circ Cardiovasc Interv. 2013;6:184–97.

13. Kumbhani DJ, Steg PG, Cannon CP, Eagle KA, Smith SC, Crowley K, et al. Resistant hypertension: a frequent and ominous finding among hypertensive patients with atherothrombosis. Eur Heart J. 2013;34:1204–14.

14. Daugherty SL, Powers JD, Magid DJ, Tavel HM, Masoudi FA, Margolis KL, et al. Incidence and prognosis of resistant hypertension in hypertensive patients. Circulation. 2012;125:1635–42.

15. Egan BM, Zhao Y, Axon RN, Brzezinski W, Ferdinand KC. Uncontrolled and apparent treatment resistant hypertension in the United States, 1988 to 2008. Circulation. 2011;124:1046–58.

16. De la Sierra A, Segura J, Banegas JR, Gorostidi M, de la Cruz JJ, Armario P, et al. Clinical features of 8295 patients with resistant hypertension classified on the basis of ambulatory blood pressure monitoring. Hypertension. 2011;57:898–902.

17. Pimenta E, Calhoun DA. Resistant hypertension: incidence, prevalence, and prognosis. Circulation. 2012;125:1594–6.

18. Esler M. The sympathetic nervous system through the ages: from Thomas Willis to resistant hypertension. Exp Physiol. 2011; 96:611–22.

19. DiBona GF, Esler M. Translational medicine: the antihypertensive effect of renal denervation. Am J Physiol Regul Integr Comp Physiol. 2010;298:R245–53.

20. Oliveria SA, Lapuerta P, McCarthy BD, L'Italien GJ, Berlowitz DR, Asch SM. Physician-related barriers to the effective management of uncontrolled hypertension. Arch Intern Med. 2002;162:413–20.

21. Banegas JR, Messerli FH, Waeber B, Rodríguez-Artalejo F, de la Sierra A, Segura J, et al. Discrepancies between office and ambulatory blood pressure: clinical implications. Am J Med. 2009;122:1136–41. Elsevier Inc.

22. National Institute for Health and Clinical Excellence. Percutaneous transluminal radiofrequency sympathetic denervation of the renal artery for resistant hypertension. NICE Interventional Procedure Guidance 418. 2012. p. 1–10.

23. Mancia G, Bombelli M, Facchetti R, Madotto F, Quarti-Trevano F, Polo Friz H, et al. Long-term risk of sustained hypertension in white-coat or masked hypertension. Hypertension. 2009;54: 226–32.

24. Fagard RH. Resistant hypertension. Heart. 2012;98:254–61.

25. Sarafidis PA, Bakris GL. Resistant hypertension: an overview of evaluation and treatment. J Am Coll Cardiol. 2008;52:1749–57. American College of Cardiology Foundation.

26. Acelajado MC, Calhoun D, Oparil S. Reduction of blood pressure in patients with treatment-resistant hypertension. Expert Opin Pharmacother. 2009;10:2959–71.

27. Ishikawa J, Carroll DJ, Kuruvilla S, Schwartz JE, Pickering TG. Changes in home versus clinic blood pressure with antihypertensive treatments: a meta-analysis. Hypertension. 2008;52:856–64.

28. Mancia G, Parati G. Office compared with ambulatory blood pressure in assessing response to antihypertensive treatment: a meta-analysis. J Hypertens. 2004;22:435–45.

29. Mancia G, Sega R, Bravi C, De Vito G, Valagussa F, Cesana G, et al. Ambulatory blood pressure normality: results from the PAMELA study. J Hypertens. 1995;13:1377–90.

30. Dolan E, Stanton A, Thijs L, Hinedi K, Atkins N, McClory S, et al. Superiority of ambulatory over clinic blood pressure measurement in predicting mortality: the Dublin outcome study. Hypertension. 2005;46:156–61.

31. Pickering TG, White WB. When and how to use self (home) and ambulatory blood pressure monitoring. J Am Soc Hypertens. 2008; 2:119–24.

32. Salles GF, Cardoso CRL, Muxfeldt ES. Prognostic influence of office and ambulatory blood pressures in resistant hypertension. Arch Intern Med. 2008;168:2340–6.

33. Yakovlevitch M, Black HR. Resistant hypertension in a tertiary care clinic. Arch Intern Med. 1991;151:1786–92.

34. Garg JP, Elliott WJ, Folker A, Izhar M, Black HR. Resistant hypertension revisited: a comparison of two university-based cohorts. Am J Hypertens. 2005;18:619–26.

35. Pimenta E, Gaddam K, Oparil S. Mechanisms and treatment of resistant hypertension. J Clin Hypertens. 2008;10:239–44.

36. Verloop WL, Vink EE, Voskuil M, Vonken E-J, Rookmaaker MB, Bots ML, et al. Eligibility for percutaneous renal denervation: the importance of a systematic screening. J Hypertens. 2013;31:1662–8.

37. Schlaich MP, Sobotka P, Krum H, Lambert E, Esler MD. Renal sympathetic-nerve ablation for uncontrolled hypertension. N Engl J Med. 2009;361:932–4.

38. Krum H, Schlaich M, Whitbourn R, Sobotka P, Sadowski J, Bartus K, et al. Catheter-based renal sympathetic denervation for resistant hypertension: a multicentre safety and proof-of-principle cohort study. Lancet. 2009;373:1275–81.

39. Krum H, Schlaich MP, Böhm M, Mahfoud F, Rocha-Singh K, Katholi R, et al. Percutaneous renal denervation in patients with treatment-resistant hypertension: final 3-year report of the Symplicity HTN-1 study. Lancet. 2013;383:622–9.

40. Esler MD, Krum H, Sobotka PA, Schlaich MP, Schmieder RE, Böhm M. Renal sympathetic denervation in patients with treatment-resistant hypertension (The Symplicity HTN-2 Trial): a randomised controlled trial. Lancet. 2010;376:1903–9.

41. Symplicity HTN-1 Investigators. Catheter-based renal sympathetic denervation for resistant hypertension: durability of blood pressure reduction out to 24 months. Hypertension. 2011;57:911–7.

42. Esler MD, Krum H, Schlaich M, Schmieder RE, Böhm M, Sobotka PA. Renal sympathetic denervation for treatment of drug-resistant hypertension: one-year results from the symplicity HTN-2 randomized, controlled trial. Circulation. 2012;126:2976–82.

43. Medtronic. Symplicity™ RDN System Clinical Trial Data [Internet]. 2014. Available from: http://www.medtronicrdn.com/intl/healthcare-professionals/symplicity-rdn-system/symplicity-clinical-trial-data/index.htm.

44. Virmani R. Perirenal nerve distribution, density and quantification: implications for the evaluation of device safety and efficacy disclo-

sure statement of financial interest. Transcatheter Cardiovascular Therapeutics, Miami; 2012.

45. Johns EJ. Resistant hypertension and renal denervation: 3 years on. Lancet. 2014;383:583–4.

46. Doumas M, Douma S. Interventional management of resistant hypertension. Lancet. 2009;373:1228–30.

47. Doumas M, Anyfanti P, Bakris G. Should ambulatory blood pressure monitoring be mandatory for future studies in resistant hypertension: a perspective. J Hypertens. 2012;30:874–6.

48. Vonend O, Antoch G, Rump LC, Blondin D. Secondary rise in blood pressure after renal denervation. Lancet. 2012;380:778.

49. Kaltenbach B, Id D, Franke JC, Sievert H, Hennersdorf M, Maier J, et al. Renal artery stenosis after renal sympathetic denervation. J Am Coll Cardiol. 2012;60:2694–5.

50. Mahfoud F, Cremers B, Janker J, Link B, Vonend O, Ukena C, et al. Renal hemodynamics and renal function after catheter-based renal sympathetic denervation in patients with resistant hypertension. Hypertension. 2012;60:419–24.

51. Böhm M, Mahfoud F, Ukena C, Bauer A, Fleck E, Hoppe UC, et al. Rationale and design of a large registry on renal denervation: the Global SYMPLICITY registry. EuroIntervention. 2013;9: 484–92.

52. Bohm M. The global SYMPLICITY registry: safety and effectiveness of renal artery denervation in real world patients with uncontrolled hypertension. Washington, DC: American College of Cardiology Scientific Sessions; 2014.

53. Benamer H, Mylotte D, Garcia-Alonso C, Unterseeh T, Garot P, Louvard Y, et al. Renal denervation a treatment for resistant hypertension: a French experience. Ann Cardiol Angiol (Paris). 2013;62:384–91.

54. Bhatt DL, Bakris GL. The promise of renal denervation. Cleve Clin J Med. 2012;79:498–500.

55. Persu A, Renkin J, Asayama K, O'Brien E, Staessen J. Renal denervation in treatment-resistant hypertension: the need for restraint and more and better evidence. Expert Rev Cardiovasc Ther. 2013;11:739–49.

56. Kandzari DE, Bhatt DL, Sobotka P, O'Neill WW, Esler M, Flack JM, et al. Catheter-based renal denervation for resistant hypertension: rationale and design of the SYMPLICITY HTN-3 trial. Clin Cardiol. 2012;35:528–35.

57. Bhatt DL, Kandzari DE, O'Neill WW, D'Agostino R, Flack JM, Katzen BT, et al. A controlled trial of renal denervation for resistant hypertension. N Engl J Med. 2014;370:1393–401.

58. Messerli F, Bangalore S. Renal denervation for resistant hypertension? N Engl J Med. 2014;370:1454–7.

59. Medtronic. Medtronic completes first-in-man study for investigational next-generation multi-electrode renal denervation system in patients with treatment-resistant hypertension [Internet]. 2012. Available from: http://newsroom.medtronic.com/phoenix.zhtml?c= 251324&p=irol-newsArticle&ID=1772019&highlight=.

60. Whitbourn RJ, Harding S, Rothman MT, Walton T. TCT-491 renal artery denervation with a new simultaneous multielectrode catheter for treatment of resistant hypertension: results from the Symplicity Spyral(tm) first-in-man study. J Am Coll Cardiol. 2013;62:B150.

61. Worthley S, Tsioufis C. Safety and efficacy of a multi-electrode renal sympathetic denervation system in resistant hypertension: the EnligHTN I trial. Eur Heart J. 2013;34:2132–40.

62. Boston Scientific. Vessix global clinical program REDUCE HTN FIM and post market study [Internet]. 2014 [cited 2014 Mar 24]. Available from: http://www.bostonscientific.com/renal-denervation/ Data_Cases/Clinical_Data/clinical-data.html.

63. Mabin T, Sapoval M, Cabane V, Stemmett J, Iyer M. First experience with endovascular ultrasound renal denervation for the treatment of resistant hypertension. EuroIntervention. 2012;8:57–61.

64. Kona Medical. Clinical data reported for WAVE I and WAVE II studies of renal denervation therapy for hypertension at transcatheter cardiovascular therapeutics conference [Internet]. 2014 [cited 2014 Mar 25]. Available from: http://konamedical.com/ renal-denervation-therapy-studies/.

65. Neuzil P, Whitbourn RJ, Starek Z, Esler MD, Brinton T, Gertner M. TCT-61 optimized external focused ultrasound for renal sympathetic denervation – wave II trial. J Am Coll Cardiol. 2013;62:B20.

66. Neuzil P, Petru J, Vondrakova D, Kopriva K, Chovanec M, Sediva L, et al. TCT-356 circumferential therapeutic ultrasound for the treatment of resistant hypertension: preliminary results of human feasibility study (SOUND-ITV). J Am Coll Cardiol. 2012;60: B101–2.

67. Davis MI, Filion KB, Zhang D, Eisenberg MJ, Afilalo J, Schiffrin EL, et al. Effectiveness of renal denervation therapy for resistant hypertension: a systematic review and meta-analysis. J Am Coll Cardiol. 2013;62:231–41.

68. Howard JP, Nowbar AN, Francis DP. Size of blood pressure reduction from renal denervation: insights from meta-analysis of antihypertensive drug trials of 4,121 patients with focus on trial design: the CONVERGE report. Heart. 2013;99:1579–87.

69. Howard JP, Cole GD, Sievert H, Bhatt DL, Papademetriou V, Kandzari DE, et al. Unintentional overestimation of an expected antihypertensive effect in drug and device trials: mechanisms and solutions. Int J Cardiol. 2014;172:29–35.

70. Václavík J, Sedlák R, Plachy M, Navrátil K, Plásek J, Jarkovsky J, et al. Addition of spironolactone in patients with resistant arterial hypertension (ASPIRANT): a randomized, double-blind, placebo-controlled trial. Hypertension. 2011;57:1069–75.

71. De Souza F, Muxfeldt E, Fiszman R, Salles G. Efficacy of spironolactone therapy in patients with true resistant hypertension. Hypertension. 2010;55:147–52.

72. Chapman N, Dobson J, Wilson S, Dahlöf B, Sever PS, Wedel H, et al. Effect of spironolactone on blood pressure in subjects with resistant hypertension. Hypertension. 2007;49:839–45.

73. Calhoun DA, White WB. Effectiveness of the selective aldosterone blocker, eplerenone, in patients with resistant hypertension. J Am Soc Hypertens. 2008;2:462–8. American Society of Hypertension.

74. Lane DA, Shah S, Beevers DG. Low-dose spironolactone in the management of resistant hypertension: a surveillance study. J Hypertens. 2007;25:891–4.

75. Corrao G, Nicotra F, Parodi A, Zambon A, Heiman F, Merlino L, et al. Cardiovascular protection by initial and subsequent combination of antihypertensive drugs in daily life practice. Hypertension. 2011;58:566–72.

Catheter-Based Technology Alternatives for Renal Denervation: An Overview

6

Stefan C. Bertog and Horst Sievert

In the aforementioned chapters, the role of the renal sympathetic nervous system in blood pressure control has been outlined. The effect of renal sympathetic denervation on blood pressure in an animal model has been described and it has been demonstrated that renal denervation in humans causes what it intends to, a reduction in overall sympathetic tone (as demonstrated by norepinephrine spillover and muscle sympathetic nerve activity). Finally, human data on renal denervation has been summarized. In line with physiological plausibility, the promising early results of radiofrequency renal denervation have led to a surge in interest in the sympathetic nervous system and renal denervation coupled with significant investment in new technology design. Importantly, at the time of this writing, it has been announced that the Symplicity-3 trial did not meet the predefined primary endpoint. Specifics regarding the outcome of the trial are not available, yet.

Though initial technology has a proven and longer standing track record, it has theoretical and practical shortcomings: the potential for renal artery injury beyond that of the adventitia and renal sympathetic nerves, unreliability in achieving circumferential denervation and procedural time investment and pain.

These shortcomings have prompted modifications in current catheter design, invention of new catheters and exploration of entirely new concepts (Table 6.1). The original Symplicity™ renal denervation system (Medtronic, Minneapolis, MN, USA) has been redesigned by the manufacturer into a spiral catheter (Spyral) with multiple electrodes that can be delivered over the wire into the renal artery (discussed in Chap. 7). This design has undergone a first-in-man study (the 1-month results of which were presented at 2013 Transcatheter Therapeutics [TCT]).

A number of companies have explored the use of catheters using multiple electrodes to facilitate radiofrequency energy delivery in a more reliable fashion and to significantly shorten the procedure duration. Cordis (Bridgewater, NJ, USA) has designed a spiral catheter (Thermocool) similar to the new generation Medtronic catheter with irrigated multiple electrodes (discussed in Chap. 20). It has undergone extensive animal testing with human trials planned. A multi-electrode catheter (EnlighTEN) with electrodes arranged in a basket-like fashion has been designed by St. Jude Medical (St. Paul, MN, USA) and human studies have been completed (discussed in Chap. 8). In addition, Covidien (Dublin, Ireland) has designed a balloon-tipped catheter (Covidien One-Shot™) that harbors multiple electrodes on its surface that appose to the renal artery wall upon inflation and allows irrigation during the procedure (discussed in Chap. 12). Human data have recently been shown. Similarly, the Vessix™ Renal Denervation System (Boston Scientific, Natick, MA, USA) is a balloon tipped non-irrigated multi-electrode catheter (discussed in Chap. 19) that has been tested in human trials with data presented at international meetings. In addition, to radiofrequency application, the use of ultrasound energy has been explored. In this context, the Paradise catheter from Recor is a balloon-tipped catheter with an ultrasound transducer positioned in its center that emits ultrasound energy to the renal artery wall in a circumferential manner while cooling is provided by balloon irrigation (discussed in Chap. 9). Other ultrasound catheters (Sound Interventions Inc., Stony Brook, NY, USA and CardioSonic Inc., Tel Aviv, Israel) will be discussed in Chaps. 10 and 11. Finally, radiation exposure to the renal arteries causes interruption of the sympathetic fibers. This concept has been explored by Best Medical Inc., Springfield, VA. It is unquestionable that application of any form of energy, radiofrequency, ultrasound or radiation, has the potential for collateral damage. The biggest concern related to it is the occurrence of renal artery stenosis [1, 2] the incidence of which fortunately appears to be low but nevertheless

S.C. Bertog, MD, FACC, FSCAI
H. Sievert, MD, FESC, FACC, FSCAI (✉)
CardioVascular Center Frankfurt,
Seckbacher, Landstrasse 65, 60389 Frankfurt, Germany
e-mail: sbertog@aol.com; info@cvcfrankfurt.de

Table 6.1 Selection of renal denervation devices including only those devices that currently have CE-mark

	Basic design	Energy application	Irrigation	Delivery system profile	Ablation time per side	Baseline office BP (mmHg)	6-month BP reduction (mmHg)	Ambulatory BP reduction (mmHg)	Responder rate
Enlighten[a]	Basket design of multiple electrodes	RF unipolar	No	8F guide	12 min	176/96	26/10 (n=45)	not reported	77 % at 18 months
Vessix[a]	Balloon-mounted multiple electrodes	RF bipolar	No	8F sheath	30 s	182/100	25/10 (n=139)	9/6 (n=67)	85 % at 12 months
Maya one shot[a]	Balloon-mounted multiple electrodes	RF unipolar	Yes	7F/8F	120 s	182/96	20/8 (n=47)	11/6 (n=37)	Not reported
Medtronic[a]	Steerable tip catheter	RF unipolar	No	6F	8–16 min	178/96	32/12 (n=49)	11/7 (n=20)	84 % at 6 months
Paradise[a]	Self-centering ultrasound transducer	Ultrasound	Yes	7F	30 s	180/109	29/15 (n=15)	16/9 (n=13)	100 % at 6 months

[a]Data presented in this table is based on updates presented at Transcatheter Therapeutics (TCT) in 10/2013

BP blood pressure

important considering that renal denervation is treatment for a silent disease and that there currently is an absence of proof that treatment will improve cardiovascular endpoints. Efforts to maximize renal sympathetic nerve interruption while minimizing renal artery injury include the use of bipolar electrodes and catheter or balloon irrigation. Theoretically, these measures may reduce the amount of injury at the catheter-vessel interface allowing higher energy delivery to deeper layers including the adventitia harboring the renal sympathetic fibers. Indeed, in a number of small clinical trials outlined in the respective device chapters, it appears that the magnitude of blood pressure reduction is comparable to that reported in the initial Symplicity trials. However, definitive statements regarding efficacy can only be made by direct comparison between devices. In an effort to avoid renal artery injury by energy delivery, the concept of chemical neurolysis has theoretical merit (discussed in Chaps. 15, 16, and 18). By this technique, injection of a neurotoxic agent via microneedles avoids vessel wall injury with subsequent fibrosis. Moreover, with this approach, pain generation may be limited as the pain fibers have been described mainly in the

media of the renal arteries rather than the adventitia [3]. Data using this concept in a limited number of patients have recently been shown (TCT 2013) with promising results. Finally, renal denervation using external application of ultrasound energy (discussed in Chap. 13) has been studied in a small number of humans. It avoids the potential for vascular access complications.

It remains to be determined if aforementioned theoretical advantages translate into equivalent or better efficacy and safety. The following chapters will, in a more detailed fashion outline devices that are either already in clinical use or on the horizon of human studies.

References

1. Kaltenbach B, Id D, Franke JC, et al. Renal artery stenosis after renal sympathetic denervation. J Am Coll Cardiol. 2012;60(25):2694–5.
2. Vonend O, Antoch G, Rump LC, Blondin D. Secondary rise in blood pressure after renal denervation. Lancet. 2012;380(9843):778.
3. Schenk EA, El-Badawi A. Dual innervation of arteries and arterioles. A histochemical study. Z Zellforsch Mikrosk Anat. 1968; 91(2):170–7.

Medtronic Ardian Symplicity™ Renal Denervation Devices

Krishna J. Rocha-Singh

7

Key Points

- The Medtronic Ardian renal denervation catheter systems, the Arch™ and Flex™ catheters (Table 7.1), were the first percutaneous monopolar single-electrode radiofrequency devices to establish safety and proof-of-concept in the treatment of patients with severe treatment resistant hypertension.
- The use of the Medtronic Ardian Symplicity catheter systems in the proof-of-concept Symplicity HTN-1 and the randomized, crossover Symplicity HTN-2 trials were associated with low rates of device related complications.
- The renal denervation procedure time averages 66.1±23 min (time from initial femoral access to catheter withdrawal). An average four ablations per artery are typically performed (range 1–6); intravenous narcotics and sedatives were used to manage pain during the delivery of RF energy.
- Results from the extended 3-year follow-up of the Symplicity HTN-1 trial established the Arch™ and Flex™ Catheters as safe and effective in providing a significant and durable BP reduction in patients with treatment resistant hypertension.
- Rapid iteration of the Medtronic Ardian Spyral™ Catheter, a multi-monopolar electrode, over-the-wire catheter, allows for simultaneous electrode activation that reduces renal denervation treatment times and enables easier treatment of challenging renal artery anatomies.

Radiofrequency Ablation

Huang et al. first introduced radiofrequency (RF) catheter ablation for the disruption of the atrio-ventricular junction in 1987 [1]. Since that time, RF catheter ablation has become one of the most useful and widely accepted therapies in cardiac electrophysiology; modifications of RF energy delivery and improvements in the electrode design have resulted in significant expansion of its cardiac indication. More recently, RF technology has been used for the percutaneous sympathetic denervation of human renal arteries in the treatment of severe drug resistant hypertension [2–5].

RF energy is a form of alternating electrical current that produces a lesion by two distinct physical mechanisms: (1) direct resistive heating of the tissue in contact with the catheter electrode and (2) thermal conduction or passive heat transfer to deeper tissue layers. Resistive heating in regions close to the RF current source is rapid while passive heat transfer into deeper tissue layers is a slower process [6]. The transfer of heat continues after the discontinuation of RF current delivery and results in the lesion expansion. While RF electrical current can be delivered by a bipolar mode (i.e., between two closely placed electrodes), the more frequent use is via a monopolar mode with completion of the electrical circuit via the second electrode placed on the patient's skin at a distant location (typically the back or thigh). In the case of renal denervation, RF current is delivered to specific sites along the renal artery intimal surface through percutaneous arterial approach.

Radiofrequency Lesion Formation

The effects of RF energy on vascular tissue depends on several factors which include power (wattage), duration of its application, temperature, electrode size, quality of the electrode/tissue contact (impedance), the histological characteristics of the tissue and the blood flow over the electrode/tissue interface which determines the degree of heat dissipation [7, 8]. The RF electrode surface temperature is impacted

K.J. Rocha-Singh, MD
Department of Cardiology, Prairie Heart Institute at
St. John's Hospital, 619 E. Mason St., Springfield, IL, USA
e-mail: krs@krsingh.com

R.R. Heuser et al. (eds.), *Renal Denervation: A New Approach to Treatment of Resistant Hypertension*,
DOI 10.1007/978-1-4471-5223-1_7, © Springer-Verlag London 2015

Table 7.1 Medtronic Ardian renal denervation devices (2007–2014)

Catheter name	Electrode size	Ablation time	Catheter configuration	Guiding catheter F size compatible
Arch™ and $$$;	Single (2 mm)	2 min/site	Non-steerable	8F
Flex™ and $$$;	Single (2 mm)	2 min/site	Non wire-based steerable	6F
Spyral™ and $$$;	Multi-electrode (4.2 mm)	Simultaneous firing 50 s/treatment	Over-the-wire	6F

by the blood flow over the electrode and the temperature of the heated tissue decreases in a hyperbolic manner as the distance from the RF electrode increases, both of which are important factors in the use of the monopolar electrodes in renal denervation [9]. At temperatures above 100 °C, irreversible damage occurs to tissues surrounding the electrode [10]. This results in plasma protein degeneration and coagulation of blood elements resulting in charring or coagulum formation, which are typically noted in cardiac ablation. An important sign indicating charring or coagulant formation is the sudden rise in impedance rather than the gradual decrease that typically accompanies successful RF delivery.

Impedance, Power and Duration of RF Application

Measuring baseline impedance is used to assess the effectiveness of the contact between the RF electrode and tissue surface. As the tissue is heated, there is a temperature dependent drop in electrical impedance [9]. A positive correlation between the pre-ablation impedance and heating efficacy and a similar association between the decline in impedance during energy delivery and heating efficacy has been established [11]. Therefore, monitoring tissue surface temperature is essential and provides useful information as to the quality of the electrode/tissue interface [12]. Although temperature rise is greater and faster with properly engaged electrodes, a gradual increase in temperature as opposed to an abrupt rise may provide for a more homogeneous RF lesion [9].

The duration of steady state RF energy delivery is also an important variable and typically ranges from between 30 and 45 s in clinical practice. The optimal duration of RF energy application to effect optimal renal denervation remains a topic of debate as it reflects the extent of axonal ablation and the potential clinical effectiveness (i.e., blood pressure reduction) of the procedure and currently ranges from 30 to 120 s. However, the duration of energy application and electrode temperature must be balanced against the potential for renal intimal damage and subsequent renal artery lesion formation [13]. The degree of successfully ablated tissue is also proportional to the applied power of the RF source. In general, energy delivery is regulated by temperature control determined by default target temperatures with adjustment of energy to maintain a specific temperature. The algorithm associating

power, temperature, impedance and duration of energy exposure are all specific to individual monopolar renal denervation devices. The Medtronic Ardian renal denervation system uses a non-balloon, non-occlusive design with the initial Arch™ catheter uses a platinum electrode tip, providing adequate renal intimal contact to ensure transfer of adequate energy and impedance. The denervation procedure is performed using non-overlapping ablations spaced in a helical pattern to minimize intimal damage (4–6 ablations/renal artery) with the application of 5–8 W per ablation site while the generator algorithm monitors temperature and impedance and adjusts power to prevent tissue over-heating and potential intimal damage. If the surface temperature exceeds the pre-specified value, the power is terminated; likewise, if the temperature is too low, the system generates an "error code" telling the operator that the surface contact in likely insufficient.

Electrode size influences the volume of the ablation lesion and may also impact the clinical effectiveness of ablation. In general, larger electrodes result in larger lesions, which may produce greater ablative efficacy [13, 14]. However, in the case of renal denervation, the ideal relationship between lesion size, treatment efficacy and safety is yet to be fully understood and reported.

The blood supply and proximity to major blood vessels determines the degree of heat dissipation (i.e., the "heat sink") and represents another important factor that influences optimal ablative lesion formation. Convective heat dissipation through blood flow occurs at the tissue level and at the electrode tip [14]. At the tissue level, convective heat dissipation removes heat from the tissue limiting the penetration depth of the RF current. In the case of renal denervation, an appropriately sized renal artery and adequate renal artery blood flow is essential in delivering the appropriate amount of energy to affect renal denervation. In the case of accessory renal arteries and patients with end-stage renal disease (ESRD) with small renal arteries, the reduction in the caliber of the renal artery diameter and blood flow is an important factor which reduces the effectiveness of the monopolar technology.

During the application of RF energy for renal denervation, duration of energy application and impedance are typically the only parameters available for direct observation by the operator. Newer iterations of the monitoring systems may provide feedback regarding the rate of rise of temperature and provide the operator with feedback if an ideal combination of impedance drop and temperature rise has not been achieved, which in the case of the Medtronic Ardian Flex™ Catheter monitor system, an "error 50" may be recorded. Beyond this limited procedural feedback, the application of RF energy to the renal intima may cause substantial visceral pain with the ablation of afferent sympathetic nerves and type A and C nerve fibers that mediate pain via the dorsal root ganglia of the central nervous system.

Both efferent and afferent nerves are ablated during RF denervation; however, the effectiveness of the RF ablative lesion relates to the depth and distribution of these nerve fibers along the renal artery. In postmortem studies of nine renal arteries, over 90 % of the sympathetic nerves were located within 2 mm of the renal lumen [15]. The methodology of this study by Atherton et al., has centered on the fixation process involved in assessing renal nerves. In these nine specimens, nerves were distributed equally around the artery but tended to arborize and become more superficial when analyzed proximal in the renal artery through its distal segment. Thus, the optimal procedure is to perform treatment at the proximal through the distal part of the renal artery. Additionally, the depth of the ablative RF energy and the resultant death of renal sympathetic nerves and its potential influence on subsequent near and long-term blood pressure effect has been a point of speculation [16, 17].

In another assessment of renal denervation, Steigerwald performed renal artery ablation in seven pigs [18]. These pigs were followed up by repeat angiography, optical coherence tomography (OCT) and complete histological examination of both kidneys. This evaluation demonstrated that renal denervation leads to loss of renal artery endothelium but this is almost completely reversed by 10 days without having detrimental effect on renal parameters (renal function). The ablated segments of the renal artery demonstrate transmural tissue coagulation; ablation caused an immediate reduction in the number of autonomic nerve fascicles in the adventitia of these arteries and declined further through 10 days. OCT

of the artery performed immediately pre- and post- ablation revealed evidence of thrombus. Similar observations have been noted in human renal arteries treated with another RF monopolar catheter [19]. This has prompted a European expert panel to suggest the potential use of antiplatelet therapy during the procedure and for 4 weeks follow-up [20].

Finally, the potential negative impact on the effectiveness of the RF ablation by unapparent atherosclerosis and/or vessel wall calcification has caused some controversy with regards to the relevance of RF parameters drawn from normal renal arteries in pigs. Nevertheless, the appropriate balance of RF energy induced tissue temperature, duration of applied power and the resulting lesion depth may influence the subsequent blood pressure response; however, this is balanced by potential safety concerns of RF induced renal intimal lesions.

The Medtronic Ardian Renal Denervation Catheters

The first generation Ardian renal denervation catheter, the Arch™ catheter (Fig. 7.1), had a uni-electrode configuration that required a point-by-point application of RF energy to the renal artery wall by the operator. This allowed for greater operator flexibility as to the number and location of applied ablations (minimum 4–6 ablation sites per renal artery) and allowed the operator to avoid sites of obvious fluoroscopically evident calcium and/or atheroma. It is not recommended that a complete circumferential ablation be performed in a single plane due to the potential risk of inducing a renal artery stenosis. The second generation Flex™ catheter (Fig. 7.2) is also uni-electrode, but with a smaller shaft size and markedly improved flexibility, providing greater catheter maneuverability, which is particularly helpful in complex or tortuous renal anatomies.

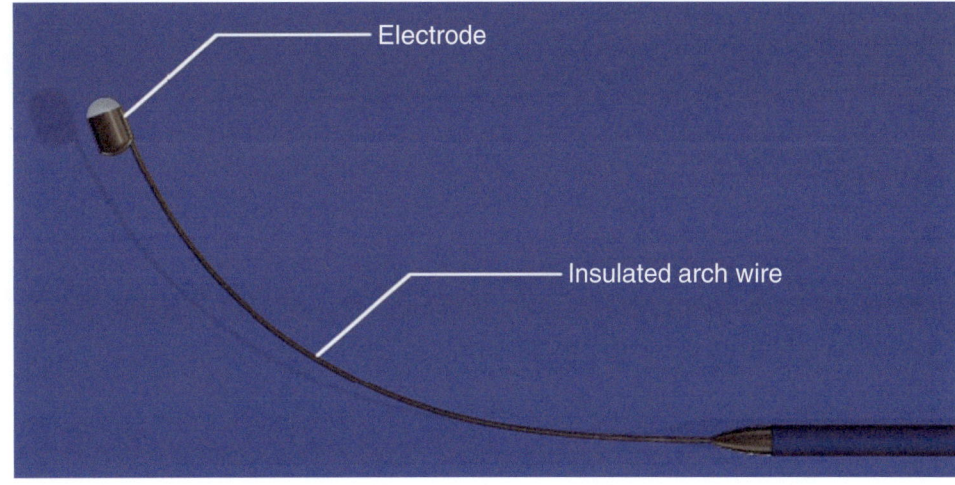

Fig. 7.1 The first generation Symplicity Arch™ was constructed of a platinum uni-electrode tip on a insulated nitinol wire, compatible with an 8F guide catheter. Careful retraction and rotation of the entire catheter was required to obtain the optimal spiral ablation pattern

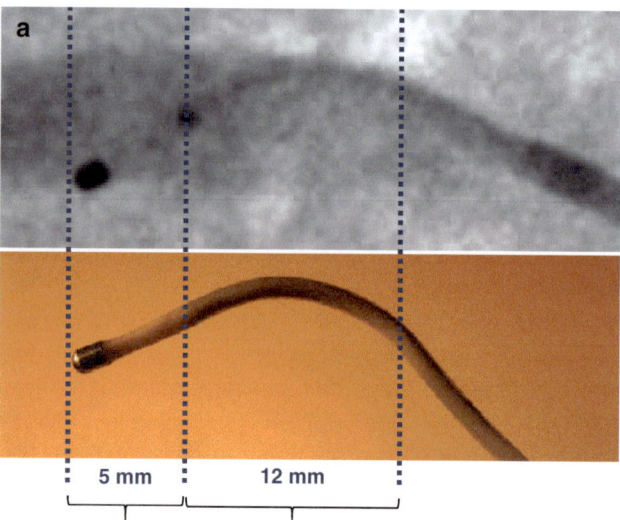

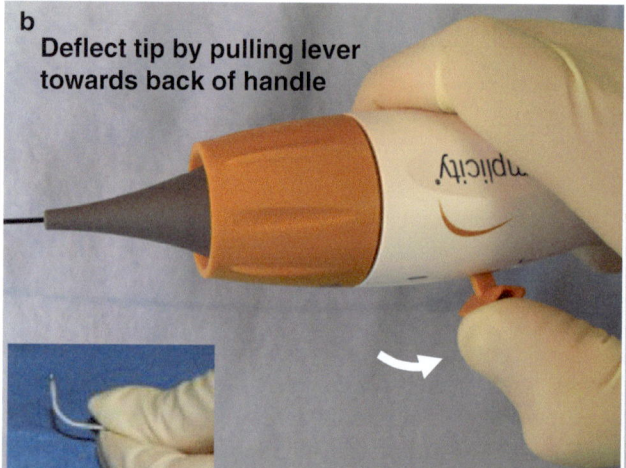

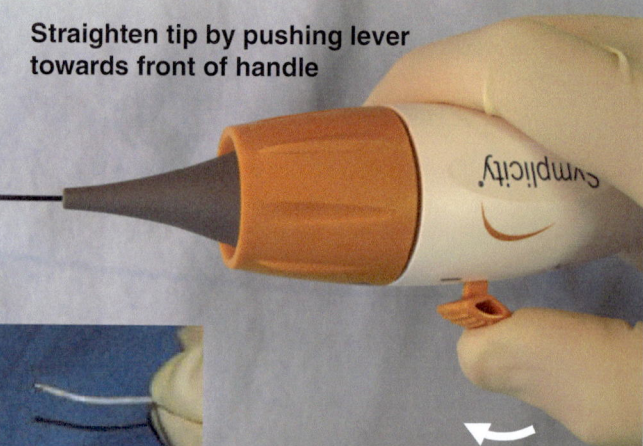

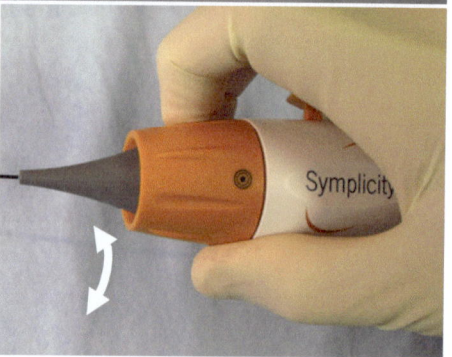

Fig. 7.2 (**a**) The second generation Symplicity Flex™ Renal Denervation Catheter is constructed of a uni-electrode, 6F guiding catheter compatible catheter with a self-orienting, flexible tip. The catheter is constructed of a 12 mm deflectable terminal distal end. (**b**) *Upper panel*, *left* and *right* demonstrates deflection of the electrode tip by either pulling (deflection) or pushing (straightening) the electrode lever. *Lower panel*: The Symplicity Flex™ catheter shaft and electrode can rotate independent of the handle body; the handle rotator has a tactile "click" every 45°; the dot on the rotator provides the relative rotational reference. (**c**) *Upper panels*, *right* and *left*, demonstrate appropriate electrode/intima wall contact seen under fluoroscopy. Impedance feedback provided by the control console should also be used to assess optimal electrode/intima contact. The *lower panel* demonstrate excessive wall contact, shown distending the vessel wall with the electrode. (**d**) Repositioning for retreatment: In repositioning the Flex™ electrode for the next treatment, the entire catheter is retracted proximally; if needed, the catheter tip is straightened using the handle lever. The electrode is then deflected to make contact with the vessel wall, using visual and impedance feedback. The electrode may be rotated to the to obtain the optimal spiral ablation configuration. A distant between ablation sites ≥5 mm (approximately 3 electrode lengths) is optimal; the secondary shaft marker may assist in identifying 5 mm spacing

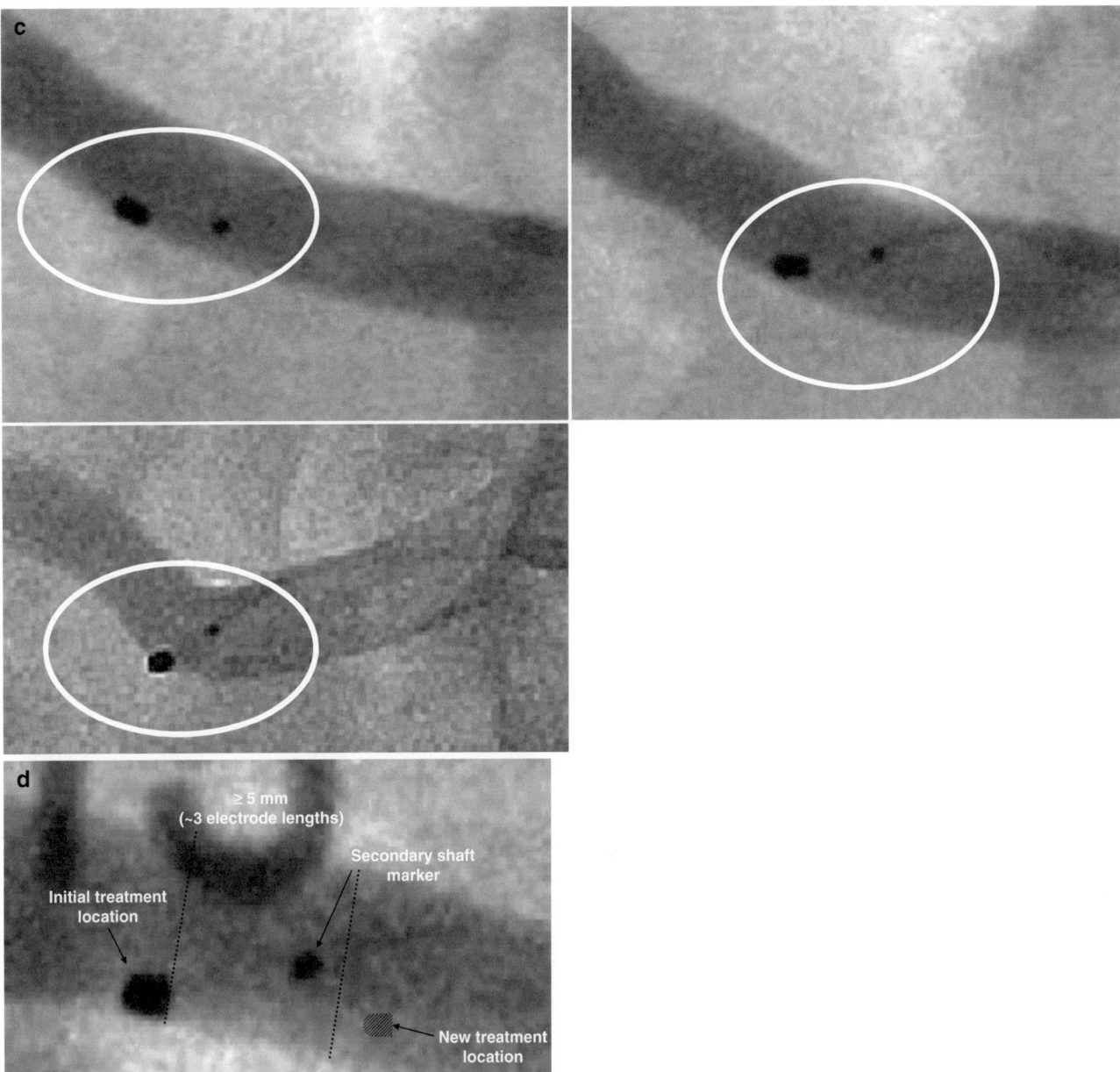

Fig. 7.2 (continued)

The third generation Spyral™ catheter (Fig. 7.3) is a multi-electrode configuration in a spiral, over-the-wire design. The theoretical advantages of the Spyral™ are its associated reduced procedural time due to simultaneous firing of all four electrodes and the resulting less patient pain, reduced contrast use and radiation exposure. Each electrode, the length of an angioplasty balloon radiopaque marker band, is able to provide specific information regarding temperature and impedance and may be turned on or off independently by the operator. The Spyral™ design includes an atraumatic tip and is able to treat vessels diameters from 3 to 8 mm, with the four radiopaque electrodes able to ablate simultaneously in each vessel quadrant, applying sufficient radial force to the renal intima to maximize impedance. The wire-based design is a important safety iteration, allowing the operator to address both routine and complex renal artery

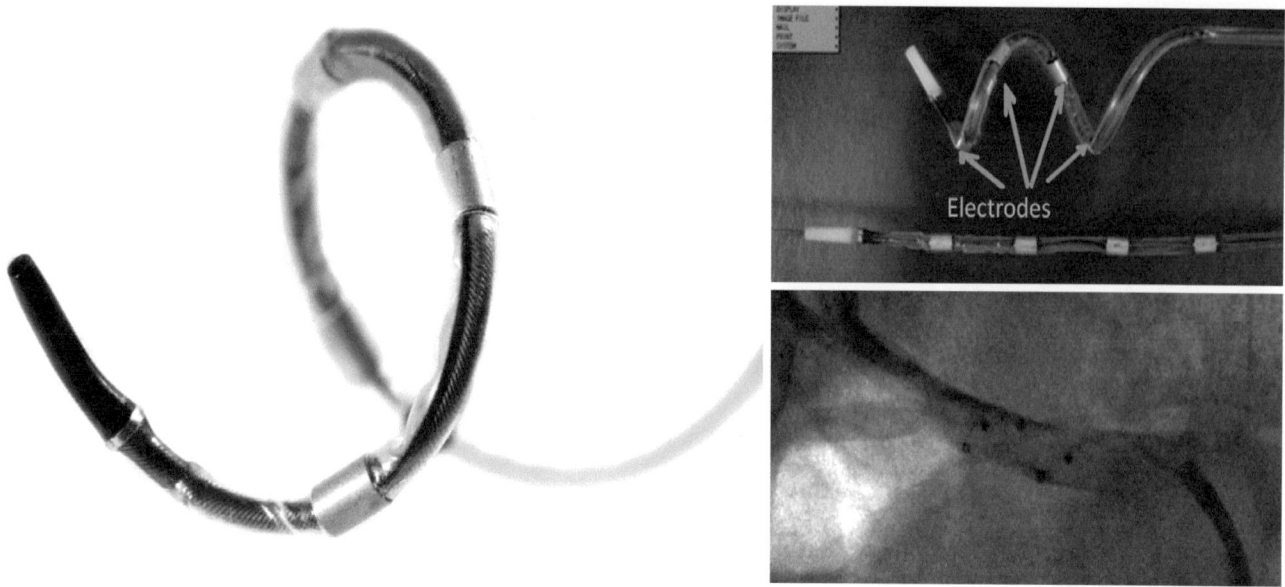

Fig. 7.3 The third generation Symplicity Spyral™ Renal Denervation Catheter is four electrode monopolar 6F compatible catheter constructed of an elastomeric shaft and radiopaque tip (*left panel*). The catheter shaft is straightened by the introduction of a 0.014″ guidewire which is used to insert the Spyral™ catheter into the renal artery. Careful traction or forward pressure on the Sypral™ while removing the guidewire allows for optimal electrode positioning (*lower right panel*). Each of the four electrodes can be operated independently and provides the operator with impedance readings

anatomies. After passage of the 0.014″ wire and advancing of the Spyral™, the wire is slowly withdrawn allowing the Spyral™ to assume its designed shape. Applying gentle forward pressure on the Spyral™ as the wire is withdrawn allows the catheter to assume a more compressed configuration and thereby treat shorter main renal arteries. The safety and clinical effectiveness associated with the use of the multi-electrode Spyral™ catheter awaits the results of an on-going prospective European and Australian registry.

Device Related Complications

The application of monopolar RF energy to the renal intima with the Medtronic Ardian renal denervation devices is frequently associated with intense visceral pain during the 2-minute ablation period. Therefore, it is mandatory to provide the patients with adequate intravenous analgesics administered throughout the procedure in order to avoid excessive patient movement that may negatively affect electrode/intimal contact and result in a suboptimal ablations. In the Symplicity HTN-2 trial, atropine was required, however, this frequently resulted in bradycardia during the procedure and its use was subsequently abandoned. Among 50 patients in the Symplicity HTN-1 and Symplicity HTN-2 trials, only one case of renal artery dissection associated with the use of the Arch™ catheter and one case of common femoral artery pseudoaneurysm were reported [2, 3].

In the Symplicity HTN-2 trial one of the 52 patients who underwent the initial procedure, overall procedures were appropriately low. One patient experienced arterial pseudoaneurysm and one patient experienced arterial hypotension requiring the reduction of blood pressure medications. Additionally, one device unrelated case of urinary tract infection and post-procedure parenthesis and lumbar pain 1-month post procedure were reported. In this randomized crossover trial design, among the 35 patients who were crossed over there was 1 renal artery dissection following guide catheter insertion during angiography that was stented without further complications. One hospitalization due to post renal denervation hypotension necessitating intravenous fluids likewise occurred. In this case, the antihypertensive medications were reduced and the patient subsequently discharged home without further sequelae. Three hypertensive events requiring hospitalization occurred in two patients.

Six-month anatomic follow-up of renal arteries of 43 patients enrolled in the Symplicity-HTN 2 trial and 81 patients included in the open label sub-study using computer tomographic angiography (CTA) revealed no evidence of vascular lesions. There was one case of a moderate renal artery stenosis that was avoided during the application of RF energy that was felt to progress to a significant renal artery stenosis during the 6-month follow-up. This patient presented with accelerating hypertension and renal artery duplex ultrasonography demonstrated a severe renal artery stenosis, which was subsequently stented and the patient improved.

In the Symplicity HTN-2 trial, renal function (glomerular infiltration rate, GFR) of 49 patients with a baseline value greater than 45 mm per minute/1.73 m² remained stable through 6 months after the denervation procedure. Subsequent trials have noted similar maintenance of GFR. Additionally, in patients who undergo renal denervation with established Chronic Kidney Disease Stage 3–4 and a mean GFR of 31 ml/1.73 m2 showed no worsening of their renal function through 6-month follow-up [21]. No long-term data in CKD patients beyond this time point are currently available.

There have been no deaths reported in the Symplicity HTN-1 and 2 cohorts. Two deaths were reported in the study cohort who reached 24 months (one due to myocardial infarction and sudden cardiac death) and were not attributed to denervation procedure. Therefore, overall, early adverse events were reported in <4 % of patients enrolled in these studies.

The Future

Numerous medical device companies have recently introduced new renal denervation technologies into proof-of-concept clinical trials. These technologies involve various iterations of RF energy technology (i.e., multi-electrode monopolar and bipolar RF), focused and non-focused high-frequency ultrasound, beta-radiation and the use of a variety of neurotoxins injected directly into the renal intima to reach the adventitia. This technology explosion may potentially broaden the regulatory indications for renal denervation to include diabetes and metabolic syndromes, chronic renal failure, heart failure, cardiac arrhythmias and obstructive sleep apnea. Indeed, hypertension specialists and interventionalists will likely be faced with a multitude of trial data including hypothesis generating large, prospective registries of variable quality and follow-up, large shammed, randomized controlled trial and first-in-man trial data exploring novel catheter designs to improve ease of use, procedural time, patient comfort and reduce cost. Nonetheless, device acceptance will likely be driven by the quality of independently adjudicated safety and effectiveness data. In this regard, the large, randomized, sham controlled pivotal Symplicity-HTN 3 trial will establish a high bar regarding the quality data required to drive regulatory approval, reimbursement and physician and patient acceptance.

Nonetheless, additional clinical investigative work is required to better identify the hypertensive patient most likely to obtain a clinically relevant response to renal denervation. The potential to transform an interventional procedure (monopolar RF renal denervation) into one that provides the operator with more targeted feedback for the application of RF energy in order to assure a complete anatomic denervation would be an important step forward. Given the concerns of the variable "non-responder" rates, which have been reported as high as 38 % [3], it would be important to know whether a successful "on-the-table" anatomic denervation has been performed so that any subsequent suboptimal blood pressure response to this successful anatomic denervation would reflect the simple disassociation between the influence of renal sympathetic nerves and treatment resistant hypertension. Indeed, early observational data would suggest that not all patients respond with a substantial drop in blood pressure despite an observed regression in left ventricular hypertrophy and a decrease in heart rate response to exercise [22] which are considered surrogates for successful renal denervation. This has important clinical implications as evolving experience in the treatment of patients who fail to adequately respond after RF denervation may be subjected to repeat renal denervation procedures, either with RF or other energy sources (i.e., ultrasound). Importantly, case reports have documented that vessel retreatment has been associated with the development of renal artery lesions [23], irrespective of an improvement in BP control. As such, exploring potential biomarkers to assist in identifying appropriate patients in which renal denervation may not substantially impact blood pressure control is important. This would allow the consideration of evolving sympathetic modulators, which are currently being evaluated in pre-clinical trials, specifically iliac arterio-venous artery-venous anastomosis formation (Coupler™, ROX Medical. San Clemente, CA), carotid sinus stent implantation for carotid sinus stimulation (Mobius HD™, Vascular Dynamics, Inc. Mountain View, CA) or carotid baroreceptor stimulation via an implantable single lead patch electrode and generator (BaroStim™ neo™, CVRx, Minneapolis, MN). Indeed, patients who fail renal denervation may, in the future, be appropriate patients for more invasive therapies in an attempt to reduce cardiovascular risks.

References

1. Huang S, Bharati S, Grahman A, Lev M, Marcus F, Odell R. Closed chest catheter desiccation of the atrioventricular junction using radiofrequency energy—a new method of catheter ablation. J Am Coll Cardiol. 1987;9:349–58.
2. Krum H, Schlaich M, Whitbourn R, et al. Catheter-based renal sympathetic denervation for resistant hypertension: a multicenter safety and proof-of-principle cohort study. Lancet. 2009;373:1275–81.
3. Symplicity HTN-2 Investigators, Esler MD, Krum H, Sobotka PA, et al. Renal sympathetic denervation in patients with treatment-resistant hypertension (The Symplicity HTN-2 Trial): a randomized controlled trial. Lancet. 2010;376:1903–9.
4. Symplicity HTN-2 Investigators, Esler MD, Krum H, Schlaich M, et al. Renal sympathetic denervation for treatment of drug-resistant hypertension: one-year results from the Symplicity HTN-2 randomized, controlled trial. Circulation. 2012;126:2976–82.

5. Krum H, Schlaich M, Bohm M, Rocha-Singh K, Katholi R, Esler M. Percutaneous renal denervation in patients with treatment-resistant hypertension: final 3-year report of the Symplicity HTN-1 study. Lancet. 2013. doi:10.1016/S0140-6736(13)63192-3.

6. Whayne J, Nath S, Haines D. Microwave catheter ablation of myocardium in vitro. Assessment of the characteristics of tissue heating and injury. Circulation. 1994;89:2390–5.

7. Ammar S, Ladich E, Steigerwald K, Deishenhofer I, Joner M. Pathophysiology of renal denervation procedures: from nerve anatomy to procedural parameters. Eurointervention. 2013;9:R85–95.

8. Patel H, Dhillon P, Mahfoud F, Lindsay A, Hayward C, Ernst S, Lyon A, Rosen S, di Mario C. The biophysics of renal sympathetic denervation using radiofrequency energy. Clin Res Cardiol. 2013. doi:10.1007/s00392-013-0618-6.

9. Haines E. The biophysics of radiofrequency catheter ablation in the heart: the importance of temperature monitoring. Pacing Clin Electrophysiol. 1993;16:586–91.

10. Erez A, Shitzer A. Controlled destruction and temperature distribution in biological tissues subjected to monoactive electro-coagulation. J Biomech Eng. 1980;102:42–9.

11. Ko W, Huang S, Lin J, Shau W, Lai L, Chen P. New method for predicting efficiency of heating by measuring bio-impedance during radiofrequency catheter ablation in humans. J Cardiovasc Electrophysiol. 2001;12:819–23.

12. Avitall B, Mughal K, Hare J, Helms R, Krum D. The effects of electrode-tissue contact on radiofrequency lesion generation. Pacing Clin Electrophysiol. 1997;20:2899–910.

13. Otomo K, Yamanashi W, Tondo C, Antz M, Bussey J, Pitha J, Arruda M, Nakagawa H, Wittkampf F, Lazzara R, Jackman W. Why a large tip electrode make s a deeper radiofrequency lesion: effects of increase n electrode cooling and electrode-tissue interface area. Pacing Clin Electrophysiol. 1998;9:47–54.

14. Nakagawa H, Wittkampf F, Yamanashi W, Pitha J, Imai S, Campbell D, Arruda M, Lazzara R, Jackman W. Inverse relationship between electrode size and lesion size during radiofrequency ablation with active electrode cooling. Circulation. 1998;98:458–65.

15. Atherton D, Deep N, Mendelsohn F. Micro-anatomy of the renal sympatheticnervous system: a human postmortem histologic study. Clin Anat. 2012;25:628–33.

16. Tellez A, Rousselle S, Palmieri T, Rate W, Wicks J, Degrange A, Hyon C, Gongora C, Hart R, Grundy W, Kaluza G, Granda J. Renal artery nerve distribution and density in the porcine model: biologic implications for the development of radiofrequency ablation therapies. Trans Res. 2013;162:381–9.

17. Rippy M, Zarins D, Barman N. Catheter-based renal sympathetic denervation: chronic preclinical evidence for renal artery safety. Clin Res Cardiol. 2011;100:1095–101.

18. Steigerwald K, Titova A, Malle C, Kennerknecht E, Jilek C, Hausleiter J, Nahrig J, Laugwitz K, Loner M. Morphological assessment of renal arteries after radiofrequency ablation catheter-based sympathetic denervation in a porcine model. J Hypertens. 2012;30:2230–9.

19. Templin C, Jaguszewski M, Ghadri J, Sudano I, Gaehwiler R, Hellermann J, Schoenenberger-Berzins R, Landmesser U, Erne P, Noll G, Luscher T. Vascular lesions induced by renal nerve ablation as assessed by optical coherence tomography: pre- and post-procedural comparison with the Symplicity catheter system and the EnligHTN multi-electrode renal denervation catheter. Eur Heart J. 2013. doi:10.1093/eurheasrtj/eht141.

20. Mahfoud F, Luscher T, Anderson B, Baumgartner I, Cifkova R, DiMario C, Doevendans P, Fagard R, Komajda M, Fajadet J, LeFevre T, Lotan C, Sievert H, Volpe M, Widimsky P, Wijns W, Williams B, Windecker S, Witkowski A, Zeller T, Bohm M. Expert consensus document from the European Society of Cardiology on catheter-based renal denervation. Eur Heart J. 2013;34:2149–57.

21. Hering D, Mahfoud F, Walton S, Krum H, Lambert G, Lambert E, Sobotka P, Bohm M, Cremers B, Esler M, Schlaich M. Renal denervation in moderate to severe CKD. J Soc Nephrol. 2012;23:1250–7.

22. Schirmer S, Sayed M, Reil JC, Ukena C, Linz D, Kindermann M, Laufs U, Mahfoud F, Bohm M. Improvements of left-ventricular hypertrophy and diastolic function following renal denervation—effects beyond blood pressure and heart rate reduction. J Am Coll Cardiol. 2013;63:1916–23. doi:10.1016/jacc2013.10.073.

23. Kaiser L, Beister T, Wiese A, von Wedel J, Meincke F, Kreidel F, Busjahn A, Kuck K, Bergmann M. Results of the ALSTER BP real-world registry on renal denervation employing the Symplicity system. Eurointervention. 2014;10:157–65.

Sympathetic Renal Denervation Using the EnligHTN Multi-electrode Ablation System: The St Jude Experience

Costas Tsioufis, Michael Doumas, Charles Faselis, and Vasilios Papademetriou

Introduction

The role of the sympathetic nervous system (SNS) in the pathophysiology of hypertension and cardiovascular disease has long been recognized, and efforts to inhibit sympathetic overactivity date several decades back. The SNS was first depicted during the seventeenth century by Willis, who provided in 1664 the anatomy of sympathetic nerves from the brain to the periphery [1]. The detailed anatomy of sympathetic fibers was described in the twentieth century, mainly due to the work of Barahas and others [2–5]. The identification of the functional role of SNS in animal and human physiology and pathophysiology was a very difficult and time consuming task. Pourfois de Petit, Stelling, Brown-Sequard, Waller, and Bernard during the eighteenth and nineteenth century described the vasomodulating effects of sympathetic fibers [6, 7] and von Euler won the Nobel prize for the discovery of noradrenaline as sympathetic neurotransmitter in 1946 [8]. The seminal role of the SNS in hypertension was highlighted by the development of ganglionic blockers in the 1950s, the first effective antihypertensive drugs through sympathetic blockade [9].

Bradford described the role of renal sympathetic fibers as early as 1889 through meticulous animal research [10]. Recent work by DiBona, Esler, Victor, Campese, Zanchetti, Mancia and others provided significant information about the functional role of renal sympathetic innervation in health and disease, unveiling a reciprocal association of the brain and the kidneys [11–14]. Renal efferent sympathetic nerves course from the brain through the spinal cord and arrive at the kidneys, innervating the renal cortex, the juxtaglomerular apparatus and glomerular arterioles. Efferent sympathetic stimulation results in enhanced renin release, increased sodium and water reabsorption, as well as reduced renal blood flow and glomerular filtration rate [15]. Renal afferent sympathetic nerves respond to renal injury and transmit signals from the kidneys to the brain, which stimulate sympathetic activity [16]. This reciprocal association of central and peripheral sympathetic activity is implicated in the pathogenesis of hypertension and several other disease conditions, including chronic kidney disease, congestive heart failure, obstructive sleep apnea, polycystic ovary syndrome, sympathetically-driven tachyarrhythmias, and cirrhosis [17–20].

The inhibition of renal sympathetic activity was achieved through surgical sympathectomy, an extensive operation that became popular during the first half of the twentieth century. Surgical sympathectomy for the management of malignant hypertension, a devastating and lethal condition, was first performed by Adson in 1925 [21]. Bilateral renal sympathetic denervation was first performed by Papin and Ambard in 1924 for the management of renal pain [22], and by Page in

C. Tsioufis, MD
Kapodestrian University, Athens, Greece

Department of Interventional Cardiology/Hypertension,
Department of Veterans Affairs Medical Center,
50 Irving str NW-151-E, Washington, DC 20422, USA
e-mail: ktsioufis@gmail.com

M. Doumas, MD
Aristotle University, Thessaloniki, Greece

Department of Interventional Cardiology/Hypertension,
Department of Veterans Affairs Medical Center,
50 Irving str NW-151-E, Washington, DC 20422, USA
e-mail: michalisdoumas@yahoo.co.uk

C. Faselis, MD
Veteran Affairs Medical Centre and George Washington
University, Washington, DC, USA

Department of Interventional Cardiology/Hypertension,
Department of Veterans Affairs Medical Center,
50 Irving str NW-151-E, Washington, DC 20422, USA
e-mail: Charles.faselis@va.gov

V. Papademetriou, MD (✉)
Veteran Affairs Medical Center and Georgetown University,
50 Irving str NW-151-E, Washington, DC 20422, USA

Department of Interventional Cardiology/Hypertension,
Department of Veterans Affairs Medical Center,
50 Irving str NW-151-E, Washington, DC 20422, USA
e-mail: vasilios.papademetriou@va.gov

R.R. Heuser et al. (eds.), *Renal Denervation: A New Approach to Treatment of Resistant Hypertension*,
DOI 10.1007/978-1-4471-5223-1_8, © Springer-Verlag London 2015

1934 for the management of malignant hypertension in a young girl with severe hypertension and target organ damage [23]. However, the results were not very satisfactory and a wider surgical disruption of splanchnic sympathetic nerves (splanchnicectomy) dominated. From the 1930s until the 1950s splanchnicectomy was performed in several specialized centers all over the States and became the treatment of choice for the management of malignant hypertension unresponsive to conservative therapy [24–29]. The operation was found to be effective and even life saving in many patients; however it was associated with substantial operative risk and was poorly tolerated with significant adverse events severely impairing patients' quality of life. With the advent of effective and well-tolerated oral anti-hypertensive drugs in the mid 1950s the prevalence of malignant hypertension was substantially reduced and splanchnicectomy was abandoned [30].

The concept of interventional management of hypertension was revived recently due to a combination of two factors: (a) the need of an effective management of patients with resistant hypertension, and (b) the technological advent which enabled a transvascular, minimally-invasive approach for renal nerve disruption. Resistant hypertension is defined as the failure to achieve blood pressure goals despite the use of at least three antihypertensive drugs, one of which is a diuretic [31, 32]. The exact prevalence of resistant hypertension remains uncertain; however, recent data indicates that approximately 12 % of hypertensive patients are resistant to treatment [33, 34]. This translates to an estimated number of about 120 million patients worldwide suffering from resistant hypertension. Sympathetic fibers follow the renal arteries and the majority lie within 2–3 mm from the inner layer of the renal artery [35]. Therefore, sympathetic fibers can be easily reached and interrupted transvascularly using various forms of energy, such as thermal radiofrequency (RF) ablation, cryoablation, and ultrasound ablation. Several devices have been developed for renal nerve ablation and so far six devices received European approval, five of them using radiofrequency energy and one using ultrasound technology. The Symplicity (Ardian/Metronic) was the first device tested in humans and used a single-tip electrode for energy delivery. The EnligHTN (St. Jude's) is a multi-electrode ablation system with four electrodes mounted on a basket for an easy and predictable circumferential energy delivery. The Vessix V2 system (Vessix Vascular-Boston Scientific) and the OneShot system (Covidien) have the electrodes mounted on a balloon. The Iberis system (Terumo) has a 4 French shaft, which is appropriate for radial access. The Paradise system (ReCor Medical) uses ultrasound technology as an energy source.

In this chapter we will describe the St Jude device, we will present the experimental and human experience with this device, we will critically address the advantages and disadvantages of renal nerve ablation, and finally we will provide future perspectives of this innovative interventional technique for the management of resistant hypertension and other conditions characterized by sympathetic overactivity.

The St Jude Experience

EnligHTN Renal Denervation System

The EnligHTN Ablation System consists of a generator and an ablation catheter. The St Jude Medical EnligHTN™ renal denervation system (Fig. 8.1a) consists of the EnligHTN Ablation Catheter and the EnligHTN Generator (Model 1500 T11.5 with Software 3.011). The EnligHTN Ablation Catheter (St Jude Medical, St Paul, MN, USA) has an expandable basket with four Platinum–Iridium (Pt–Ir) electrodes that can deliver low-level RF energy to the renal arterial wall. The expandable feature of the basket and the deflectable distal catheter section allow good apposition between the ablation electrodes and the target ablation sites in the renal artery. Each electrode has a temperature sensor to monitor the temperature at the ablation site. The Ablation Generator delivers RF energy to the EnligHTN Renal Artery Ablation Catheter using a proprietary algorithm. Each electrode on the ablation catheter has a corresponding display channel on the generator. The generator channels facilitate control and monitoring of the ablation process. It consists of four independent channels, which simultaneously monitor the temperature of each of the four ablation electrodes and adjusts the magnitude of the RF output based on a proprietary algorhythm. The target temperature on the first generation device was 75 °C. The generator has built-in safety features, which include a self-test at power-up and automatic RF power shut-off if the measured tissue impedance was $<50\,\Omega$ or exceeds $400\,\Omega$ or the temperature exceeds the setting by >5 °C for >3 s or exceeds 80 °C. The EnligHTN™ Ablation Catheter was available in two sizes for use in the study. The small size basket was designed for renal artery diameters between 4 and 5.5 mm, and the large size basket size for renal artery diameters between 5.5 and 8 mm.

The second generation generator is slimmer and has updated futures (Fig. 8.1b). It can be operated via a touch screen and features allow simultaneous activation of all electrodes. The new algorithm aims at a target temperature of 70 °C and burning time of 60 s, thus substantially shortening procedure time. A new ablation catheter that is 6F is in preparation.

The first generation ablation system was used in the early animal studies and EnligHTN I study. The second generation system is being used in EnligHTN III and EnligHTN IV studies.

Fig. 8.1 (**a**) First generation ablation system. Generator and 8 F ablation catheter. (**b**) Second generation generator with a touch screen

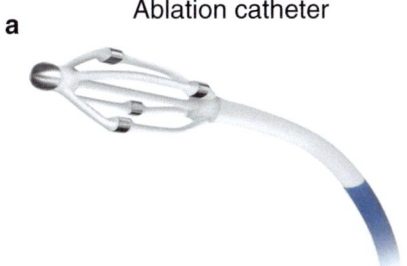

Ablation catheter

- Multi-electrode
- Radiopaque electrodes
- 8 F compatible
- Deflectable, Atraumatic tip
- Easily inserted via common femoral access

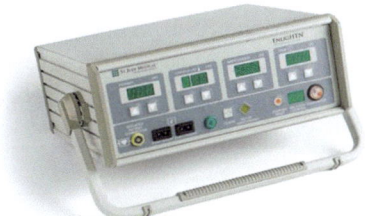

Generator

- Default settings:
  - Power output (6 W)
  - Impedance (400 Ω)
  - Electrode temperature set at 75° C°
  - Energy delivery -90 s per ablation
- Electrodes are temperature controlled

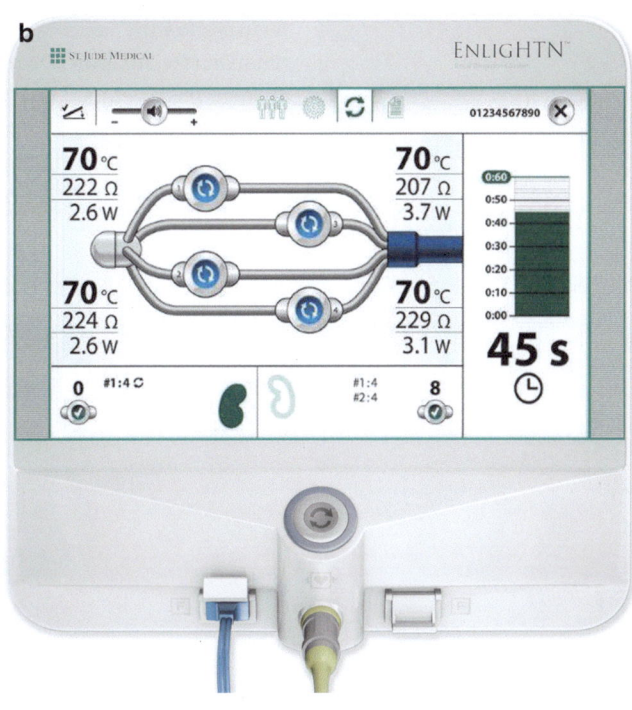

Procedure

The first generation ablation system is utilizing an 8F guide catheter which is advanced and engages each renal artery sequentially. Renal angiography is performed to confirm renal artery anatomy. An appropriate basket size is chosen based on the renal artery diameter (small basket 4.0–5.5 mm diameter/large basket 5.5–8.0 mm diameter). The ablation procedure is being standardized as follows: The ablation catheter is introduced to the renal artery and advanced so the tip is situated before the first major renal artery branch. The basket is then expanded, and after assuring good contact with the arterial wall, each electrode is activated sequentially for 90 s (the second generation system will be using simultaneous activation of all four electrodes, aiming at 70 °C and burning time of 60 s). The basket is then collapsed, pulled back, turned and re-expanded to repeat the ablation procedure. A total of 4–8 discrete ablation lesions are delivered. The ablation catheter is then withdrawn and a renal angiogram is repeated to assess safety. The same procedure is repeated in the contralateral renal artery. Heparin is given during the procedure (3,000–7,000 U) as per protocol, to avoid clot formation. Visceral pain occurring during the ablation procedure is managed with intravenous analgesics, sedatives and/or narcotics.

Animal Data

The early animal experiments were carried out in miniature swine (Fig. 8.2) and the objective was primarily the feasibility and safety of the procedure. The early results showed that

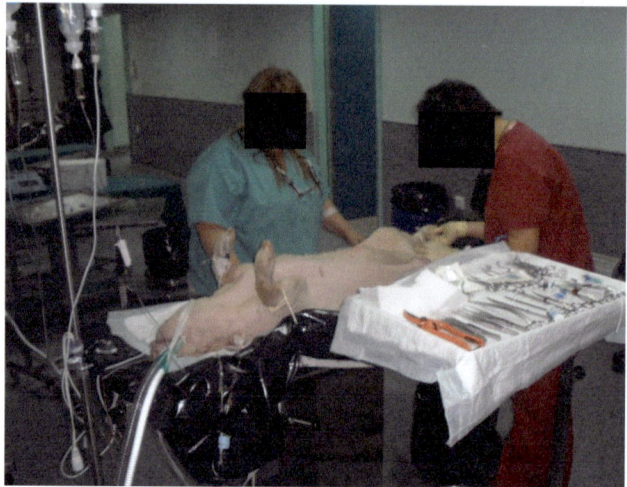

Fig. 8.2 Swine animal model for renal denervation

it was feasible to place radiofrequency ablation lesions transvascularly through the arterial wall and ablate the fibers coursing through the adventitia of the renal artery. The lesions were transmural and reached up to 3 mm from the endothelium of the artery. It was also shown that the procedure was safe, there was no aneurysm formation or perforation. One month after the procedure it was shown that the lesions would heal with no residual findings. Acutely however, it was found that a clot could be formed at the ablation site, but it could be prevented using heparin and aspirin. The ablation catheter allowed placement of the electrodes in a pre-determined manner and geometric distribution that would ensure circumferential interruption of the sympathetic fibers (Fig. 8.3).

The first animal study was designed to further assess feasibility and safety, but also to evaluate the effects of renal denervation on renal hemodynamics [36]. In this study we investigated the acute and chronic effects of catheter-based renal nerve ablation on renal hemodynamics assessed by average peak velocity (APV), renal blood flow (RBF), renal flow reserve (RFR) and resistive index (RI). The aims of this study were based on the premise that sympathetic overdrive is accompanied by impaired RBF and renal denervation

Transmurality

Acute lesion formation*

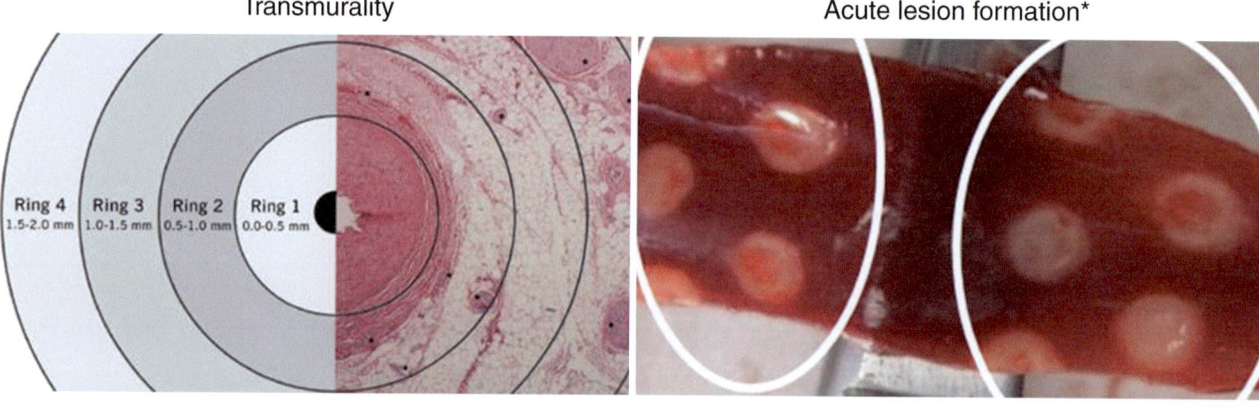

Predictable pattern

After one month*

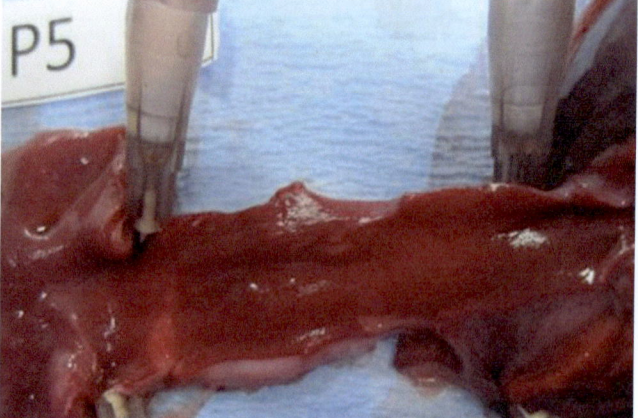

*Animal study. Results on file at St. Jude Medical

Fig. 8.3 The ablation procedure, acute and chronic ablation lesions of the dissected renal artery

would result in improvement in renal blood flow. Experiments were performed in nine farm swine. APV was measured by a 0.014-in. Doppler flow wire placed in the stem of the renal artery under baseline and hyperemic conditions, induced by intrarenal dopamine (50 µg/kg). RFR was calculated as the ratio of hyperemic to basal peak velocity, and RI was estimated as peak systolic velocity − end-diastolic velocity)/ peak systolic velocity. RSD was achieved via the lumen of the main renal artery with a specifically designed catheter connected to a radiofrequency generator according to pre-specified algorithm. APV and RBF increased acutely post ablation in all animals, compared to APV and RBF before ablation (61.44 ± 32.6 versus 20.44 ± 6.38 cm/s, $p < 0.001$; and 407.4 ± 335.1 versus 161.1 ± 76.6 ml/min, $p = 0.003$; respectively), whereas RFR and RI were reduced (1.51 ± 0.59 versus 2.85 ± 1.33, $p < 0.001$; and 0.67 ± 0.07 versus 0.74 ± 0.07, $p = 0.005$; respectively). One month post ablation APV and RBF compared to APV and RBF before ablation remained significantly higher whereas RFR and RI remained lower as compared to baseline. From these experiments we concluded that catheter-based renal nerve ablation exerts acute and chronic effects on renal hemodynamics in a large animal model.

Human Data

EnligHTN I Study

EnligHTN I was the first in human study, using the multi-electrode SD Jude EnligHTN ablation system [37]. The study was designed to assess the safety and efficacy of the procedure. The primary efficacy objective was reduction of office blood pressure from baseline to 6 months. Blood pressure was measured at baseline, pre-discharge, 1-, 3-, and 6-month post-procedure. Additional efficacy data collection included changes in anti-hypertensive medication, home BP monitoring, and 24-h ambulatory BP. The primary safety objective was the rate of AEs. Other data collection included blood analysis: complete blood count, basic metabolic profile, serum creatinine concentration, eGFR using the modified diet in renal disease (MDRD) formula and serum cystatin C, urine analysis (albumin-to-creatinine ratio), 12-lead ECG, and renal artery evaluation (using duplex ultrasonography and/or CT scan).

The study enrolment was conducted from October 2011 to March 2012. A total of 62 patients were consented for enrolment. Sixteen patients were excluded during the screening process. One of the 16 patients was excluded from the study due to multiple renal arteries found on the screening renal angiogram. In total, 46 patients completed baseline evaluation and underwent the renal denervation procedure. Forty four of the 46 patients (96 %) met all the inclusion and no exclusion criteria. The baseline characteristics of study participants are depicted in Table 8.1.

Table 8.1 Baseline characteristics

	n = 46*
Gender (female)	15 (33 %)
Ethnic origin (white)	45 (98 %)
Body mass index (kg/m²)	32 (5)
Coronary artery disease	9 (20 %)
Hyperlipidemia	27 (59 %)
Type II diabetes mellitus	15 (33 %)
Sleep apnea	14 (30 %)
eGFR (mL/min/1.73 m²)	87 (19)
Serum creatinine (µmol/L)	78 (17)
Cystatin C (mg/L)	1.14 (0.29)
Number of anti-hypertensive medications	4 (0.6)
Office systolic blood pressure (mmHg)	176 (16)
Office diastolic blood pressure (mmHg)	96 (14)
Heart rate (bpm)	71 (12)

The procedure was generally performed with conscious sedation at the operators' discretion. This was not mandated in the protocol. It included, but was not limited to the combination of intravenous midazolam and fentanyl, titrated as appropriate. Most patients experienced back pain during the denervation procedure, which was generally well controlled with sedation and analgesia. The median procedure time (from initiation to completion of RF energy delivery) was 34.0 min and the mean (+SD) number of ablations delivered was 7.7 (+0.8) for the right and 7.4 (+1.4) for the left renal arteries. One patient had the renal denervation procedure performed on a single side only due to difficulty engaging the other renal artery. The mean fluoroscopic time was 11.0 ± 7.1 min and the mean contrast volume used was 139.5 ± 93.2 ml. All the AEs were collected in the study.

A CEC adjudicated the events for seriousness and relatedness to the procedure and device. No serious vascular AEs occurred during the procedure, including no renal artery damage (i.e. no renal artery dissections, aneurysms, or flow limiting renal artery vasospasms) or serious vascular access site complications. Minor peri-procedural events which were attributed to either the device or procedure were reported and include: non-flow limiting vasospasms, vascular access site haematomas, hypotension, vasovagal episodes, bradycardia, transient haematuria, pain, and nausea. Vasospasm was reported as an AE although no specific threshold was established for reporting the event. An independent CEC reviewed all vasospasms and determined none were flow limiting (>50 % reduction in vessel lumen diameter). All minor peri-procedural events were reported to have resolved without further clinical sequelae. Serious AEs that were deemed possibly related to the procedure and/or device were reported in three (6.5 %) patients over 6 months of follow-up. Events include hypotension, progression of pre-existing renal artery stenosis, and a progression of hypertensive renal disease with an increase in serum creatinine.

Table 8.2 Renal function

	Baseline n=46	Month 1 n=46	p value	Month 3 n=46	p value	Month 6 n=45
eGFR, mL/min/1.73 m²	87 (19)	85 (20)	0.32	84 (22)	0.21	82 (20)
Serum creatinine, μmol/L	78 (17)	79 (19)	0.26	81 (20)	0.19	83 (20)
Cystatin C, mg/l	1.14(0.29)	1.00 (0.25)	<0.0001	0.97 (0.20)	<0.0001	1.00 (0.23)

Renal artery evaluation was conducted on all patients by CT imaging at 6 months. No patients developed a new haemodynamically significant renal artery stenosis. Two patients with pre-existing renal artery stenosis at baseline experienced asymptomatic progression of their renal artery stenosis at 6 months. One was adjudicated as serious (>50 % occlusion in artery diameter) and one was non serious.

No patient required clinical intervention at 6 months and their renal function parameters (eGFR, serum creatinine, and cystatin C values) remained stable. Renal function was evaluated by repeated measurements of eGFR, serum creatinine and cystatin C from baseline through 6 months of follow-up (Table 8.2). No patient experienced a reduction in eGFR >50 %, a twofold increase in serum creatinine, or progressed to end-stage renal disease. While the eGFR decreased (baseline mean of 87–82 mL/min/1.73 m² at 6 months, p=0.004) and serum creatinine increased (baseline mean of 78–83 mmol/L at 6 months, p=0.004), the mean cystatin C decreased (baseline mean of 1.14–1.00 mg/L at 6 months, p=0.00013). To further evaluate changes in renal function, a more meaningful assessment of eGFR with a clinically relevant cut-off of <60 mL/min/1.73 m² was also undertaken. At baseline, three patients had an eGFR level of <60 mL/min/1.73 m². One of these patient's eGFR remained <60, while the other two improved to 60 or greater at 6 months. In contrast, two other patients with baseline eGFR values >60 (63 and 61) experienced an eGFR reduction <60. The urine albumin-to-creatinine ratio decreased significantly throughout the course of the study, with absolute results at baseline 169.4 mg/g, 1 month 142.9 mg/g, 3 months 141.2 mg/g, and 6 months 139.3 mg/g (p=0.007).

Compared with baseline, office and ambulatory systolic blood pressure of the entire cohort significantly decreased at all-time points (p<0.0001). The average office blood pressure (mmHg) at baseline was 176/96 mmHg. The resulting average office blood pressure reductions from baseline at 1 month, 3 months, and 6 months were 22.8/21.0, 22.7/21.0, and 22.6/21.0 mmHg. Over the follow-up period, as many as 80 % of patients had a reduction in office systolic blood pressure of at least 10 mmHg or greater and up to 41 % had an office blood pressure of <140 mmHg. Baseline systolic blood pressure was a strong predictor of response (p<0.0001). In addition, the in-office resting heart rate was collected at baseline (71 beats/min), 1 month (69 beats/min), 3 months (67 beats/min), and 6 months (66 beats/min) and demonstrated a decrease over time (P=0.007 at 6 months). The

baseline HR was a predictor of change in office systolic blood pressure (r=0.31, p=0.039). In addition, the reduction in HR was correlated with reduction in office systolic blood pressure (r=0.33, P=0.025). The average 24-h ambulatory BP at baseline was 150/83 mmHg. The average 24-h ambulatory blood pressure reduction from baseline to 1 month, 3 months, and 6 months was 10/5, 10/5, and 10/6 mmHg, respectively. The change in average 24-h ambulatory blood pressure correlated with both the change in office systolic blood pressure (r=0.56, p<0.0001) and office diastolic blood pressure (r=0.55, p<0.0001). These reductions in office and ambulatory blood pressures were achieved with minimal modifications to the cohort's antihypertensive medical regimen during the follow-up period. Over the 6-month follow-up period, six (13.0 %) patients had a decrease in their antihypertensive medications and four (8.7 %) had an increase in antihypertensive medications. For patients that did not have an increase or decrease in their antihypertensive medications the 6-month office BP reduction was similar to the entire cohort at 22.5/21.0 mmHg, as well as mean ambulatory blood pressure (ABPM) reductions of 10/5 mmHg.

Effect of Renal Nerve Ablation on LVH and Heart Failure Variables

The beneficial effects of renal nerve ablation in resistant hypertension may extend beyond blood pressure. In a substudy we assessed whether multi-electrode catheter-based renal nerve ablation has favorable effects on left ventricular structural and functional indices, as well as on neurohormonal activation reflected by N-terminal pro B-type natriuretic peptide (NT pro-BNP). This hypothesis was tested in twenty patients with resistant hypertension (age: 57 ± 10 years, 13 males, office blood pressure: 180/96±19/16 mmHg receiving 4.4±0.61 drugs) that underwent renal denervation and were followed for 6 months. A full transthoracic echocardiographic study was performed in all patients at both baseline and follow-up. Left ventricular mass was calculated using the Devereux formula and was indexed for body surface area and height, while tissue Doppler imaging indices of diastolic function were measured. Moreover, blood sampling was performed in order to estimate metabolic profile and NT pro-BNP levels.

At 6 months following renal nerve ablation, office systolic and diastolic blood pressure was significantly reduced and the mean interventricular septal thickness and left ventricular mass index substantially decreased. Left atrial diameter and volume were reduced from and LV function improved. Renal nerve ablation resulted in an increase of mitral valve E'/A' ratio and a decrease in the E/E', whereas isovolumic relaxation time was shortened. Furthermore, renal denervation resulted in a statistically significant reduction in NT pro-BNP levels. From these data we concluded that in patients with resistant hypertension and left ventricular hypertrophy, renal nerve ablation besides blood pressure reduction leads to favorable cardiac remodeling and attenuation of neurohormonal overdrive.

Effect of Renal Nerve Ablation on Arrhythmias

We assessed the effects of renal denervation on heart rate variability and cardiac arrhythmia. Fourteen patients with resistant hypertension underwent ambulatory blood pressure measurements and Holter monitoring at baseline and at 1 and 6 months after renal denervation using the EnligHTN ablation catheter. Supraventricular and ventricular ectopic activity was recorded in all patients. SyneScope analysis system calculated the recommended time- and frequency-domain parameters of heart rate variability.

Office and 24-h systolic and diastolic blood pressure were significantly reduced both at 1 and 6 months after renal denervation. The total number of premature supraventricular and ventricular contractions was significantly decreased both at 1 and at 6 months after renal denervation. A significant increase was observed in time and frequency domain indexes during the 24-h Holter monitoring both 1 and 6 months after the procedure. We concluded that renal nerve ablation in addition to blood pressure lowering, significantly reduces mean heart rate and arrhythmia burden while it restores autonomic balance in patients with resistant hypertension, providing evidence for the beneficial impact of denervation-induced neuro-modulation on heart rhythm.

The Future of RNA in Resistant Hypertension: Issues to Be Addressed

Resistant hypertension is likely to remain the main target of renal nerve ablation in the near future. Several issues however need to be addressed before getting wide application in this patient population. Unsolved issues can be categorized to procedure-related and device-related, safety-related, and efficacy-related.

Procedure-Related and Device-Related Unsolved Issues

As of today, renal nerve ablation is a 'blind' procedure. All renal ablation systems aim to achieve near-complete disruption of renal sympathetic fibers through the circumferential placement of ablating electrodes and the performance of several (4–8) discrete ablation lesions. However, there is currently no accurate method to confirm intra-procedurally the success of renal nerve ablation and guide the interventionalist to stop or continue the procedure. Recently, two tests have been proposed as markers of procedural success: electrical stimulation of renal arterial nerves [38], and renal blood flow during dopamine infusion [36]. Whether the proposed tests or other methods will actually prove to be accurate markers of procedural success remains to be validated in future studies.

The relative contribution of efferent and afferent renal sympathetic fibers in the pathogenesis of resistant hypertension remains poorly clarified. Subsequently, the effects of renal nerve ablation on efferent and afferent sympathetic nerve disruption and the contribution of each component on blood pressure reduction is not known. Furthermore, the possibility of sympathetic nerve re-generation following renal nerve ablation raises further questions. In addition, whether nerve re-generation takes place in the anatomical level alone or it is functional as well remains to be verified by future basic research in this field.

Current availability of six devices for renal nerve ablation and the active research for the development of many more devices (approximately 60 devices are under development) raises two important questions: (a) whether the source of energy plays an important role for the success of renal nerve ablation and the efficacy and safety of the procedure, and (b) whether clinically significant differences between the devices using the same energy source exist. Head-to-head trials are needed to answer these clinically meaningful questions. Until then, indirect comparisons may be useful, but special attention is needed in order to avoid inappropriate comparisons and premature conclusions.

Safety-Related Unresolved Issues

Safety issues represent another considerable concern. Up to now, no serious or life threatening adverse events have been reported. Vascular complications seem rare and are not usually irreversible. So far, minor vasospasm of the renal artery post-denervation, small hematomas, pseudo-aneurysms, minor bleeds, and one dissection requiring stenting have been reported. Endothelial injury at the site of ablation lesions seems to be transient and re-endothelization occurs soon enough. Clot formation at ablation sites can be prevented by appropriate antithrombotic and antiplatelet therapy.

Renal artery stenosis is another significant concern, since it was observed with radiofrequency ablation for the management of atrial fibrillation. Fortunately enough the probability of renal artery stenosis seems much lower than in the pulmonary and coronary arteries, possibly due to the fact that the energy delivered for renal ablation is much lower than the energy delivered for atrial ablation and the diameter of renal artery is much greater than the coronary and pulmonary vessels. Indeed, only two cases of renal artery stenosis due to renal nerve ablation have been reported so far [39, 40], while the procedure has been already performed in several thousand patients.

Renal function concerns after renal nerve ablation have been previously raised [41]. Renal function remained practically unaltered during the clinical studies performed so far [37, 42, 43]. A more detailed analysis of renal function did not raise any flags [44]. Of note, renal nerve ablation seems safe in patients with CKD, just like in patients without CKD [45]. In another study, renal function was meticulously assessed by biomarkers for functional and structural kidney damage and remained unaltered both in patients with and without CKD [46]. No major renal deterioration has been reported so far. Although a case report of renal failure following RNA in a patient with CKD was recently published, renal biopsy suggested that the deterioration of renal function was due to the progression of glomerulopathy itself and not related to RNA [47].

Efficacy-Related Unsolved Issues

A marked heterogeneity in blood pressure response is observed with renal nerve ablation. In almost all studies it can be seen that approximately one third of patients show an excessive blood pressure fall, one third of patients experiences small but significant reductions, whereas the remaining one third of patients exhibits little if any blood pressure reduction. This response heterogeneity is not unforeseen: it is observed with drug therapy as well. Hypertension is a multifactorial disease and renal nerve ablation does not modify all contributing mechanisms. Although it seems rational to assume that renal nerve ablation will be effective in patients with enhanced sympathetic activity, no accurate predictors of blood pressure response have been identified so far. Sympathetic overactivity indices (muscle sympathetic nerve activity and/or plasma noradrenaline levels) do not seem to correlate with blood pressure response [48, 49]. Office blood pressure levels before the procedure and to a lesser extend baseline heart rate have been correlated with blood pressure response to renal denervation [37], however their utility for the individual patient in everyday clinical practice remains doubtful.

The disparity between office and ambulatory blood pressure reduction represents another concern. The excessive falls in office blood pressure are not accompanied by similar reductions in ambulatory blood pressure levels. A smaller reduction of ambulatory compared to office blood pressure

has been observed with drug therapy [50, 51]; however this difference is accentuated with renal nerve ablation. The mechanisms underlying this phenomenon have not been adequately clarified. The importance of pseudo-resistance has been highlighted in a recent study by Mahfoud et al. in which no ambulatory blood pressure response was demonstrated in this population [52]. It thus seems mandatory to use 24 h blood pressure measurement in all candidates for renal nerve ablation, in order to exclude pseudo-resistance [53].

The persistence of blood pressure reduction over time and the long-term outcome of patients undergoing renal nerve ablation remain unknown, since catheter-based renal denervation has a short history. Up to now, blood pressure reduction seems to be maintained for at least 3 years following renal nerve ablation (the maximum reported follow-up period) [54]. Regarding the long-term effects of renal denervation on morbidity and mortality, no data is available so far. Although it seems rational to assume that blood pressure reduction will be accompanied by significant benefits, it remains to be seen in prospective randomized studies comparing renal nerve ablation with optimal drug therapy. The EnligHTment study aims to stratify >5,000 patients to provide relevant information.

Applications of Renal Denervation Beyond Blood Pressure Control

Renal nerve ablation might be beneficial in all disease conditions characterized by enhanced sympathetic activity, including but not limited to chronic kidney disease, heart failure with reduced or preserved ejection fraction, obstructive sleep apnea, polycystic ovary syndrome, and tachyarrhythmias. Pilot studies in these conditions have been promising so far, however appropriately designed studies are needed to confirm these primary results.

The rationale for renal nerve ablation in chronic kidney disease comes from the sympathetic overdrive observed patients with renal insufficiency [55] and the beneficial effects of surgical excision of native kidneys in hemodialysis patients and renal transplant recipients [56, 57]. Renal nerve ablation seems to be feasible, safe, and effective in patients with chronic kidney disease [58, 59]. However, available data comes from case reports or small clinical studies and requires confirmation.

Sympathetic overactivity and fluid overload is observed in patients with heart failure [60]. Renal nerve ablation exhibited beneficial effects on cardiac function in heart failure patients with either reduced or preserved ejection fraction. However, these benefits were observed in small pilot studies [61, 62]. Larger randomized outcome studies (RE-ADAPT-CHF for reduced ejection fraction and DIASTOLE for preserved ejection fraction) are underway to evaluate the efficacy and safety of renal nerve ablation in heart failure patients.

Obstructive sleep apnea is associated with sympathetic overactivity [63] and experimental data point towards benefits of renal nerve ablation [64, 65]. A small study in humans revealed that renal denervation not only decreased blood pressure levels but modified the severity of the disease itself as well [66]. Similarly, beneficial effects on blood pressure and disease severity were also observed in patients with polycystic ovary syndrome [67], a condition characterized by enhanced sympathetic activity [68]. However, the study sample was very small in both studies and verification is waited.

The sympathetic system seems to be implicated in some forms of cardiac arrhythmia, both ventricular and supraventricular. Experimental data suggests beneficial effects of renal nerve ablation in cardiac arrhythmias [69, 70] and small studies in humans point towards benefits in ventricular tachyarrhythmias and atrial fibrillation [71, 72]. The H-FIB study will evaluate the effects of renal denervation in a large number of patients with atrial fibrillation.

Finally renal nerve ablation might prove beneficial in patients with diabetes mellitus, metabolic syndrome, high cardiovascular risk, myocardial infarction, loin pain hematuria, and polycystic kidney disease. However, these theoretical benefits have to be proven in clinical studies.

References

1. Zimmer K. Soul made flesh. London: The RandomHouse (Arrow Books); 2004. p. 188–207.
2. Barajas L, Latta H. A three-dimensional study of the juxtaglomerular apparatus in the rat. Light and electron microscopic observations. Lab Invest. 1963;12:257–69.
3. Barajas L. The innervation of the juxtaglomerular apparatus. An electron microscopic study of the innervation of the glomerular arterioles. Lab Invest. 1964;13:916–29.
4. Barajas L. Renin secretion: an anatomical basis for tubular control. Science. 1971;172:485–7.
5. Barajas L, Liu L, Powers K. Anatomy of the renal innervation: intrarenal aspects and ganglia of origin. Can J Physiol Pharmacol. 1992;70:735–49.
6. Hamilton WF, Richards DW. Output of the heart. In: Fishman AP, Richards DW, editors. Circulation of the blood. Men and ideas. Bethesda: American Physiological Society; 1982. p. 87–90.
7. Bernard C. Lecons sur les proprietes physiologiques et les alterations pathologiques des liquids de l' organisme, vol. 2. Paris: Bailliere; 1859. p. 170–91.
8. von Euler US. A specific sympathetic ergone in adrenergic nerve fibres (sympathin) and its relation to adrenaline and noradrenaline. Acta Physiol Scand. 1946;12:73–97.
9. Harrington M, Kincaid-Smith P, McMichael J. Results of treatment in malignant hypertension: a seven-year experience in 94 cases. Br Med J. 1959;2:969–89.
10. Bradford JR. The innervation of the renal blood vessels. J Physiol. 1889;10:358–407.
11. DiBona GF, Kopp UC. Neural control of renal function. Physiol Rev. 1997;77:75–197.
12. Esler M. The sympathetic system and hypertension. Am J Hypertens. 2000;13:S99–105.
13. Campese V, Kogosov E. Renal afferent denervation prevents hypertension in rats with chronic renal failure. Hypertension. 1995;25:878–82.
14. Stella A, Zanchetti A. Functional role of renal afferents. Physiol Rev. 1991;71:659–82.
15. DiBona GF, Esler M. Translational medicine: the antihypertensive effect of renal denervation. Am J Physiol Regul Integr Comp Physiol. 2010;298:R245–53.
16. Campese VM, Ku E, Park J. Sympathetic renal innervation and resistant hypertension. Int J Hypertens. 2011;2011:814354.
17. Tsioufis C, Kordalis A, Flessas D, et al. Pathophysiology of resistant hypertension: the role of sympathetic nervous system. Int J Hypertens. 2011;2011:642416.
18. Doumas M, Faselis C, Papademetriou V. Renal sympathetic denervation in hypertension. Curr Opin Nephrol Hypertens. 2011;20:647–53.
19. Charkoudian N, Rabbitts JA. Sympathetic neural mechanisms in human cardiovascular health and disease. Mayo Clin Proc. 2009;84:822–30.
20. Esler M. Pathophysiology of the human sympathetic nervous system in cardiovascular diseases: the transition from mechanisms to medical management. J Appl Physiol. 2010;108:227–37.
21. Adson AW, McCraig W, Brown GE. Surgery in its relation to hypertension. Surg Gynecol Obstet. 1936;62:314–31.
22. Papin E, Ambard L. Resection of the nerves of the kidney for nephralgia and small hydronephroses. J Urol. 1924;11:337–49.
23. Page IH, Heuer GJ. The effect of renal denervation on the level of arterial blood pressure and renal function in essential hypertension. J Clin Invest. 1935;XIV:27–30.
24. Smithwick RH, Thompson JE. Splanchnicectomy for essential hypertension. JAMA. 1953;152:1501–4.
25. Peet MM, Woods WW, Braden S. The surgical treatment of hypertension. JAMA. 1940;115:1875–85.
26. Allen EV. Sympathectomy for essential hypertension. Circulation. 1952;6:131–40.
27. Freyberg RH, Peet MM. The effect on the kidney of bilateral splanchnicectomy in patients with hypertension. J Clin Invest. 1937;16:49–65.
28. Isberg EM, Peet MM. The influence of supradiaphragmatic splanchnicectomy on the heart in hypertension. Am Heart J. 1948;35:567–83.
29. Peet MM. Hypertension and its surgical treatment by supradiaphragmatic splanchnicectomy. Am J Surg. 1948;LXXV:48–68.
30. Freis ED, Wanko A, Wilson IM, Parrish AE. Treatment of essential hypertension with chlorothiazide (diuril); its use alone and combined with other antihypertensive agents. J Am Med Assoc. 1958;166:137–40.
31. Calhoun DA, Jones D, Textor S, et al. Resistant hypertension: diagnosis, evaluation and treatment. Hypertension. 2008;117:510–26.
32. Mancia G, Laurent S, Agabiti-Rossei E, et al. 2009 Reappraisal of European guidelines on hypertension management: a European Society of Hypertension Task Force document. J Hypertens. 2009;27:2121–58.
33. Persell SD. Prevalence of resistant hypertension in the United States, 2003–2008. Hypertension. 2011;57:1076–80.
34. de la Sierra A, Segura J, Banegas JR, et al. Clinical features of 8295 patients with resistant hypertension classified on the basis of ambulatory blood pressure monitoring. Hypertension. 2011;57:898–902.
35. Atherton DS, Deep NL, Mendelsohn FO. Micro-anatomy of the renal sympathetic nervous system: a human post-mortem histologic study. Clin Anat. 2012;25:628–33.
36. Tsioufis C, Papademetriou V, Dimitriadis K, Tsiachris D, Thomopoulos C, Park E, Hata C, Papalois A, Stefanadis C. Catheter-based renal sympathetic denervation exerts acute and chronic

effects on renal hemodynamics in swine. Int J Cardiol. 2012. doi:10.1016/j.ijcard.2012. 10.038. [Epub ahead of print].

37. Worthley SG, Tsioufis C, Worthley M, Sinhal A, Chew DP, Meredith IT, Malaiapan Y, Papademetriou V. Safety and efficacy of a multi-electrode renal sympathetic denervation system in resistant hypertension: the EnligHTN I trial. Eur Heart J. 2013. doi:10.1093/eurheartj/eht197.

38. Chinushi M, Izumi D, Iijima K, Suzuki K, Furushima H, Saitoh O, Furuta Y, Aizawa Y, Iwafuchi M. Blood pressure and autonomic responses to electrical stimulation of the renal arterial nerves before and after ablation of the renal artery. Hypertension. 2013;61:450–6.

39. Vonend O, Antoch G, Rump LC, Blondin D. Secondary rise in blood pressure after renal denervation. Lancet. 2012;380:778.

40. Kaltenbach B, Id D, Franke JC, Sievert H, Hennersdorf M, Maier J, Bertog SC. Renal artery stenosis after renal sympathetic denervation. J Am Coll Cardiol. 2012;60:2694–5.

41. Petidis K, Anyfanti P, Doumas M. Renal sympathetic denervation: renal function concerns. Hypertension. 2011;58:e19.

42. Krum H, Schlaich M, Whitbourn R, et al. Catheter-based renal sympathetic denervation for resistant hypertension: a multicentre safety and proof-of-principle cohort study. Lancet. 2009;373: 1275–81.

43. Symplicity HTN-2 Investigators, Esler MD, Krum H, Sobotka PA, et al. Renal sympathetic denervation in patients with treatment-resistant hypertension (the symplicity HTN-2 trial): a randomised controlled trial. Lancet. 2010;376:1903–9.

44. Mahfoud F, Cremens B, Janker J, Link B, Vonend O, Ukena C, Linz D, Schmieder R, Rump LC, Kindermann I, Sobotka PA, Krum H, Scheller B, Schlaich M, Laufs U, Böhm M. Renal hemodynamics and renal function after catheter-based renal sympathetic denervation in patients with resistant hypertension. Hypertension. 2012; 60:419–24.

45. Hering D, Esler MD, Schlaich MP. Chronic kidney disease: role of sympathetic nervous system activation and potential benefits of renal denervation. EuroIntervention. 2013;9:R127–35.

46. Dorr O, Liebetrau C, Mollmann H, et al. Renal sympathetic denervation does not aggravate functional or structural renal damage. J Am Coll Cardiol. 2013;61:479–80.

47. Schneider S, Baumann M, Lefeldt S, Laugwitz KL, Heemann U. Renal failure after renal sympathetic ablation in a patient with chronic kidney disease – which came first, the chicken or the egg? Int J Cardiol. 2013. doi:10.1016/j.ijcard.2013.04.123.

48. Brinkmann J, Heusser K, Schmidt, Menne J, Klein G, Bauersachs J, Haller H, Sweep FC, Diedrich A, Jordan J, Tank J. Catheter-based renal nerve ablation and centrally generated sympathetic activity in difficult-to-control hypertensive patients: prospective case series. Hypertension. 2012;60:1485–90.

49. Hering D, Lambert EA, Marusic P, Walton AS, Krum H, Lambert GW, Esler MD, Sclaich MP. Substantial reduction in single sympathetic nerve firing after renal denervation in patients with resistant hypertension. Hypertension. 2013;61:457–64.

50. Mancia G, Parati G. Office compared with ambulatory blood pressure in assessing response to antihypertensive treatment: a meta-analysis. J Hypertens. 2004;22:435–45.

51. Ishikawa J, Carroll DJ, Kuruvilla S, Schwartz JE, Pickering TG. Changes in home versus clinic blood pressure with antihypertensive treatments: a meta-analysis. Hypertension. 2008;52:856–64.

52. Mahfoud F, Ukena C, Schmieder R, Cremers B, Rump L, Vonend O, Weil J, Schmidt M, Hoppe UC, Zeller T, Bauer A, Ott C, Blessing E, Sobotka PA, Krum H, Schlaich M, Esler M, Böhm M. Ambulatory blood pressure changes after renal sympathetic denervation in patients with resistant hypertension: clinical perspective. Circulation. 2013;128:132–40.

53. Doumas M, Anyfanti P, Bakris G. Should ambulatory blood pressure monitoring be mandatory for future studies in resistant hypertension: a perspective. J Hypertens. 2012;30:874–6.

54. Krum H, Schlaich MP, Bohm M, et al. Percutaneous renal denervation in patients with treatment-resistant hypertension: final 3-year report of the symplicity HTN-1 study. Lancet. 2013. doi:10.1016/S0140-6736(13)62192-3. [Epub ahead of print].

55. Papademetriou V, Doumas M, Anyfanti P, Faselis C, Kokkinos P, Tsioufis K. Renal nerve ablation for hypertensive patients with chronic kidney disease. Curr Vasc Pharmacol. 2014;12(1):47–54 [Epub ahead of print].

56. Converse Jr RL, Jacobsen TN, Toto RD, et al. Sympathetic overactivity in patients with chronic renal failure. N Engl J Med. 1992;327:1912–8.

57. Hausberg M, Kosch M, Harmelink P, et al. Sympathetic nerve activity in end-stage renal disease. Circulation. 2002;106:1974–9.

58. Hering D, Mahmoud F, Walton AS, Krum H, Lambert GW, Lambert EA, Sobotka PA, Böhm M, Cremers B, Esler MD, Schlaich MP. Renal denervation in moderate to severe CKD. J Am Soc Nephrol. 2012;23:1250–7.

59. Schlaich MP, Bart B, Hering D, Walton A, Marusic P, Mahfoud F, Böhm M, Lambert EA, Krum H, Sobotka PA, Schmieder RE, Ika-Sari C, Eikelis N, Straznicky N, Lambert GW, Esler MD. Feasibility of catheter-based renal nerve ablation and effects on sympathetic nerve activity and blood pressure in patients with end-stage renal disease. Int J Cardiol. 2013. doi:10.1016/j.ijcard.2013.01.218. [Epub ahead of print].

60. Doumas M, Faselis C, Tsioufis C, Papademetriou V. Carotid baroreceptor activation for the treatment of resistant hypertension and heart failure. Curr Hypertens Rep. 2012;14:238–46.

61. Davies JE, Manisty CH, Petraco R, Barron AJ, Unsworth B, Mayet J, Hamady M, Hughes AD, Sever PS, Sobotka PA, Francis DP. First-in-man safety evaluation of renal denervation for chronic systolic heart failure: primary outcome from REACH-Pilot study. Int J Cardiol. 2013;162:189–92.

62. Brandt MC, Mahfoud F, Reda S, Schirmer SH, Erdmann E, Bohm M, Hoppe UC. Renal sympathetic denervation reduces left ventricular hypertrophy and improves cardiac function in patients with resistant hypertension. J Am Coll Cardiol. 2012;59:901–9.

63. Prabhakar NR, Kumar GK. Mechanisms of sympathetic activation and blood pressure elevation by intermittent hypoxia. Respir Physiol Neurobiol. 2010;174:156–61.

64. Franquini JV, Medeiros AR, Andrade TU, Araújo MT, Moysés MR, Abreu GR, Vasquez EC, Bissoli NS. Influence of renal denervation on blood pressure, sodium and water excretion in acute total obstructive apnea in rats. Braz J Med Biol Res. 2009;42:214–9.

65. Linz D, Mahfoud F, Schotten U, Ukena C, Neuberger HR, Wirth K, Böhm M. Renal sympathetic denervation suppresses post-apneic blood pressure rises and atrial fibrillation in a model for sleep apnea. Hypertension. 2012;60:172–8.

66. Witkowski A, Prejbisz A, Florczak E, Kądziela J, Śliwiński P, Bieleń P, Michałowska I, Kabat M, Warchoł E, Januszewicz M, Narkiewicz K, Somers VK, Sobotka PA, Januszewicz A. Effects of renal sympathetic denervation on blood pressure, sleep apnea course, and glycemic control in patients with resistant hypertension and sleep apnea. Hypertension. 2011;58:559–65.

67. Schlaich MP, Straznicky N, Grima M, Ika-Sari C, Dawood T, Mahfoud F, Lambert E, Chopra R, Socratous F, Hennebry S, Eikelis N, Böhm M, Krum H, Lambert G, Esler MD, Sobotka PA. Renal denervation: a potential new treatment modality for polycystic ovary syndrome? J Hypertens. 2011;29:991–6.

68. Sverrisdóttir YB, Mogren T, Kataoka J, Janson PO, Stener-Victorin E. Is polycystic ovary syndrome associated with high sympathetic nerve activity and size at birth? Am J Physiol Endocrinol Metab. 2008;294:E576–81.

69. Linz D, Wirth K, Ukena C, et al. Renal denervation suppresses ventricular arrhythmias during acute ventricular ischemia in pigs. Heart Rhythm. 2013;10:1525–30.

70. Zhao Q, Yu S, Zou M, Dai Z, Wang X, Xiao J, Huang C. Effect of renal sympathetic denervation on the inducibility of atrial fibrillation during rapid atrial pacing. J Interv Card Electrophysiol. 2012;35:119–25.

71. Ukena C, Bauer A, Mahfoud F, Schreieck J, Neuberger HR, Eick C, Sobotka PA, Gawaz M, Böhm M. Renal sympathetic denervation for treatment of electrical storm: first-in-man experience. Clin Res Cardiol. 2012;101:63–7.

72. Pokushalov E, Romanov A, Corbucci G, Artyomenko S, Baranova V, Turov A, Shirokova N, Karaskov A, Mittal S, Steinberg JS. A randomized comparison of pulmonary vein isolation with versus without concomitant renal artery denervation in patients with refractory symptomatic atrial fibrillation and resistant hypertension. J Am Coll Cardiol. 2012;60:1163–70.

Marc Sapoval, Atul Pathak, Leslie A. Coleman,
Austin R. Roth, Helen L. Reeve, and Thomas Zeller

Introduction

Sympathetic nervous system over-activity has been linked to numerous pathophysiologic conditions affecting the cardiovascular, renal, and metabolic systems. Specific conditions wherein sympathetic over-activity has been described include essential hypertension, heart failure, arrhythmias, diabetes, sleep apnea syndrome, obesity, and chronic kidney disease [1, 2]. Increased sympathetic nervous system efferent activity to the renal system contributes to blood pressure homeostasis by promoting sodium and water retention, renin secretion and vasoconstriction of renal arterioles. Further, renin release stimulates the production of angiotensin II and thereby mineralocorticoids, mediating vasoconstriction and sodium and water retention, respectively. In addition, afferent

M. Sapoval, MD, PhD
Interventional Radiology, Hopital Européen Georges Pompidou,
20 Rue Leblanc, Paris 75015, France
e-mail: marc.sapoval2@egp.aphp.fr

A. Pathak, MD, PhD, DACLAM
Clinical Pharmacology and Cardiovascular Medicine,
University Hospital and Faculty of Medicine,
37 Allees Jules Guesde, Toulouse 31073, France
e-mail: atul.pathak@univ-tlse3.fr

L.A. Coleman, DVM, MS (✉)
ReCor Medical Inc., 1049 Elwell Court,
Palo Alto, CA 94303, USA
e-mail: lcoleman@recormedical.com;
hreeve-stoffer@recormedical.com

H.L. Reeve, PhD
VP Clinical, ReCor Medical BV, Herengracht 124–128,
1015 BT Amsterdam, The Netherlands
hreeve-stoffer@recormedical.com

A.R. Roth, BS, MS
ReCor Medical, 1049 Elwell Court,
Palo Alto, CA 94303, USA
e-mail: aroth@recormedical.com

T. Zeller, MD
Department Angiology, Universitäts-Herzzentrum Freiburg – Bad Krozingen, Südring 15, Bad Krozingen 79189, Germany
e-mail: Thomas.zeller@universitaets-herzzentrum.de

signals from the kidneys communicate with sympathetic centers in the central nervous system and play an important role in the regulation of overall sympathetic tone [3]. Chronic elevation in sympathetic activity contributes to the development of chronic hypertension, and potential end organ damage [4].

Chronic hypertension is managed by a combination of lifestyle changes and medications. Despite the use of multiple classes of anti-hypertensive medications, hypertension remains uncontrolled in a significant number of patients. Resistant hypertension is defined as blood pressure above goal despite the concurrent use of three different anti-hypertensive medication classes, one ideally being a diuretic with all agents prescribed at doses that provide optimal benefit [5, 6]. Catheter-based renal denervation is a novel approach to disrupt renal sympathetic nerve activity in order to reduce blood pressure in patients with resistant hypertension [7, 8]. The premise is that targeted denervation of the renal efferent and afferent nerves leads to a decrease in local and central sympathetic activity resulting in a reduction in arterial blood pressure while simultaneously impacting numerous other systemic disorders affecting the cardiovascular, renal, and metabolic systems.

To date, there are two primary approaches for catheter based delivery of energy for renal denervation: (1) radiofrequency energy delivered to the renal arterial wall, transmurally, in a spiral fashion to focally ablate sympathetic nerves [9–12] (2) ultrasound energy delivered circumferentially to the adventitia and peri-adventitia, sparing the arterial wall, to ablate the sympathetic nerves [13].

Therapeutic Ultrasound

Therapeutic ultrasound energy consists of high-frequency sound waves (i.e. rapid mechanical oscillations) that generate frictional heating in soft tissues [14]. Due to the physics of sound propagation, direct tissue contact with the ultrasound source is not required for energy transmission. Importantly, ultrasound energy absorption in liquids (i.e. water, blood) is negligible reducing the risk of blood coagulation and the potential for thrombogenicity.

Ultrasound for Renal Denervation

The Paradise System utilizes a cylindrical ultrasound source which creates uniform toroidal lesions with controllable geometries, allowing for optimized treatment parameters that reduce the number of treatment sites and the overall treatment duration. By optimizing the size, shape and location of the lesion, denervation can be maximized while completely protecting the arterial intimal and medial layers.

Advantages of Ultrasound Over Radiofrequency Ablation

Ultrasound ablation offers distinct advantages over radiofrequency ablation for renal denervation due to the way in which energy is delivered to the tissue and due to the ability to control the resultant tissue heat profile. The ability to ablate without the energy source making direct contact with the arterial wall is one of the main distinctions between ultrasound and radiofrequency devices. Radiofrequency devices require impedance measurements to ensure proper contact with tissue, a step that is unnecessary when using ultrasound. Since direct tissue contact is necessary to ablate tissue with radiofrequency electrodes, the tissue receiving the highest influx of energy is immediately adjacent to the electrode, and cannot be cooled. In contrast, ultrasound devices do not require direct tissue contact and balloon cooling of the arterial wall can be implemented while maintaining stabilization and position of the device within the artery. Balloon cooling allows for the maintenance of physiologic temperatures at the surface. Another important distinction is that radiofrequency relies on thermal conduction alone to heat nerves residing away from the arterial wall. In contrast, ultrasound propagates into tissues, depositing energy in a predictable and controllable pattern that defines the size, shape and location of the thermal lesion. This allows for very precise energy deposition that can take place in short time periods, reducing the unpredictability that is inherent in heat conduction through heterogeneous biological media.

The ReCor Medical Paradise® Renal Denervation System

The CE Marked Paradise System is a next generation catheter-based renal denervation device that delivers ultrasound energy to perform targeted circumferential denervation to the renal afferent and efferent sympathetic nerves

with the goal of achieving a reduction in systemic arterial blood pressure, and mitigating end organ effects due to sympathetic over-activity.

The Paradise System currently consists of a single use 6-French ultrasound delivery catheter (5-French catheter will be launched in 2014) and an automated, portable customized generator working together to manage precise and uniform energy delivery with the aim of ablating the sympathetic nerves that surround the renal artery, while simultaneously cooling the endothelial and medial layers of the arterial wall to preserve the integrity of the arterial wall during the energy delivery process. The Paradise Catheter is introduced via femoral, or radial access, under fluoroscopic guidance and advanced into the renal artery. Bilateral renal denervation is achieved by delivering ultrasound energy within each renal artery. The specific components of the Paradise System are described in more detail below.

Description of the Paradise System Components

Paradise Transducer

The ultrasonic energy source, transducer, is the core component of the Paradise System. The transducer is a cylindrical ceramic ultrasound transducer that produces circumferentially uniform sound waves that propagate into, and are absorbed by, the tissue surrounding the renal artery. The Paradise Generator manages the delivery of the circumferential ultrasound energy to the renal nerves located within and beyond the arterial wall.

Paradise Catheter

The Paradise Catheter has a distal balloon which is pressurized by the Paradise System to a range of 1.5–2.0 ATM using sterile circulating water (Fig. 9.1c). The ultrasound transducer is located within the balloon (Fig. 9.1b). The transducer converts electrical energy to acoustic energy, which is then delivered radially from the balloon into the renal artery. The pressurized balloon manages the location of the ultrasound transducer within the artery and allows fluid circulation that serves to cool the wall of the renal artery.

Paradise Generator

The Paradise Generator contains a touch screen which allows users to operate the Paradise System in a stepwise fashion to prepare the balloon for insertion, to inflate and/or deflate the balloon and also to deliver energy (Fig. 9.1a). This manner of operation, combined with a series of sensors,

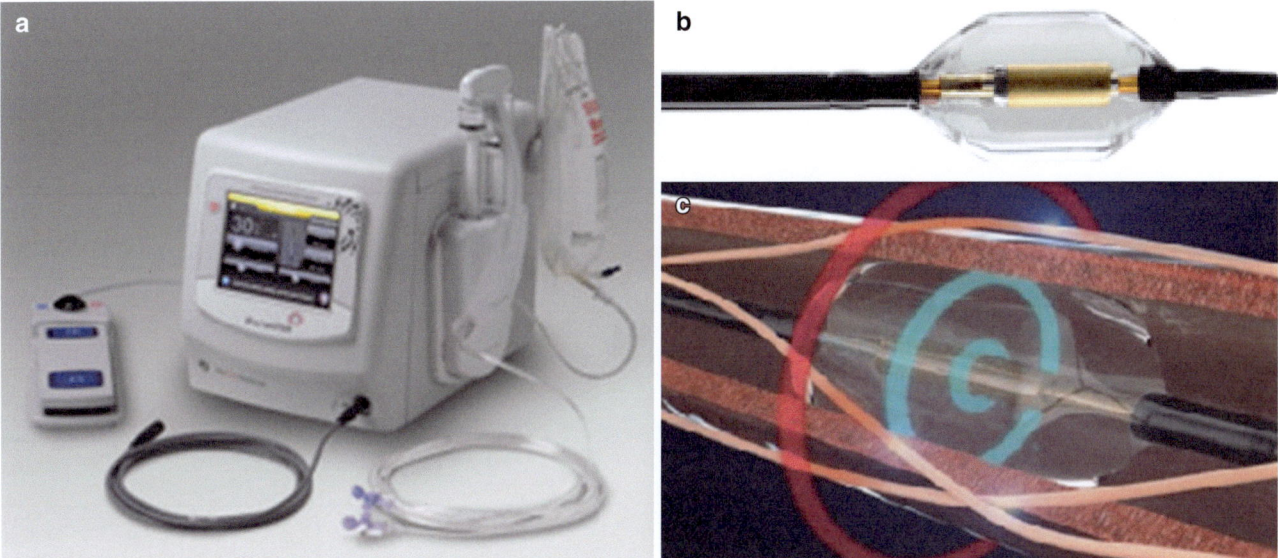

Fig. 9.1 The paradise renal denervation system. (**a**) Paradise generator. (**b**) Paradise catheter: ultrasound transducer within cooling balloon. (**c**) The paradise system in situ (artistic rendering)

both internally and within the disposable cartridge allows the main central processing unit within the generator to monitor and control the state of the Paradise System at any moment in time. The dosage settings of the Paradise Generator are fixed and based on the efficiency of the transducer and the balloon size. Each catheter has an embedded chip that communicates to the generator the specific power settings to be applied.

Paradise Cartridge

The Paradise Cartridge when used in conjunction with the Paradise Generator controls the fluid flow into and out of the Paradise Catheter. Fluid flows in a closed-loop through the Paradise Cartridge and the Paradise Catheter.

Paradise Connection Cable

The Paradise Connection Cable allows for the communication of transducer information from the Paradise Catheter to the Paradise Generator as well as the transfer of electrical energy during the procedure.

Preclinical Results

The Paradise System has been developed to optimize safety and effectiveness by creating a cooled zone to ensure safety, and an ablation zone, to optimize effectiveness. Extensive in vitro and in vivo testing has been conducted to evaluate system functionality, device deliverability, thermal and

cooling settings, treatment parameters and the overall safety and effectiveness of the system.

Thermal Profile

The target thermal profile for energy delivery determined by ReCor Medical Inc. includes a cooled zone wherein tissue temperatures are maintained between 37 and 55 °C to minimize endothelial or medial cell damage; a target ablation zone 1–6 mm from the arterial lumen wherein tissue temperatures should reach >60 °C for short durations to achieve immediate neural cell death; and a far field cooled zone wherein tissue temperatures do not exceed physiologic temperatures to ensure there is no damage to non-target tissues (Fig. 9.2). Optimization of the tissue thermal profile can be achieved through management of the power of energy delivered, the duration of energy delivery, and the cooling flow rate.

In vitro and in vivo studies have been conducted to optimize the thermal profile of the Paradise System to effectively ablate the renal nerves. The cooling flow rate, power, and duration of energy delivered were varied in preclinical studies (in vitro initially and subsequently confirmed in vivo). Optimization of the thermal profile/thermal dose, and optimization of the number of ablations, was performed in vivo.

Computer Simulations

Computer simulation models were developed to characterize and optimize the thermal profile of the system. Simulations provide information regarding the heating pattern and depth of thermal energy delivered from the transducer. The model demonstrates the heating pattern emanating from the length

Fig. 9.2 Target thermal profile for ablation of renal nerves while preserving renal arterial wall

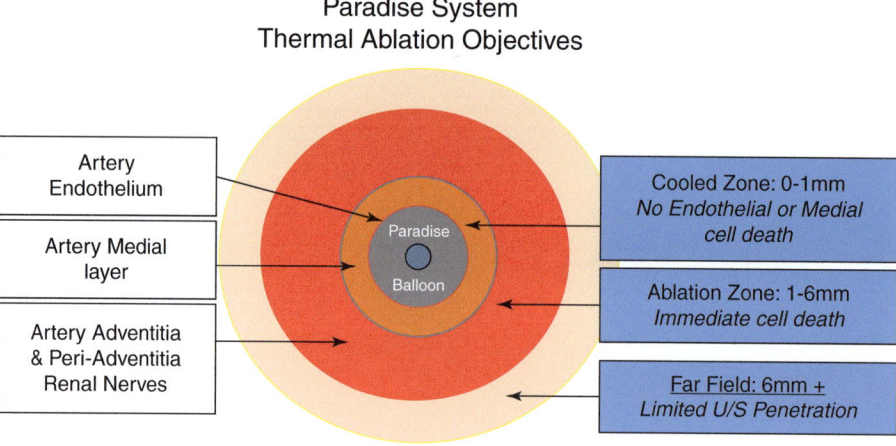

Paradise System
Thermal Ablation Objectives

Fig. 9.3 In vitro gel model demonstrating target thermal profile (average temperature achieved with the paradise system) for ablation of renal nerves while preserving renal arterial wall

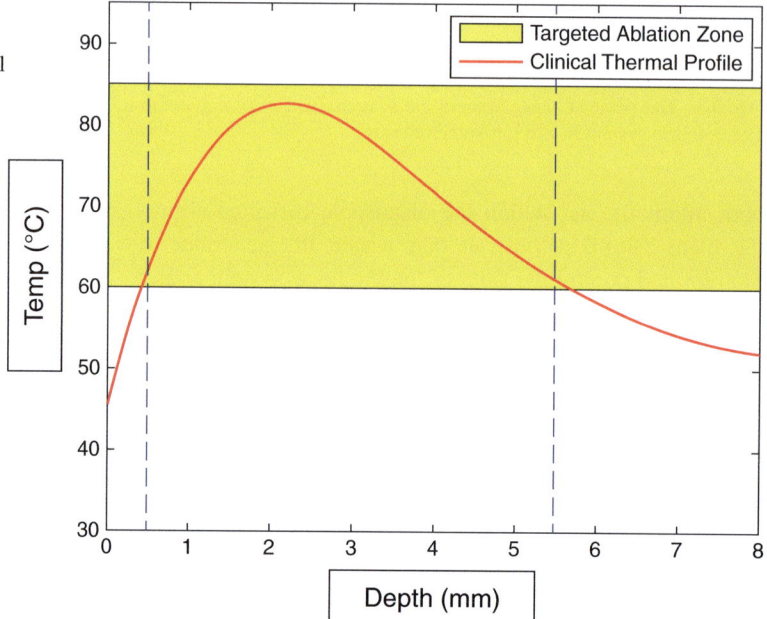

of the transducer and the depth of heating with peak temperatures reached at several millimeters of depth with cooling on the surface.

Bench Models

In vitro studies confirmed the thermal profile observed in computer simulations. A gel model was utilized which mimics characteristics of tissue. The Paradise Catheter was inserted into the gel and thermocouples were placed at specific depths surrounding the balloon/transducer to measure the energy (heat) delivered. A temperature curve was generated based on the thermocouple readings. Based on this model and animal data, treatment parameters have been optimized for clinical use. At near depths (0–0.5 mm) temperatures remained below 60 °C and then reached ablation temperatures in the 0.5–6 mm range. Beyond 6 mm, the temperatures dropped off again below ablation levels. Figure 9.3 shows the average temperature at specific depths (thermal profile) in the gel model.

In Vivo Studies

Animal studies were performed in either porcine or ovine models due to similarities in renal anatomy with humans. These in vivo studies have demonstrated the ability of the system to allow for appropriate insertion of the device and positioning of the transducer in the renal arteries. Bilateral renal ablation was performed in all studies and the safety and effectiveness of the system evaluated via histologic assessment of the renal arteries, kidneys, and abdominal peripheral organs. Additionally, effectiveness was assessed via measurement of kidney norepinephrine levels.

Effectiveness

The animal studies have demonstrated that the target thermal profile has been achieved in vivo with preservation through cooling of the arterial wall, and ablation of nerves at the target ablation zone of 1–6 ± 2 mm. The actual tissue ablation zone varies depending on the biological structures present.

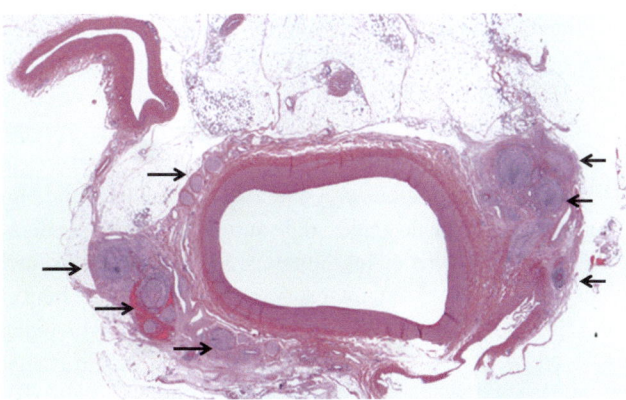

Fig. 9.4 Paradise system ablation zone in vivo. Photomicrograph of a histologic cross-section of a porcine renal artery treated with the paradise system (H&E). The renal arterial intimal and medial layers are preserved through system cooling whereas the renal sympathetic nerves (←) within the adventitia and peri-adventitia are ablated

The renal vein, arterioles, and lymph nodes serve as heat sinks, preventing adjacent tissues from reaching ablation temperatures. Effective ablation of the nerves, characterized by irreversible necrosis, has been demonstrated histologically. A decrease in nerve function has further been demonstrated by immunohistochemical staining for specific nerve proteins; and by measurement of norepinephrine levels in the kidney, the end organ target of the renal sympathetic nerves.

Figure 9.4 is a representative histologic image of a porcine renal artery treated with the Paradise System at 7 days. As indicated, the renal artery (first millimeter of tissue) is spared whereas the ablation zone extends out to 6 mm, to target the majority of sympathetic nerves surrounding the renal artery. Quantification of affected nerves determined that on average 75 % of the nerves along the length of the artery were ablated with the Paradise System in animal models. In contrast, radiofrequency ablation ablates in a noncircumferential manner and heats at depths of 0–3 mm thereby potentially missing a large percentage of nerves.

Further confirmation of the effectiveness of the Paradise System was demonstrated through specific immunostaining of the renal nerves for structural nerve and functional nerve proteins. Positive staining was observed for two structural proteins [neurofilament protein, NFP, and S-100, nervous system specific protein] whereas reduced staining was observed for tyrosine hydroxylase (TH), a functional nerve protein. These data illustrate that in nerves (clearly identified through the structural proteins), function was greatly diminished consistent with thermal ablation.

Further evidence for a decrease in nerve function is demonstrated by kidney norepinephrine levels (Table 9.1). Eight animals were selected to get either one (n=3), two (n=3), or three (n=2) 30 s treatments in the proximal, mid, and/or distal regions of both renal arteries. A significant decrease in norepinephrine levels was evident at 7 days for 1, 2 or 3 treatment emissions per artery when compared to

Table 9.1 Percentage reduction of kidney norepinephrine levels and percent of ablated nerves based on number of ultrasound emissions

Ultrasound emissions	Mean norepinephrine level	Percent reduction of norepinephrine vs. control	Percent of ablated nerves
0 Emission (control)	969 ± 44 ng/g	–	–
1 Emission	435 ± 217 ng/g	55 %	44 %
2 Emissions	104 ± 164 ng/g	89 %	76 %
3 Emissions	30 ± 36 ng/g	97 %	76 %

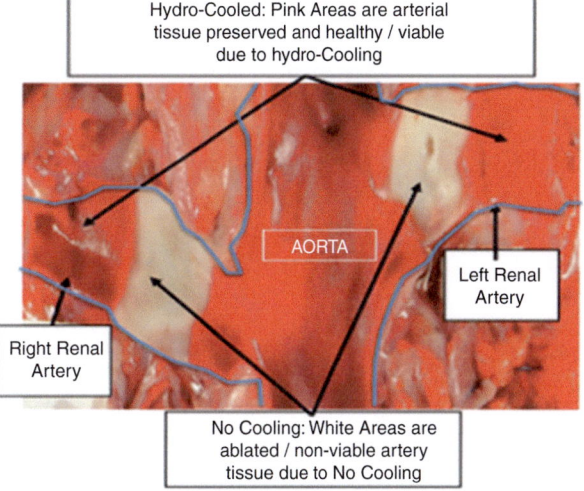

Fig. 9.5 Tetrazolium staining of the porcine aorta and bilateral renal arteries demonstrating the benefit of the cooling balloon feature of the paradise system

control animals (n=2), which correlated with the percentage of ablated nerves. Two or three emissions resulted in far greater reduction than one emission, consistent with the current clinical protocol.

Renal Artery Safety

In addition, in vivo animal studies confirmed that the Paradise System does not cause clinically significant renal artery damage or functional impairment. As illustrated in the histology image in Fig. 9.4, the renal arterial wall (endothelium and medial layer) is preserved with minimal to no injury, which is important in minimizing any risk of renal stenosis. Preservation of the arterial wall is primarily due to the cooling feature of the system. Further, there is no evidence of ultrasound related damage to the renal vein, ureter, or kidney detected.

An acute animal study illustrated the benefit of the cooling feature. Porcine renal arteries were treated bilaterally with the Paradise System with the cooling feature turned on, per clinical use in the distal renal artery, and with the cooling feature turned off, in the proximal renal artery. The arteries were then immersed in Tetrazolium chloride (TTC) which differentiates viable (red) tissue from non-viable (white) tissue within the treatment area. The results are clearly delineated in Fig. 9.5, wherein the treatment emissions with the cooling feature turned off are white (non-viable) and those in which the system is used as intended with the cooling feature are viable.

Clinical Experience

The ReCor Paradise System received CE mark on December 23, 2011. First in human evidence of the clinical safety and efficacy of the system was evaluated in the first-in-man REnal Denervation by Ultrasound transCatheter Emission (REDUCE) Trial, a single-center feasibility study conducted at Vergelegen Medi-Clinic, South Africa. Subsequently, two multi-center, ReCor Medical Inc. sponsored post-market evaluations (the REALISE and ACHIEVE studies) have also been undertaken as well as an investigator-led study (the RETREAT study) to evaluate patients who have not adequately responded to a previous renal nerve ablation treatment with radiofrequency.

The REDUCE Study

Patients were treated in the REDUCE study between October 2011 and February 2012; 1-year follow-up is complete on all patients. Preliminary results from the REDUCE study were published in May 2012 by Mabin et al.

Patients enrolled in the REDUCE study were diagnosed with resistant hypertension as defined by the 2007 European Society of Hypertension and the European Society of Cardiology [15], with a minimum blood pressure of 140/90 mmHg (office), 135/85 mmHg (home) and 130/80 mmHg (ambulatory) despite being treated with at least three anti-hypertensive medications including a diuretic. Patients under the age of 18 years, pregnant, allergic to contrast media, or with any known cause of secondary hypertension were excluded. A CT-scan was performed at screening to further exclude patients with vascular abnormalities (including renal artery stenosis and iliac or femoral artery stenosis precluding insertion of the Paradise catheter) or not meeting the anatomical criteria (renal artery of more than 20 mm in length and 4 mm in diameter).

Baseline and follow-up evaluations (scheduled at 2 weeks, 1, 2, 3, 6, and 12 months) included physical examination, blood and urine analysis, and medication intake. Office (three measurements), home (three measurements twice daily over 3 days) and 24-h ambulatory blood pressures were recorded at regular time intervals during the course of the study. Baseline and follow-up (6 months) CT-scan images were reviewed by an independent radiological core laboratory. Patients were asked to continue their anti-hypertensive medications unless otherwise indicated by the investigator.

Fifteen patients with resistant hypertension underwent renal denervation in the REDUCE study. All patients met the ESH-ESC criteria for resistant hypertension at baseline. Average office blood pressure was $182\pm22/110\pm15$ mmHg, average home blood pressure $169\pm14/101\pm13$ mmHg, and average 24-h ambulatory blood pressure $168\pm16/98\pm15$ mmHg. Patients took, on average, 4.5 antihypertensive medications, with 100 % receiving diuretics, 91 % calcium-channel blockers, and 82 % angiotensin-converting enzyme inhibitors. Treated patients were 64 % female and 36 % male, 64 % white and 36 % colored, and 55 ± 14 years old (range 32–80 years). Baseline co-morbidities and cardiovascular risk factors included hyperlipidemia (64 %), coronary artery disease (36 %), and diabetes (27 %).

A 12-French treatment catheter was used for the first three cases, while the subsequent 12 subjects were treated with a 6-French catheter. Up to three ultrasound emissions were delivered in each renal artery at variable energies and with variable cooling flow rate. The majority of emissions were for 50 s (range 14–55). Eight patients were treated with low cooling flow of either 8 ml/min (n = 5) or 5 ml/min (n = 3). Of these, two patients developed clinically significant renal artery stenosis noted at their 6-month follow up visit, requiring angioplasty and stenting. In subsequent procedures, the cooling flow rate was increased to 41–50 ml/min with no further reports of stenosis.

Office blood pressure was measured at 2 weeks, 1, 3, 6 and 12 months post treatment. Ambulatory blood pressure was measured at 3, 6 and 12 months post treatment. Pretreatment, the mean office systolic blood pressure was 182 ± 22 mmHg (n = 15). By 180 days post treatment the average blood pressure was reduced to 149 ± 17 mmHg (n = 15) or an average drop of 33 mmHg which was sustained through the 12-month follow-up (153 ± 17 mmHg). Ambulatory blood pressure also decreased post procedure with a mean change of $-14/-7$ mmHg at 6 months (Fig. 9.6).

A responder has been defined as ≥10 mmHg drop in office systolic blood pressure or a ≥5 mmHg drop in ambulatory systolic blood pressure [16]. Based on this definition, 13/15 (87 %) REDUCE patients met the criteria of a responder by office blood pressure at 6 months; all patients met the criteria within the 12-month follow-up period. 9/13 (69 %) of REDUCE patients met the criteria of a responder by ambulatory blood pressure at 6 months, and 11/13 (85 %) met the criteria within the 12-month follow-up period.

Pain (back; abdominal; groin) associated with the procedure was reported in 9/15 patients. This type of procedural pain has been previously reported associated with radiofrequency renal denervation and is usually transient and mild. A total of three device-related events requiring intervention were reported: two cases of stenosis discussed above and one case of procedural renal artery dissection.

Fig. 9.6 REDUCE blood pressure measurements over time. (**a**) Mean office blood pressure over time (n = 15 per timepoint). (**b**) Mean office blood pressure change from baseline over time (n = 15 per timepoint)

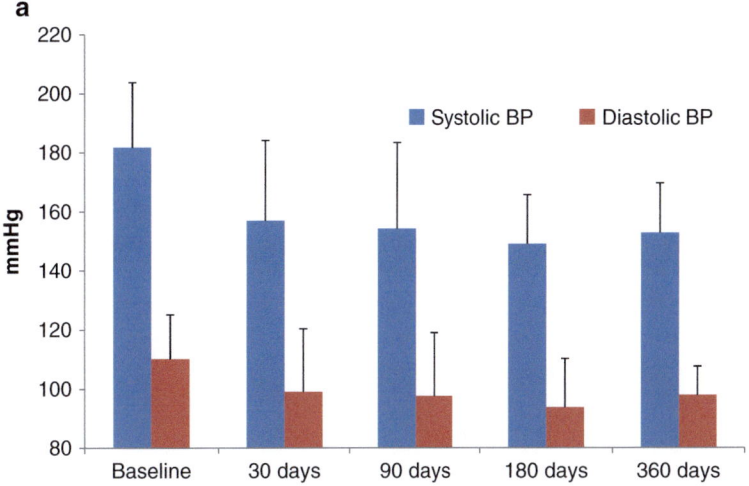

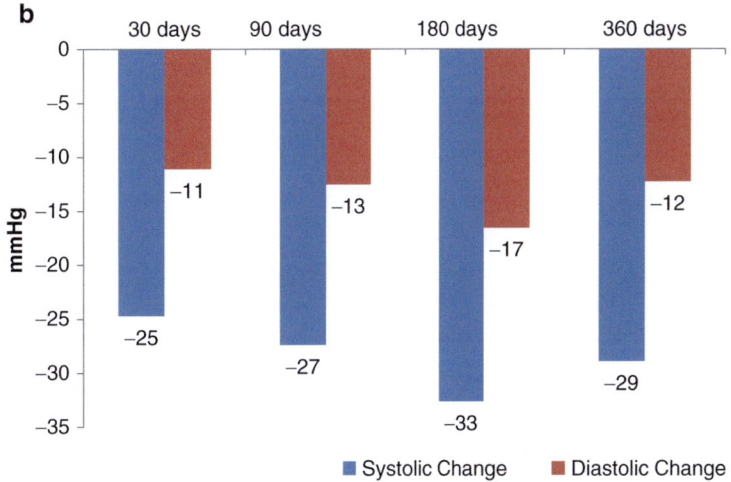

In summary the REDUCE study was designed to document the safety and effectiveness of the Paradise® System in the setting of a first-in-man feasibility study. The efficacy of the treatment despite the small study sample size was encouraging, with an overall mean drop in blood pressure of approximately 30 mmHg recorded over 12 months follow-up.

The REALISE Study

The REALISE Study was designed as an adjunct confirmatory clinical study based on the REDUCE protocol to further evaluate the Paradise System, and to further evaluate refinements in treatment parameters.

The study is a single-arm, open label prospective study conducted in France at two clinical sites. Patients enrolled in the study had moderate resistant hypertension as defined by the 2007 ESH/ESC guidelines. Moderate resistant hypertension is defined as office blood pressure >140/90 mmHg despite the use of a minimum of three anti-hypertensive medications, including a diuretic on maximally tolerated doses. All patients enrolled in the study were managed by a multi-disciplinary team which includes a hypertension specialist. The majority of patients were on five anti-hypertensive medications at baseline, and approximately two third of patients were taking spironolactone at baseline yet met the criteria of resistant hypertension.

The first eligible patient was treated on May 22, 2012. Enrolment in the REALISE study was completed in March 2014. One year follow up will be completed in 2015.

All patients enrolled in REALISE to date were treated at the higher cooling flow rate (41–50 ml/min) to ensure minimal damage to the arterial wall. The amount of energy (power) and duration of energy delivery was varied slightly in this patient group. For patients enrolled in 2012, two balloon sizes were available (6 and 8 mm diameter); however, in 2013, the full range of four balloon sizes was available.

Baseline and follow-up evaluations (scheduled at 1, 2, 3, 6, and 12 months) included physical examination, blood and urine analysis, and medication intake. Office (three measurements), home (three measurements twice daily over 3 days) and 24-h ambulatory blood pressures were recorded at regular time intervals during the course of the study. Baseline and follow-up (6-month) CT-scan images will be reviewed by an independent radiological core laboratory. Patients were asked to continue their anti-hypertensive medications unless otherwise indicated by the investigator.

Preliminary results on the complete patient cohort (n = 20) were presented at TCT, 2014 [17]. The mean age of enrolled patients was 55 years; 70 % were males. Baseline comorbidities and cardiovascular risk factors included hyperlipidemia (45 %), type II diabetes mellitus (35 %), history of peripheral vascular disease (30 %), history of stroke (30 %), history of myocardial infarction (30 %), history of obstructive sleep apnea (20 %), and prior renal denervation (5 %). The mean office blood pressure at baseline was 167/96 mmHg, and mean ambulatory blood pressure at baseline was 157/92 mmHg. Preliminary results demonstrate a mean office blood pressure drop of –13/–9 at 6 months (n = 20) and –17/–5 at 12 months (n = 7); and a mean ambulatory blood pressure drop of –12/–5 at 12 months (n = 8). Additionally, post treatment, the mean anti-hypertension medication burden decreased from 5.4 to 4.4 with an overall reduction in medication burden of 21 %.

System related safety events included the following: procedural pain (n = 5); access related vascular injury (n = 2); and systemic blood pressure effects including: hypotension (n = 2), dizziness (n = 1), hypertension (n = 1). There have been no reports of new onset renal artery stenosis.

In summary, preliminary results from the REALISE study demonstrate progressive decreases in office and ambulatory blood pressure at 6 and 12 months following treatment with the Paradise System in patients with moderate resistant hypertension despite optimal medical management, including spironolactone, in the majority of patients at baseline. The REALISE study provides additional confirmatory evidence of the effectiveness of ultrasound renal denervation.

The ACHIEVE Study

The TrAnsCatHeter Intravascular ultrasound Energy delivery for rEnal denervation (ACHIEVE study) is currently enrolling in Sweden, Germany, and the Netherlands. This study is designed to document the post-market performance and clinical effectiveness of the Paradise System in patients with resistant hypertension under standardized treatment parameters of fixed cooling flow, short duration of emission, and consistent energy delivery (automatically calculated based on balloon size).

Patients with resistant hypertension, defined as baseline office blood pressure of 160/90 mmHg and ambulatory blood pressure of 130/80 mmHg are eligible to participate in the ACHIEVE study. Patients with documented pre-existing renal stenosis anatomical abnormalities are excluded. Measurement of office blood pressure is made at all follow-up visits and recordings of 24-h ambulatory blood pressure are required for all patients at 6 and 12 months post treatment.

A total of 100 patients will be enrolled in the ACHIEVE study. Enrolment in the ACHIEVE study is estimated to be complete by early 2015 with follow up complete early 2016. At the time of this writing, there are no reports of stenosis or other major procedural or device-related events in over 80 patients treated.

The RETREAT Study

The RETREAT (Redo of transcatheter Renal Denervation) study is an investigator sponsored study on-going in Germany to document the effect of treating radiofrequency non-responders with the Paradise® System. Patients are considered eligible if they underwent unsuccessful catheter-based radiofrequency renal denervation ≥6 months prior to study participation with a systolic office based blood pressure ≥140 mmHg despite the use of ≥3 anti-hypertensive medications. The primary endpoints of the study include a change in office blood pressure at 6 months, a change in ambulatory blood pressure at 6 months, and a decrease in anti-hypertensive medications. Safety events will be collected and analyzed. To date, 7 patients, out of a target of 20 patients, have been enrolled and there have been no reports of adverse events, or any safety issues. Results are expected in the second half of 2015.

Conclusions

The ReCor Medical Paradise® System is the first CE marked percutaneous endovascular system to use ultrasound energy for renal denervation. The early clinical results with the Paradise System are compelling and demonstrated the acute safety and effectiveness of the device. The unique design features of the Paradise System offer significant advantages over first-generation radiofrequency renal denervation systems: direct tissue contact is not required to deliver energy, eliminating the need for catheter manipulation, and thereby improving consistency of treatment; self-centering tip of the Paradise Catheter allows for uniform energy delivery in every treatment site, and a fluid-filled low pressure balloon surrounding the catheter cools the endothelium and medial layers of the artery during energy delivery thereby minimizing damage to non-target tissues.

Ongoing and future clinical studies with the Paradise System will help confirm the durability and efficacy of this novel therapy.

References

1. Fisher, et al. Central sympathetic overactivity: maladies and mechanisms. Auton Neurosci. 2009;148:5–15.
2. Esler M. The 2009 Carl Ludwig lecture: pathophysiology of the human sympathetic nervous system in cardiovascular diseases: the transition from mechanisms to medical management. J Appl Physiol. 2010;108:227–37.
3. DiBona G, Kopp U. Neural control of renal function. Physiol Rev. 1997;77:75–197.
4. Mancia G, et al. Sympathetic activation in the pathogenesis of hypertension and progression of organ damage. Hypertension. 1999;34:724–8.
5. Calhoun D, et al. Resistant hypertension: diagnosis, evaluation, and treatment: a scientific statement from the American Heart Association Professional Education Committee of the Council for High Blood Pressure. Circulation. 2008;117:e510–26.
6. Mancia G, et al. 2013 ESH/ESC guidelines for the management of arterial hypertension: the task force for the management of arterial hypertension of the European society of hypertension (ESH) and of the European society of cardiology (ESC). Eur Heart J. 2013;34:2159–219.
7. Schlaich M, et al. Renal denervation and hypertension. Am J Hypertens. 2011;24:635–42.
8. Schlaich M, et al. International expert consensus statement: percutaneous transluminal renal denervation for the treatment of resistant hypertension. JACC. 2013. doi:10.1016/j.jacc.2013.08.1616.
9. Krum H, et al. Catheter-based renal sympathetic denervation for resistant hypertension: a multicentre safety and proof-of-principle cohort study. Lancet. 2009;373:1275–81.
10. Symplicity HTN-1 Investigators. Catheter-based renal sympathetic denervation for resistant hypertension: durability of blood pressure reduction out to 24 months. Hypertension. 2011;57:911–7.
11. Esler M, et al. Renal sympathetic denervation in patients with treatment-resistant hypertension (the symplicity HTN-2 trial): a randomized controlled trial. Lancet. 2010;376:1903–9.
12. Esler M, et al. Renal sympathetic denervation for treatment of drug-resistant hypertension: one-year results from the symplicity HTN-2 randomized controlled trial. Circulation. 2012;126:2976–82.
13. Mabin T, et al. First experience with endovascular ultrasound renal denervation for the treatment of resistant hypertension. EuroIntervention. 2012;8:57–61.
14. Kennedy, et al. High intensity focused ultrasound: surgery of the future? Br J Radiol. 2003;76:590–9.
15. Mancia G, et al. 2007 guidelines for the management of arterial hypertension: the task force for the management of arterial hypertension of the European Society of Hypertension (ESH) and of the European Society of Cardiology (ESC). Eur Heart J. 2007;28:1462–536.
16. Mahfound, et al. Ambulatory blood pressure changes after renal sympathetic denervation in patients with resistant hypertension. Circulation. 2013. doi:10.1161/CIRCULATIONAHA.112.000949.
17. Montelescot G, et al. REALISE trial: Renal Denervation by Ultrasound Transcatheter Emission. TCT 2014.

Therapeutic Intra Vascular Ultrasound (TIVUS)

10

Sharad V. Shetty and Sandeep Chopra

Introduction

Sympathetic nerve modulation as a therapeutic strategy in hypertension had been considered long before the advent of modern pharmacological therapies. Radical surgical methods for thoracic, abdominal, or pelvic sympathetic denervation had been successful in lowering blood pressure in patients with so-called malignant hypertension. However, these methods were associated with high perioperative morbidity and mortality and long-term complications including bowel, bladder, and erectile dysfunction, in addition to severe postural hypotension [4, 8, 9]. Recently developed endovascular catheter technology enables selective denervation of the human kidney, with radiofrequency (RF) energy delivered in the renal artery lumen, targeting the renal nerves located in the adventitia of the renal arteries.

Clinical studies have been done to assess the safety and efficacy of a percutaneous, catheter-based approach using RF designed to ablate renal sympathetic nerves specifically, via the lumen of the main renal artery (Symplicity™; Medtronic, Palo Alto, CA, USA). This approach was shown to reduce blood pressure successfully, without serious adverse events in patients with resistant hypertension [3, 5] which was shown to be maintained through 24 months [10]. Procedural limitations of the RF based renal denervation (RDN) include the catheter instability which triggers frequent treatment interruptions regardless of physician skill, the overall duration of the procedure and the associated patient discomfort or pain necessitating sedation and analgesia with bradycardia reported in 13 % of cases [1].

S.V. Shetty, MBBS, MD, FRACP (✉)
S. Chopra, MBBS, MD, DM
Department of Cardiology,
Royal Perth Hospital,
197 Wellington Street, Perth,
WA 6000, Australia
e-mail: sharad.shetty@health.wa.gov.au;
drsandeepchopra@gmail.com

Ultrasound Catheter Based Denervation

Ultrasound (US) energy consists of high-frequency sound waves (i.e., rapid mechanical oscillations), which are emitted by a piezoelectric transducer, and pass through the surrounding fluids. This generates frictional heating in soft tissues resulting in temperature increase at a depth from the vascular lumen. A novel modality of using ultrasonic energy for catheter-based renal denervation has been recently developed. This CE-marked PARADISE™ technology (Percutaneous Renal Denervation System by ReCor Medical, Ronkonkoma, NY, USA) uses a catheter with a cylindrical transducer that emits ultrasound energy circumferentially [7] This innovative technology endeavours to overcome the limitations of the currently used percutaneous RF-based RDN including the need for adequate vessel wall contact, requirement for longitudinal separation of ablation points and hence the need for long renal artery length to achieve adequate ablation points.

The TIVUS™ System

The Therapeutic Intra Vascular Ultrasound (TIVUS™) System for neural ablation using transluminal ultrasound has been developed by Cardiosonic Ltd. (Tel Aviv, Israel). The TIVUS™ System is a high intensity, non-focused, ultrasound catheter system, which enables remote, localized and controlled thermal modulation of nerves adjacent to renal arterial adventitia in order to perform safe therapeutic renal sympathetic denervation.

Device and Procedure Description: Renal Denervation Using the TIVUS™ System

The TIVUS™ System comprises of two main parts: the TIVUS™ Console and the TIVUS™ Catheter. The first generation catheter, a unidirectional one, consists of a single

R.R. Heuser et al. (eds.), *Renal Denervation: A New Approach to Treatment of Resistant Hypertension*,
DOI 10.1007/978-1-4471-5223-1_10, © Springer-Verlag London 2015

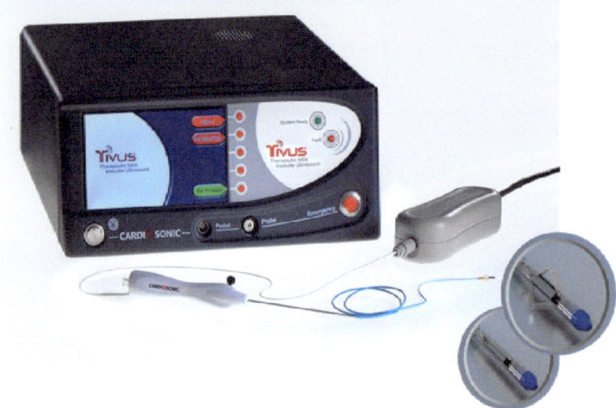

Fig. 10.1 The TIVUS™ System (Console and Multidirectional Catheter) (Printed with permission from Cardiosonic)

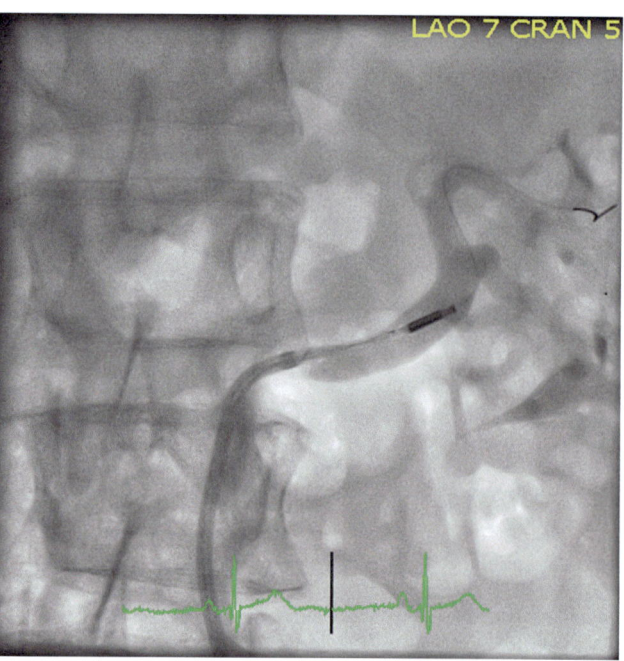

Fig. 10.2 Fluoroscopic image of the multidirectional TIVUS™ Catheter in the renal artery introduced over a 0.014″ guidewire (Printed with permission from Cardiosonic)

ultrasonic element. The Multidirectional TIVUS™ Catheter is an alteration of the Unidirectional TIVUS™ Catheter and both these catheters are powered by the Modular TIVUS™ Console or the TIVUS™ Console (Fig. 10.1). Both catheters are 6 French compatible and passed over a 0.014″ wire. The Unidirectional and the Multidirectional TIVUS™ Catheters developed by Cardiosonic are similar in terms of mechanical and biocompatibility characteristics. Interventions are performed under fluoroscopic guidance and the TIVUS™ Catheter is introduced into each renal artery via femoral arterial access. The catheter can be delivered either through a guiding catheter sheath or steerable introducer sheath, over a 0.014″ guidewire, which is left in place during the ablation (Fig. 10.2). With the steerable guiding sheath, there is an ability to manipulate the catheter tip to facilitate optimal positioning and delivery. It also has the additional capability of steering the catheter away from the vessel wall if required. The transducer can be distanced away from the vessel wall by rotation of a knob on the handle which deflects the distal tip of the catheter shaft.

The Multidirectional TIVUS™ Catheter is composed of three ultrasonic elements, which emit ultrasonic energy simultaneously. A gradual distancing mechanism is operated via a designated lever on the handle. The lever deploys three petals between the ultrasonic elements, and thus positions the ultrasonic elements at a safe distance from the renal artery wall. The catheter design (multiple ultrasonic elements and the distancing mechanism) facilitates and simplifies the procedure. Bilateral denervation is achieved by delivering US energy in up to three locations within each renal artery.

The TIVUS™ System contains several integrated safety mechanisms as part of the TIVUS™ console, for example:

1. Temperature Sensor (thermistor): Measures the blood temperature near the catheter tip and turns off the excitation if the blood temperature exceeds the maximal pre-set temperature.

2. Distance Sensor and Control: The ultrasound transducer receives ultrasonic echo feedback from the tissue and evaluates the distance from artery wall; this prevents potential thermal damage to the artery wall. If the ultrasound transducer is sensed to be too close to the artery wall, excitation will not be enabled.

In accordance with the general advantages of ultrasonic hyperthermia, the TIVUS™ System may offer several beneficial characteristics:

- Inducing a remote thermal effect in tissues adjacent to vascular lumen.
- The TIVUS™ transducer is positioned intra-luminally and does not touch the arterial wall, thus preventing direct thermal or mechanical effect.
- The catheter system allows continuous cooling of the transducers and the vessel wall by preserving uninterrupted maintenance of renal blood flow.
- Real-time feedback enables a monitored yet robust treatment.
- The flexibility of the Multidirectional TIVUS™ enables circumferential treatment in short renal arteries.
- Absence of any interaction of the ultrasound waves with metal allows treatment of previously stented segments, not otherwise possible with RF energy.

Mechanism of Action

The TIVUS™ System uses high intensity US to induce thermal effect to target nerves, and is intended for renal denervation. US is a widely accepted energy source for hyperthermia

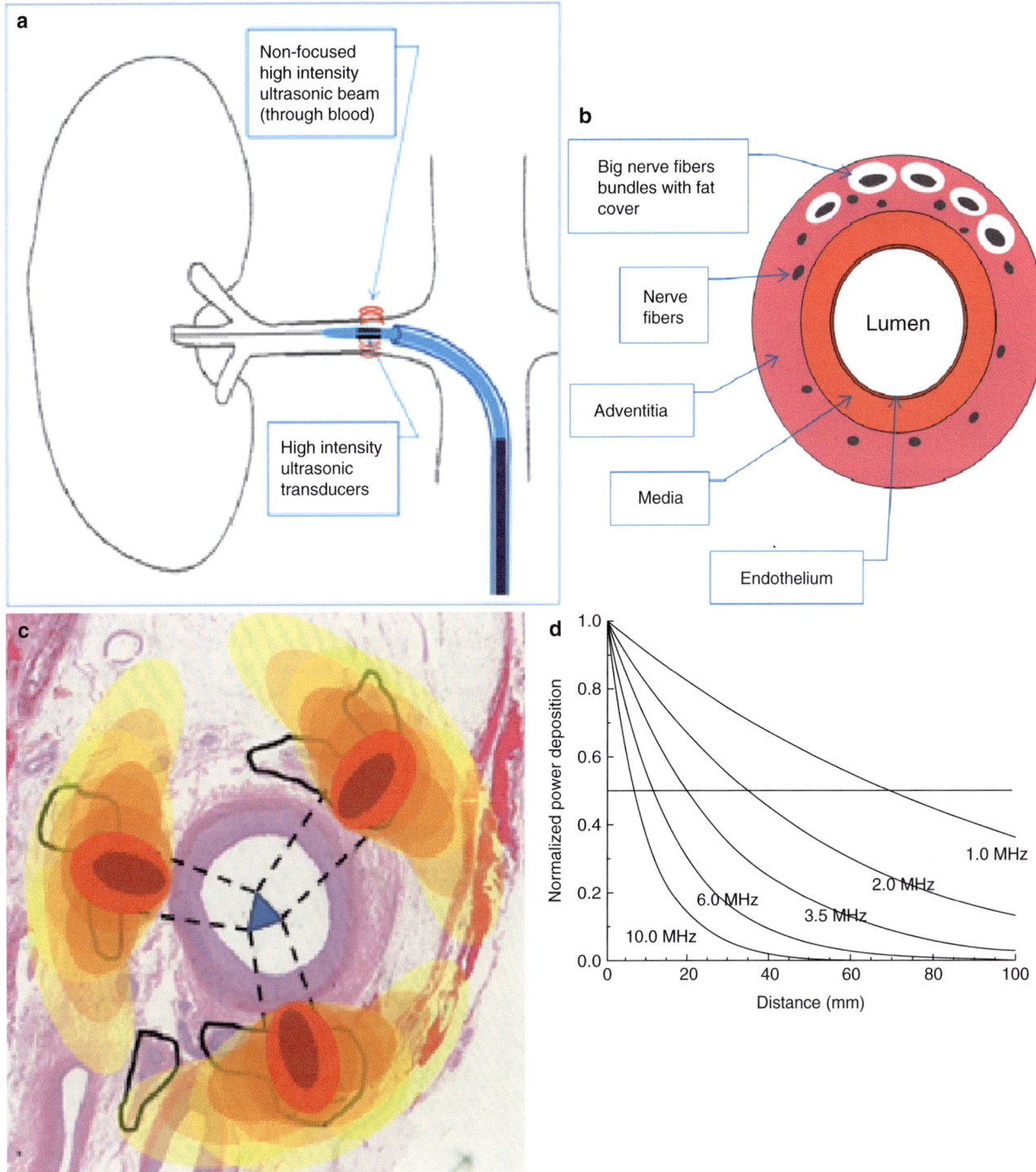

Fig. 10.3 Renal denervation using the TIVUS™ system: (**a**) Catheter positioning in a renal artery. (**b**) Transverse section of a peripheral artery. (**c**) Thermal effect to connective tissue and nerves following TIVUS™ treatment (*dark line*), illustration of the TIVUS™ ultrasonic transducers and the path of the ultrasonic energy beam, as well as the inner artery spared layers and intact endothelium. (**d**) Thermal effect distance per ultrasonic beam frequency (Printed with permission from Cardiosonic)

therapy in various organs [2]. The TIVUS™ System, comprised of a catheter-mounted ultrasonic transducer and a console, generates high intensity, non-focused ultrasonic energy which can be delivered percutaneously to tissues adjacent to blood vessels of varying diameters (Fig. 10.3a).

In contrast to low intensity US applied for imaging, where tissue heating is negligible, the US energy generated by the TIVUS™ System is absorbed into the tissue and transformed into heat, thus resulting in a thermal effect on the target tissue and nerves. The other ultrasonic effects on tissue (such as

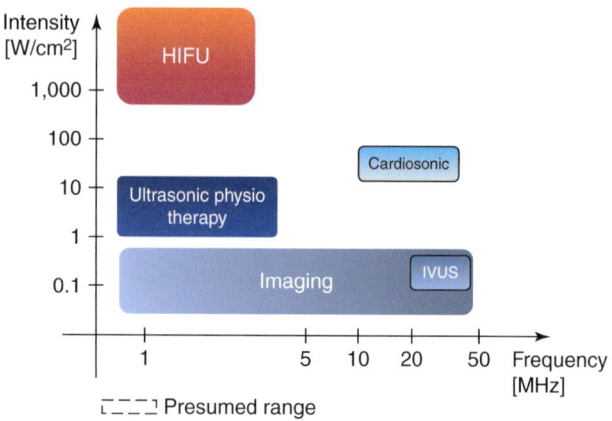

Fig. 10.4 Medical ultrasonic modalities (Printed with permission from Cardiosonic)

cavitation or streaming) are insignificant. Figure 10.4 illustrates the intensity and frequency range of the TIVUS™ system in comparison to other ultrasonic medical modalities. It is noteworthy that while Cardiosonic's US element frequency is at a higher range similar to imaging modalities, the intensity is somewhat higher than physical therapy devices and significantly lower than High Intensity Focused Ultrasound (HIFU) products, mostly used in oncological therapies. During treatment, the catheter is placed at a distance from the artery wall, therefore preventing mechanical damage to the artery wall and allowing cooling of the ultrasonic transducer as well as vascular intima by renal blood flow. The ultrasonic energy is absorbed by the tissues adjacent to the artery, which is heated to 50–80 °C. Heating a tissue beyond 50 °C causes irreversible denaturation of protein (eg. collagen) and other thermal effects, resulting in remote damage to the outer artery wall layers and perivascular tissue, while avoiding damage to the vessel's intimal layer. Thermal damage to the media, if present, is negligible. When US is applied to nerves located in the adventitial and perivascular layers, heating of nerve cells and their supporting tissue results in axonal degeneration and cell death (Fig. 10.3c) [2, 6, 11]. Heating causes irreversible damage and blockage of unmyelinated nerve fibres above 47 °C and of myelinated nerve fibres above 58 °C [11]. The depth of penetration and hence absorption of US energy, depends on the beam frequency; as the frequency rises, the depth of penetration decreases (Fig. 10.3d).

TIVUS™ Pre-clinical and Clinical Data

Animal Studies

Cardiosonic conducted a series of feasibility experiments (swine model) followed by seven animal studies which included 34 treated animals testing various sets of treatment parameters. The animal testing included assessments of safety and performance as well as comparison to an existing RF based technol-

ogy. 30-day and 45-day safety and performance controlled studies were conducted which included a total of 19 animals treated with different sets of treatment parameters. Analysis revealed no statistically significant renal function alteration, normal angiographic appearance of the renal arteries, and mostly no treatment related renal artery luminal narrowing of >20 % or other abnormalities on histopathological examination. Performance measures resulted in Nor-Epinephrine (NE) concentration lowered by approximately 50 % compared with a standardized reference level (range: 42–93 %).

Clinical Experience-Unidirectional TIVUS

TIVUS I is a First-In-Man (FIM) multicenter study conducted across centres in Australia, Europe and Israel in order to evaluate the TIVUS™ System safety and performance. The study included patients with essential hypertension with Office Systolic Blood Pressure (OSBP) ≥160 mmHg, despite treatment with more than three antihypertensive medications, including a diuretic. In addition, the clinical experience includes patients treated under a compassionate use program for severe resistant hypertension associated with impaired renal function or previously implanted renal artery stent. Overall a total of 18 patients were successfully treated at six investigational sites worldwide. Safety and feasibility have been demonstrated by virtue of absence of device related complications and reduction in blood pressure measurements.

Compassionate Use

Two additional patients underwent this procedure under a compassionate use indication, each approved by the local Ethics Committee as required by national law and regulation. Both patients were male presenting with OSBP of ≥160 mmHg. Demographic data for these patients is summarized in Table 10.1. Both procedures were uncomplicated, with no periprocedural or device related adverse events. These patients were noted to have significant reductions in BP post TIVUS™ procedure, as demonstrated in Fig. 10.5 and Table 10.2.

Current and Future Direction of Clinical Research

TIVUS II Trial

The TIVUS II trial is being conducted in order to further assess the safety, efficacy and performance of the TIVUS™ system using the Multidirectional TIVUS™ Catheter. It is a prospective, multicenter, non-randomized, single-arm, open-label clinical study that was launched in 2013. The trial consists of three

Table 10.1 Baseline data (compassionate use)

Baseline variables	999-001	999-002
Age (years)	69	70
BMI	29.76	32.25
No. of anti-hypertensive meds	5	4
Year diagnosed with HTN	1997	2007
eGFR (mL/min/1.73 m²)	50	44
Serum creatinine (μmol/L)	Up to 2	1.67
Diabetes mellitus	Yes	Yes
Hyperlipidemia	Yes	Yes
Office BP at baseline (SBP/DBP mmHg)	170/69	178/68
24 h ABPM (SBP/DBP mmHg)	160/62	160/47
Reason for companionate use	Moderate decreased renal function	Rt. renal artery stenting (2007)

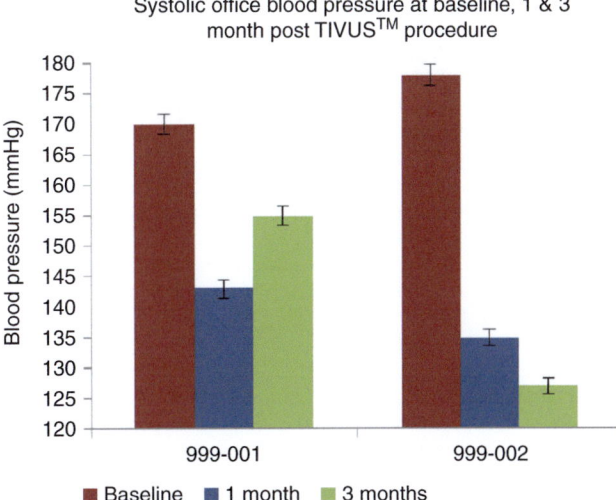

Fig. 10.5 SBP reduction post TIVUS™ procedure per patient (compassionate use) (Printed with permission from Cardiosonic)

Table 10.2 BP reductions (compassionate use)

Patient #	999-001	999-002
Baseline SBP (mmHg)	170	178
1 month follow up	143	135
3 month follow up	155	127

Table 10.3 Baseline characteristics (TIVUS II)

Baseline variables	Mean ± SD or % (n/N)
Age (years)	63.3 ± 11.6
Male gender	56 % (14/25)
Ethnic origin (white)	100 % (25/25)
BMI	33.0 ± 8.3
No. of anti-hypertensive meds	4.6 ± 1.1
eGFR (mL/min/1.73 m²)	80.2 ± 28.9
Serum creatinine (μmol/L)	88.6 ± 29.4
Diabetes mellitus	76 % (19/25)
Hyperlipidemia	44 % (11/25)
Office SBP at baseline (mmHg)	173.7 ± 22.2
Office DBP at baseline (mmHg)	90.7 ± 18.6
24 h ABPM (SBP)	152.9 ± 15.1

concurrent cohorts with a total of 80 patients anticipated to be enrolled. These patients should have adhered to a stable drug regimen including maximally tolerated doses of three or more antihypertensive medications of different classes, of which one must be a diuretic.

Cohort A: TIVUS™ Severe Resistant HTN: A minimum of 58 patients presenting with resistant hypertension and OSBP of 160 mmHg (150 mmHg for DM) or greater.

Cohort B: TIVUS™ Moderate Resistant HTN: About 12 patients presenting with resistant hypertension and OSBP of 140 mmHg (130 mmHg for DM) or greater.

Cohort C: TIVUS™ Failed RF Therapy: About ten patients presenting with resistant hypertension and OSBP of 150 mmHg (140 mmHg) or greater, who underwent RF

renal denervation at least 12 month prior to screening. This cohort will include patients in whom:

- RF renal denervation was done and patient is a non-responder
- RF renal denervation was done, patient responded initially but then systolic BP rose to >150 mmHg (140 mmHg for DM).

This ongoing multicenter study is being conducted in Australia, Europe and Israel. The duration of participation for each patient will be approximately 3 years. Patients will be evaluated post-procedure at hospital discharge, 1-, 3-, 6-, 9- and 12-months. Follow up protocol at these time points will be the same as in TIVUS I study. Surveillance follow-up will then take place semi-annually through 3-years post-procedure. At these time points, record of three blood pressure measurements will be performed.

Preliminary Clinical Data-TIVUS II

To date, a total of 25 patients have undergone renal denervation using the TIVUS™ System as described in Table 10.3. Eighteen were enrolled in cohort A, five in cohort B and two post RF ablation in cohort C.

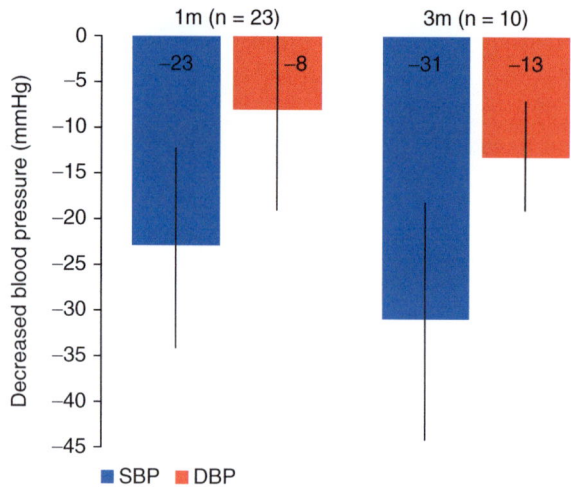

Fig. 10.6 Mean office BP reduction 1 and 3 months post TIVUS™ Procedure (Printed with permission from Cardiosonic)

Fifty six percent of the patients in the TIVUS II study were male, with a mean age of 63.3 years and mean BMI of 33.0. The study patients were on an average number of 4.6 antihypertensive medications. Mean baseline OSBP was 173.7/90.7 mmHg and mean baseline 24-h Ambulatory Blood Pressure 152.9/82.4 mmHg (See Table 10.3 for demographic data). Figure 10.6 demonstrates graphically the mean office blood pressure reduction at 1 and 3 months from TIVUS™ procedure. Patients demonstrated significant reduction in blood pressure over time, most of them showing a substantial decrease. Additionally, patients within cohort A had pronounced reductions of 26/8 mmHg and 32/13 mmHg at 1 and 3 months, respectively.

Conclusion

US based renal denervation is a safe and effective treatment for resistant hypertension. Renal denervation using the TIVUS system shows great promise for treatment of resistant hypertension. Its efficacy, safety and durability remains to be further demonstrated in a larger ongoing study and possibly a randomized controlled trial in the future.

References

1. Azizi M, Steichen O, Frank M, Bobrie G, Plouin PF, Sapoval M. Catheter-based radiofrequency renal-nerve ablation in patients with resistant hypertension. Eur J Vasc Endovasc Surg. 2012;43: 293–9.
2. Diedrierich CJ, Hynhynen K. Ultrasound technology for hyperthermia. Ultrasound Med Biol. 1999;25(6):871–87.
3. Esler MD, Krum H, Sobotka PA, Schlaich MP, Schmieder RE, Bohm M. Renal sympathetic denervation in patients with treatment-resistant hypertension (the symplicity HTN-2 trial): a randomised controlled trial. Lancet. 2010;376:1903–9.
4. Evelyn KA, Singh MM, Chapman WP, Perera GA, Thaler H. Effect of thoracolumbar sympathectomy on the clinical course of primary (essential) hypertension. A ten-year study of 100 sympathectomized patients compared with individually matched, symptomatically treated control subjects. Am J Med. 1960;28:188–221.
5. Krum H, Schlaich M, Whitbourn R, Sobotka PA, Sadowski J, Bartus K, Kapelak B, Walton A, Sievert H, Thambar S, Abraham WT, Esler M. Catheter-based renal sympathetic denervation for resistant hypertension: a multicentre safety and proof-of-principle cohort study. Lancet. 2009;373:1275–81.
6. Leighton TG. What is ultrasound? Prog Biophys Mol Biol. 2007;93:3–83.
7. Mabin T, Sapoval M, Cabane V, Stemmett J, Iyer M. First experience with endovascular ultrasound renal denervation for the treatment of resistant hypertension. EuroIntervention. 2012;8(1): 57–61.
8. Morrissey DM, Brookes VS, Cooke WT. Sympathectomy in the treatment of hypertension; review of 122 cases. Lancet. 1953;1: 403–8.
9. Smithwick RH, Thompson JE. Splanchnicectomy for essential hypertension; results in 1,266 cases. J Am Med Assoc. 1953; 152:1501–4.
10. Symplicity HTN-1 Investigators. Catheter-based renal sympathetic denervation for resistant hypertension: durability of blood pressure reduction out to 24 months. Hypertension. 2011;57(5):911–7.
11. Xu D, Pollock M. Experimental nerve thermal injury. Brain. 1994;117(2):375–84.

The "OneShot" Irrigated Balloon-Mounted Spiral Electrode Renal Denervation Device

William E.L. Ormiston and John A. Ormiston

Introduction

The reduction in office systolic blood pressure in patients with refractory hypertension (HT) using percutaneous transcatheter renal sympathetic denervation (RDN) has been mostly encouraging [1–4]. In addition improvements in renal function, sleep apnea, and heart failure are suggested [5–7]. The first generation percutaneous device (Symplicity, Medtronic, Santa Rosa, CA) achieves RDN by application of radiofrequency (RF) electrical energy in a distal-to-proximal, point-by-point spiral pattern. This typically requires five or six ablations of 2 min duration, to each renal artery. This is time-consuming and the patient may experience more than 25 min of pain.

The OneShot Renal Ablation System (Covidien, Campbell, CA, United States of America) is an irrigated RF balloon designed to deliver electrical current alternating at RF to achieve denervation using a single 2-min ablation to each renal artery. The total duration of energy application is shortened to typically 4 min hence the procedure can be shorter and the duration of pain limited [8, 9]. The spiral electrode may ensure more predictable ablation than a point by point approach.

W.E.L. Ormiston, MBChB (✉)
Department of Radiology, Auckland City Hospital,
Park Rd, Grafton, Auckland, New Zealand
e-mail: WOrmiston@adhb.govt.nz

J.A. Ormiston, MBChB, FRACP, FRACR
Department of Mercy Angiography, Mercy Hospital,
98 Mountain Rd, Epsom, Auckland 1023, New Zealand

University of Auckland School of Medicine,
Auckland, New Zealand

Cardiology, Auckland City Hospital, Auckland, New Zealand
e-mail: johno@mercyangiography.co.nz

Device Description

The major components of the OneShot Ablation System [8, 9] are the irrigated RF balloon catheter (Fig. 11.1) and a radio frequency generator (RFG) with an integrated pump. A mono-polar silver electrode mounted on the non-compliant balloon in a helical configuration (Fig. 11.1) delivers RF energy to the arterial wall, ensuring delivery in a spiral pattern without the need to manipulate the catheter. The balloon is delivered to the renal artery over a conventional 0.014 in. interventional guide wire through a guide catheter. Radio-opaque markers identify the balloon ends for positioning under fluoroscopy (Fig. 11.1). Balloons are available in 5, 6 and 7 mm diameters. The guide catheter size used for the first trial was 9F [8] but subsequent balloons are compatible with 7 and 8F guides. The balloon is inflated to nominal size at 1 atmosphere pressure with normal saline delivered by the pump integrated to the RFG. The inflated balloon stabilizes electrode contact with the renal arterial wall. Renal angiography showing occlusion of the artery by the balloon assures contact of the ablating spiral electrode with the arterial wall (Fig. 11.1). During ablation, saline seeps from the eight irrigation holes that are present in the balloon close to the electrode (Fig. 11.1). These are designed to cool and mitigate damage to non-target arterial tissue, effectively allowing the energy to penetrate deeper into the tissue. The spiral monopolar electrode in conjunction with an external dispersive electrode deliver a single, 2-min application of electrical energy alternating at RF to each artery. In long arteries several non-overlapping applications of RF energy may be possible.

The RFG features a touch screen interface for user input and displays instructional messages and procedural feedback such as power delivered, impedance, and remaining treatment time. The RFG displays warning messages and triggers automatic shut-offs to ensure safe operation of the system [8].

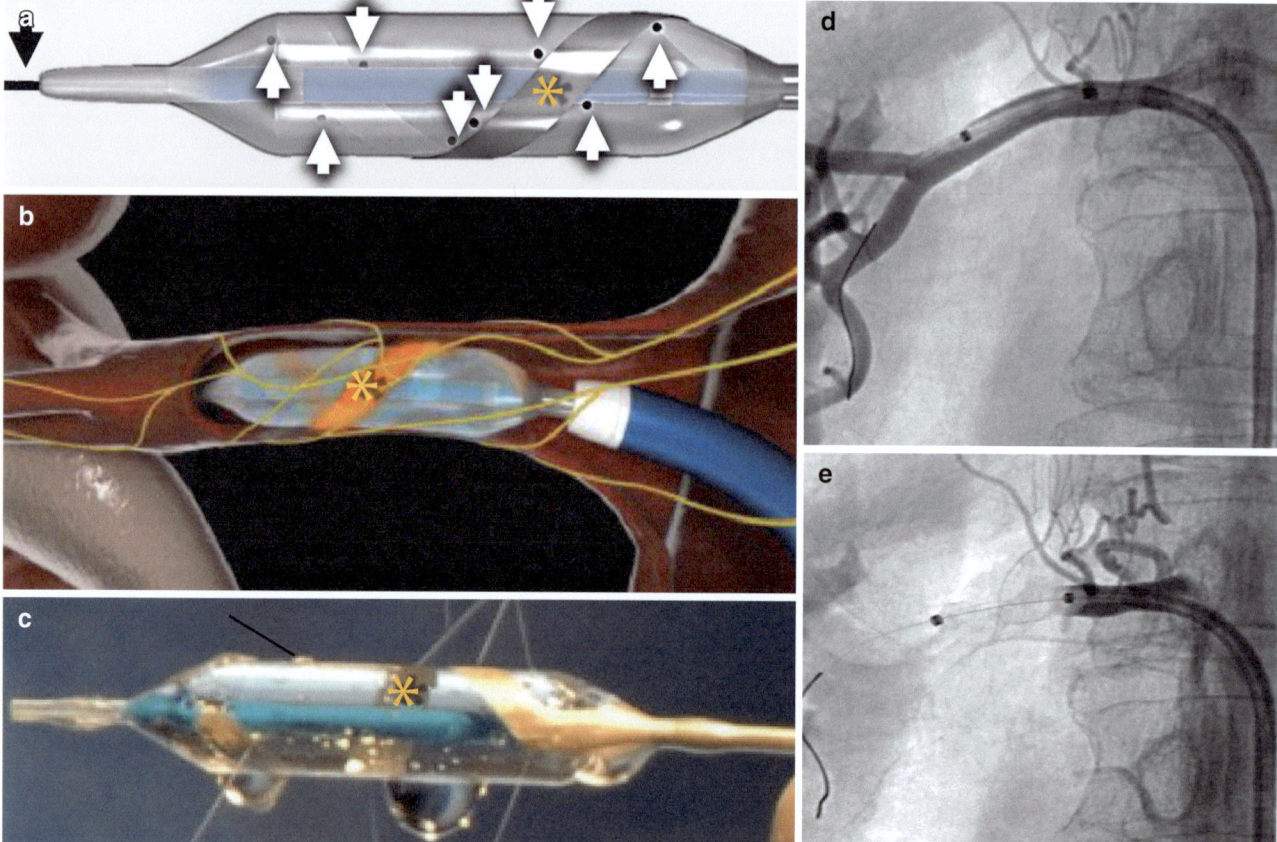

Fig. 11.1 The OneShot irrigated RF renal sympathetic denervation system In (**a**) is depicted the OneShot balloon with the spiral electrode indicated by the asterisks. The *black arrows* indicate the eight irrigation holes in the balloon adjacent to the electrode. The balloon is delivered over a 0.014 in. wire (*white arrow*). The diagram in (**b**) is a left renal artery cutaway showing the inflated balloon and with the spiral electrode in an orange colour. The sympathetic nerves are shown in *yellow*. Shown in (**c**) is a left renal selective angiogram showing the position of the OneShot in this artery. In (**d**) the balloon is inflated and occludes the renal artery indicating the likelihood of apposition of the electrode to the arterial wall. In (**e**) is shown saline irrigation from the balloon holes (Reprinted from Ormiston [9] with permission from Europa Digital & Publishing)

The Renal Hypertension Ablation System (RHAS) Trial [9]

The aims of this first-in-human study were to provide hypothesis generating safety and feasibility data concerning the OneShot renal denervation device.

Endpoints

The primary endpoint was the successful insertion and positioning of the OneShot balloon in each renal artery and delivery of low level radiofrequency energy. Secondary endpoints included: (1) acute procedural safety, defined as absence of serious groin complications or vascular access site complications; (2) procedural success, defined as freedom from complications associated with the delivery and/or use of the OneShot Device or the procedure; and (3) blood pressure lowering effects of the procedure measured by the reduction of office systolic blood pressure at 6 months compared with baseline.

Patients

The inclusion and exclusion criteria were similar to those of the Symplicity HTN trials [1, 2]. Patients 18 years and older were suitable for enrollment if they had a consistent office measured systolic BP greater than or equal to 160 mmHg (or greater than 150 mmHg for patients with type 2 diabetes) despite treatment with two or more antihypertensive medications and had renal artery diameters between 4 and 7 mm. Patients were excluded if they had a glomerular filtration rate less than 45 mL/min/1.73 m [2]. Before ablation, all patients underwent computed tomography angiography (CTA) to exclude those with inappropriate renal artery diameters, multiple large arteries, early arterial division, more than mild renal artery stenosis, and serious renal abnormalities.

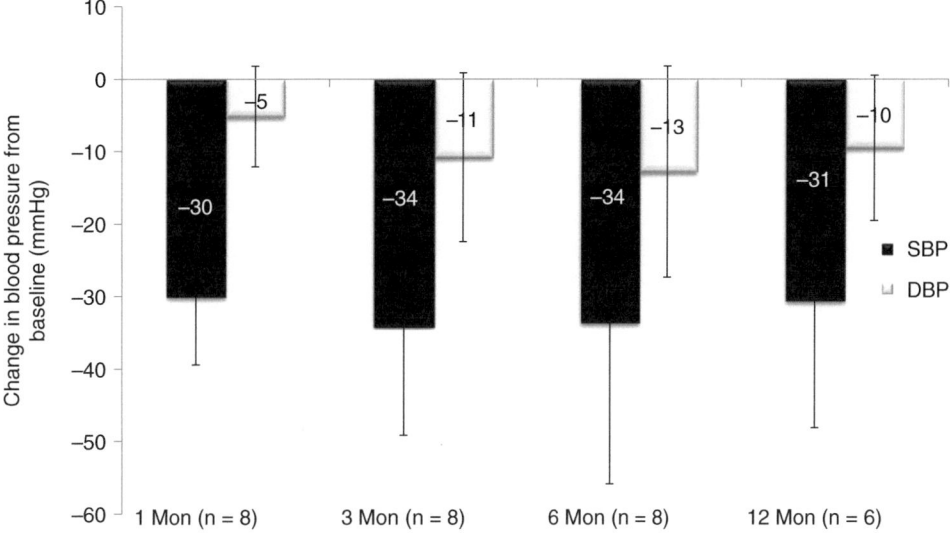

Fig. 11.2 Change in mean (with SD) office blood pressure at 1, 3, 6 and 12 months. The numbers in parenthesis indicate the number of patients with data at each visit

Follow-up

Patient assessments were carried out before the procedure and at 1, 3, 6 and 12 months follow-up. At each follow-up office blood pressure was measured, medications reviewed and potential adverse events assessed.

Study Management

Data were independently monitored to ensure compliance with the protocol and to verify that the data matched source medical records. An independent Clinical Events Committee adjudicated study endpoints and events that occurred throughout the study. The Data and Safety Monitoring Board reviewed all safety issues.

Statistical Analysis

This study was hypothesis generating and designed to provide initial performance information for the OneShot device. The sample size was not defined on the basis of an endpoint hypothesis. Descriptive statistics were provided for baseline demographics, procedural characteristics, and study outcomes. Continuous variables are expressed as mean (standard deviation) and discrete variables as percentages. Given the small sample size, changes in blood pressure were evaluated using paired t-tests. A P value of <0.05 was used as the cut-off was indicative only hence corrections for multiple t-tests were not made. All statistical analyses were performed using Statistical Analysis System (SAS) for Windows version 9.2 (SAS Institute Inc. Cary, NC).

Results

Of the 9 patients, mean age was 59.5 years, 5/9 were males, 1/9 was diabetic [9] and mean number of anti-hypertensive medications per patient was 2.9±6 [9]. The median time from insertion of the OneShot balloon to the end of treatment was 17 (interquatile range 16.0, 20.0) min. The median procedure time (arterial access to end of treatment) was 35 (30.0, 45.0) min. Median fluoroscopy time was 7.7 (7.0, 8.9) minutes and median contrast volume used was 124.0 (122.0, 130.0) min [9].

The primary endpoint of the RHAS trial, the successful insertion and positioning in each renal artery of the OneShot irrigated balloon and delivery of radiofrequency energy was achieved in 8 of 9 patients [9]. The one failure was with the first patient and was due to the high-impedance safety shut-off threshold set too low for humans. This was subsequently solved by minor generator reprogramming. The device was safe with only minor adverse events at 6 months post procedure [9].

The device was effective with over 80 % of patients having a reduction of systolic BP of >10 mmHg. The mean reduction at 12 months was 31 mmHg (Fig. 11.2). No renal artery stenosis was detected by CT angiography at 6 months. In the eight patients there was no change in renal function assessed by eGFR and serum creatinine [9].

The Rapid Trial

The Rapid renal sympathetic denervation for resistant hypertension trial using the Maya Medical OneShot system (RAPID) was a prospective, multi-center, single-arm study that enrolled 50 patients at 11 clinical sites in Europe and

New Zealand [10] abst). Patients were considered for enrollment based on an office systolic blood pressure of 160 mmHg or more despite treatment with a regimen three or more antihypertensive medications including a diuretic. Follow-up period was at 1, 3, 6, 12, 24 and 36 months. The primary safety endpoints include acute procedural safety (defined as the overall rate of serious adverse events and adverse device effects at discharge; and chronic procedural safety (defined as the overall rate of serious adverse events and adverse device events at 6 months). The primary effectiveness endpoint was the rate of office systolic blood pressure reduction >10 mmHg at 6 months compared with baseline.

Fifty patients were enrolled with a mean age of 63.0 years (58.0 % male).

Patients were on a mean of 4.9 antihypertensive drugs at baseline. The mean baseline office systolic and diastolic blood pressure measurements were 181.6 ± 20.8 and 95.5 ± 15.5 mmHg, respectively. At 1 month there was a significant reduction of systolic (-17 and -7 mmHg, $p < 0.0001$ and $p < 0.0008$ respectively) in both office systolic and diastolic blood pressures [10].

The Future of the Oneshot Program

In early January, 2014, Medtronic Corp (Santa Rosa, CA) announced that the sham controlled Symplicity III randomized trial reached is primary safety endpoint but failed to reach its primary efficacy endpoint. While the results with the OneShot appeared promising, Covidien subsequently announced that it would exit its OneShot Renal Denervation program primarily in response to slower than expected development of the renal denervation market.

References

1. Investigators SH. Renal sympathetic denervation in patients with treatment resistant hypertension (the symplicity HTN-2 trial): a randomized controlled trial. Lancet. 2010. doi:10.1016/S0140-6736(10)62039-9.
2. Investigators SH. Catheter-based renal sympathetic denervation for resistant hypertension: durability of blood pressure reduction out to 24 months. Hypertension. 2011;57:911–6.
3. Krum H, Schlaich M, Whitbourn R, Sobotka P, Sadowski J, Bartus K, Kapelak B, Walton A, Sievert H, Thambar S, Abraham W, Esler M. Catheter-based renal sympathetic denervation for resistant hypertension: a multicentre safety and proof-of-principle cohort study. Lancet. 2009;373:1275–81.
4. Esler M, Krum H, Schmieder R, Bohm M. Renal sympathetic denervation for treatment of resistant hypertension: two-year update from the Symplicity HTN-2 randomized controlled trial. J Am Coll Cardiol. 2013;61(10):A342.
5. Witkowski A, Prejbisz A, Florczak E, Kadziela J, Sliwinski P, Bielen P, Michalowska I, Kabat M, Warchol E, Januszewicz M, Narkiewicz K, Somers V, Sobotka P, Januszewicz A. Effects of renal sympathetic denervation on blood pressure, sleep apnea and glycemic control patients with resistant hypertension and sleep apnea. Hypertension. 2011;58:559–65.
6. Brandt M, Mahfoud F, Reda S, Schirmer S, Erdmann E, Bohm M, Hoppe U. Renal sympathetic denervation reduces left ventricular hypertrophy and improves cardiac function in patients with resistant hypertension. J Am Coll Cardiol. 2012;59:901–9.
7. Sobotka P, Krum H, Bohm M, Francis D, Schaiach M. The role of renal denervation in the treatment of heart failure. Curr Cardiol Rep. 2012. doi:10.1007/s11886-012-0258-x.
8. Ormiston J, Watson T, van Pelt N, Stewart R, Haworth P, Stewart J, Webster M. First-in-human use of the oneshot renal denervation system from covidien. Eurointerv. 2013;8:1090–4.
9. Ormiston J, Watson T, van Pelt N, Stewart R, Stewart J, White J, Doughty R, Stewart F, Macdonald R, Webster M. Renal denervation for resistant hypertension using an irrigated radiofrequency balloon: 12-month results from the renal hypertension ablation system (RHAS) trial. Eurointerv. 2013;9:70–4.
10. Verheye S. Preliminary result of the rapid renal sympathetic denervation for resistant hypertension using the Maya medical oneshot ablation system. www.jacctctabstracts2013.com. 2013:TCT-62.

Nevin C. Baker, Israel M. Barbash, and Ron Waksman

While radiofrequency (RF) ablation has been the predominate method for renal nerve denervation (RDN), alternative methods have now been developed and show promise for the rapidly expanding field of hypertension control. Among these novel approaches is a concept dating back to the early 1990s, vascular brachytherapy (VBT), which is currently approved by the Food and Drug Administration for the treatment of coronary artery in-stent restenosis. Similar to RF ablation, it offers the potential to cause cellular degeneration, perineural inflammation, and nerve fibrosis which are necessary for successful and complete denervation.

VBT uses a variety of clinically tested isotopes [^{192}Ir (gamma sources), ^{32}P, ^{90}Sr/^{90}Y, and ^{188}Re (beta sources)] delivered primarily via catheter-based systems for the purpose of localized radiation administration. Ideal radioisotopes for VBT include dose distribution within a few millimeters from the source with minimal dose gradient, short (<10 min) treatment times, low-dose levels to the surrounding tissues, and sufficient half-life for multiple applications when used in catheter-based systems. While both gamma and beta radiation have been utilized in clinical practice, beta radiation carries the majority of the desirable properties described above and is thus the most clinically attractive in terms of radiation exposure and safety.

For purposes of delivering beta-emitted radiation, only the Beta-Cath™ (Novoste, Norcross, GA) catheter-based system is available. A typical catheter-based VBT device consists of four parts: the transfer device, the radiation source train, the delivery catheter, and the accessories. The transfer device is used to shield, store, and transport the radiation source train to and from the treatment zone. The transfer device is a small hand-held system that hydraulically transports the train to and from the treatment zone using sterile water. Each radioactive source is 2.5 mm in length and the source train has a non-active radiopaque marker at each end. The transfer device contains 16 sources (40-mm device) to treat different injury length changes. The Beta-Cath™ 3.5F catheter (Fig. 12.1) allows the source train to be transported to the treatment zone. Treatment times are predetermined for each source train and are provided by Best Industries. The accessory pack enables the operator to use the non-sterile transfer device within the sterile field.

N.C. Baker, DO
Department of Interventional Cardiology, MedStar Washington Hospital Center, Washington, DC, USA
e-mail: Nevin.C.Baker@medstar.net

I.M. Barbash, MD
Department of Interventional Cardiology, MedStar Washington Hospital Center, Washington, DC, USA

Interventional Cardiology Department, Sheba Medical Center, Tel Aviv University, Ramat Gan, Israel
e-mail: ibarbash@gmail.com

R. Waksman, MD (✉)
Department of Interventional Cardiology, MedStar Heart Institute/MedStar Washington Hospital Center,
110 Irving St., NW, Suite 4B-1, Washington, DC 20010, USA
e-mail: ron.waksman@medstar.net

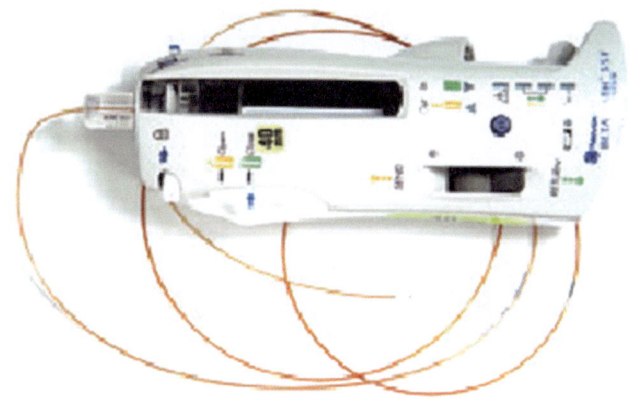

Fig. 12.1 Beta-Cath™ 3.5F system

R.R. Heuser et al. (eds.), *Renal Denervation: A New Approach to Treatment of Resistant Hypertension*,
DOI 10.1007/978-1-4471-5223-1_12, © Springer-Verlag London 2015

Limitations of RF Ablation

Ample data exists to support the concept of renal sympathetic nerve RF ablation for the treatment of resistant hypertension [1, 2]. Despite these results, an unmet need for alternative approaches still exists, mainly due to the fact that RF renal nerve ablation requires strategically placed ablations separated both longitudinally and rotationally within each renal artery to avoid adverse vascular events, particularly renal artery stenosis, and offer 'complete' denervation.

While safety results from pilot studies suggest safety with RF ablation [1], recent findings suggest that a degree of vascular injury exists that may not have initially been appreciated. Using a very sensitive tool for detection of vascular injury, Templin et al. assessed the morphological features of endothelial and vascular injury induced by RF renal nerve ablation using optical coherence tomography [3]. The authors were able to demonstrate local tissue damage that was not apparent with angiography, particularly local and diffuse vasospasm and thrombus formation following endothelial injury. Safety concerns notwithstanding, it has also been difficult to ascertain why as many as 16 % of patients undergoing RDN do not respond. While the precise failure mechanism is not entirely clear, a possible explanation may be missed ablation spots, which are the result of 'patchy' ablations or inability of the RF catheter to cause permanent nerve damage. Indeed, next generation RDN RF catheters are now being designed with this in mind. Brachytherapy for RDN may offer a method which is either as safe or perhaps improves on vascular safety, and may prove more efficacious given its large, homogenous effect.

Radiation Mediated Nerve Damage

The concept of radiation-mediated nerve injury has been studied in the animal model as well as implemented in current daily clinical practice. In 1985, after discovering that a number of their patients developed clinical signs of lumbosacral or sciatic neuropathy following wide surgical excision plus intraoperative radiotherapy at doses of 20–25 Gy, Kinsella et al. used the canine model to investigate this clinical observation. Loss of nerve fibers, particularly large myelinated fibers, were observed after treatment with 20–75 Gy of intraoperative radiation therapy to the sciatic

nerve [4]. No vascular thrombosis or occlusion was observed. A few years later, LeCouteur et al. evaluated radiotherapy on the peripheral nerves in canines and found a graded effect of radiation-induced nerve damage at doses beginning at 15 Gy [5]. Irreversible peripheral neuropathies were seen beginning around 6 months. Histopathological studies of nerves up to 2 years following irradiation demonstrated loss of axons and myelin, with a corresponding increase in endoneurial, perineurial, and epineurial connective tissue. Percentage of axon and myelin decreased to about 60 % of normal at 15 Gy and additionally at higher doses. Sindelar et al. studied pathological changes at autopsy (1–18 months after radiation therapy) for 22 patients who had been treated with intraoperative radiotherapy resulting in perineural fibrosis in the areas that were radiated [6]. Importantly, significant radiation related changes were generally not observed in major blood vessels. Clinically, stereotactic radiosurgery causes focal axonal degeneration of the trigeminal nerve. Gamma knife radiosurgery is now standard treatment for trigeminal neuralgia, showing safety and positive long-term results [7].

VBT for Renal Denervation

For many years, VBT has demonstrated to be a safe method for the treatment of coronary and renal artery in-stent restenosis [8–12]. The theoretical advantage of this approach is one of both safety and efficacy. Available histology data show that the degree of arterial damage may be smaller as compared with other reported methods, and VBT offers the ability to cover a more diffuse vascular segment, allowing, in theory, a more 'complete' denervation. This theory was tested by Waksman et al. who initially assessed the safety and feasibility of beta radiation for RDN in the animal model [13].

A total of 10 normotensive domestic swine underwent bilateral renal artery brachytherapy via the Beta-Cath™ 3.5F System (Fig. 12.1) at doses of 25 Gy (n=8) or 50 Gy (n=8) at 2 mm from the source center. Compared with untreated arteries serving as controls (n=4), the VBT procedure proved safe at both the clinical and microscopic levels with no apparent angiographic or intravascular ultrasound injuries to the vessel evident at follow up, (Figs. 12.2 and 12.3) and no thrombus or microscopic evidence of stenosis in any of the larger artery sections. Varying degrees of arteriolar changes

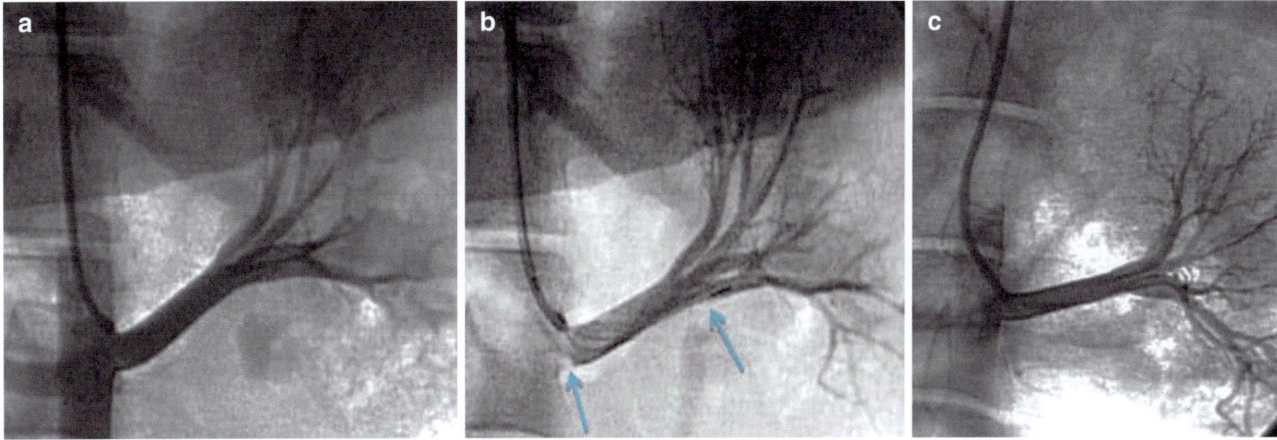

Fig. 12.2 Renal artery angiography post brachytherapy showing wide patency of the renal arteries without angiographic evidence of stenosis or aneurysm. (**a**) Baseline angiography. (**b**) Immediately following beta radiation. *Blue arrows* mark radiation source length. (**c**) Angiography at 2-month follow up (Reprinted from Waksman et al. [13] with permission from Europa Digital & Publishing)

Fig. 12.3 Intravascular ultrasound at 2-months post brachytherapy (Reprinted from Waksman et al. [13] with permission from Europa Digital & Publishing)

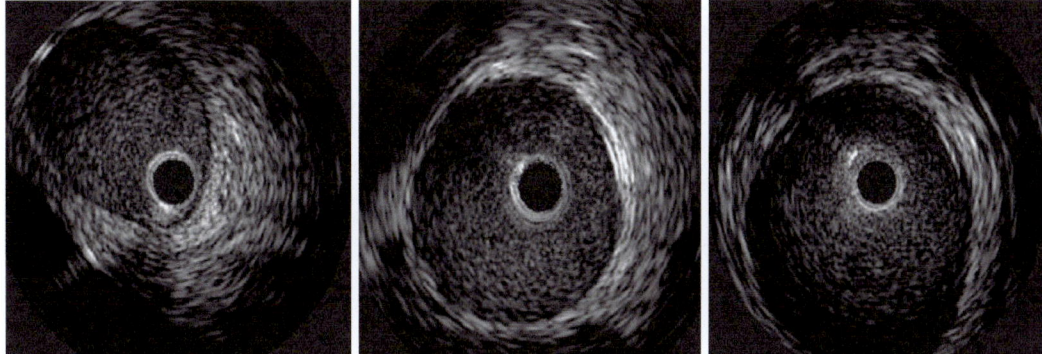

were present in the examined sections, with most showing a 2–20 % degree of endothelial cell loss. Importantly, there was no damage to adjacent body tissue or organs.

Light microscopy revealed varying degrees of histopathological neuronal changes associated with the extent of thermal injury (Fig. 12.4). At 1 month follow-up, 50 % of the nerves showed some degree of injury with a clear dose related injury-effect seen (Fig. 12.5a). Furthermore, the injury severity correlated with the radiation dose (Fig. 12.5b).

This initial safety and feasibility study of VBT for RDN indicates that this approach can cause substantial nerve fibrosis while avoiding significant damage to the renal artery. Based on these results, a first-in-man trial to assess VBT for RDN was approved by the Food and Drug Administration early in 2013 and is currently enrolling patients. The study aims to assess safety of renal artery beta irradiation VBT and to provide proof-of-concept that this approach can cause RDN and lower blood pressure in patients with resistant hypertension. Clinical efficacy and safety end points of 6-month systolic and diastolic blood pressure reduction ≥10 mmHg and renal vascular complications will be assessed, respectively.

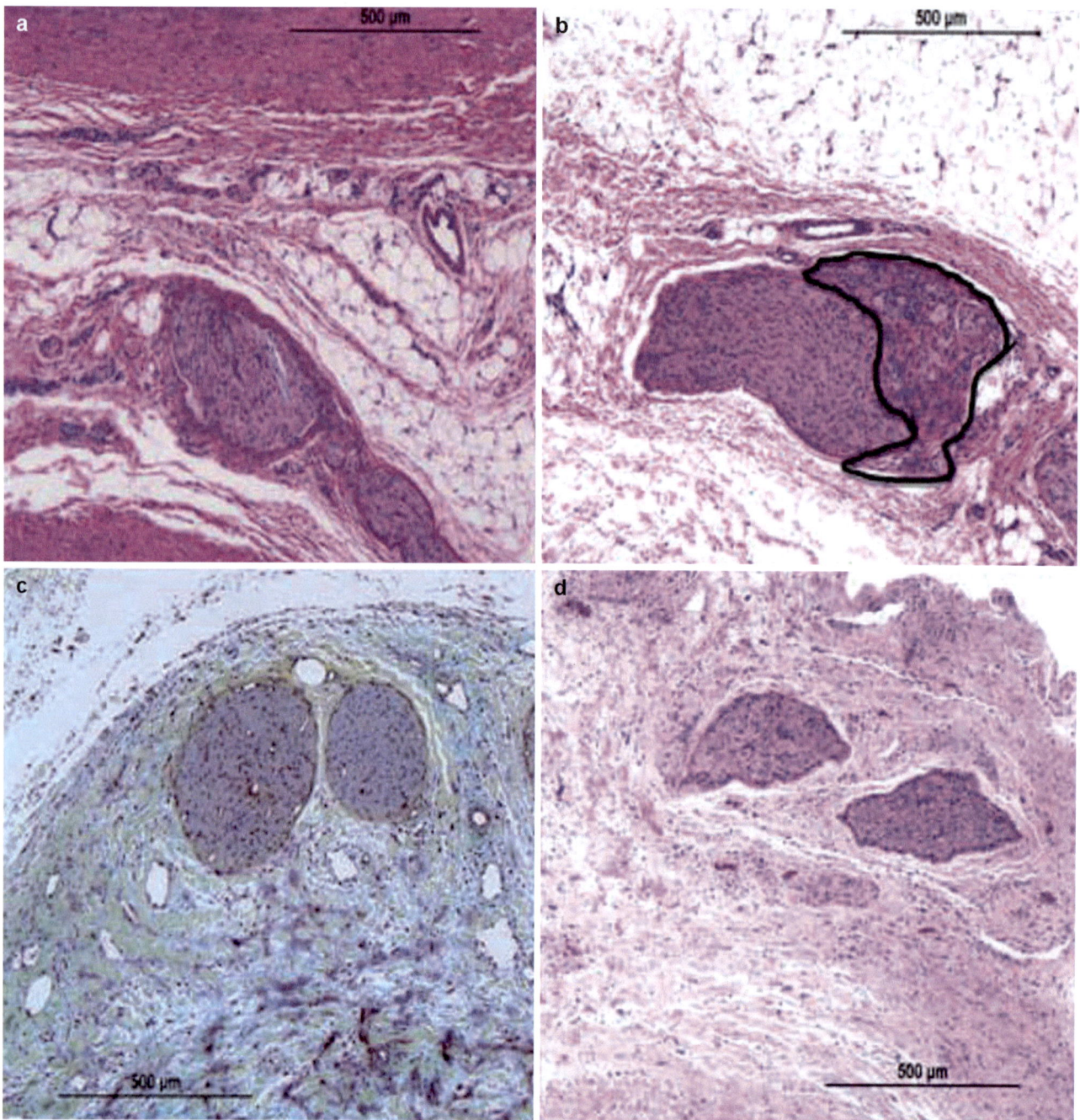

Fig. 12.4 Histological assessment of renal nerve injury. (**a**) High power image showing nerve fascicle with myxoid degeneration, H&E. (**b**) High power image showing nerve fascicles with endoneural/perineural inflammation and cellular degeneration (*blue area*), H&E. (**c**) Relation of injury to the renal artery. Focal periadventitial fat necrosis with fibrosis and myxoid degeneration, Movat. (**d**) High power image showing hypocellular fascicles with cellular degeneration, Movat (Reprinted from Waksman et al. [13] with permission from Europa Digital & Publishing)

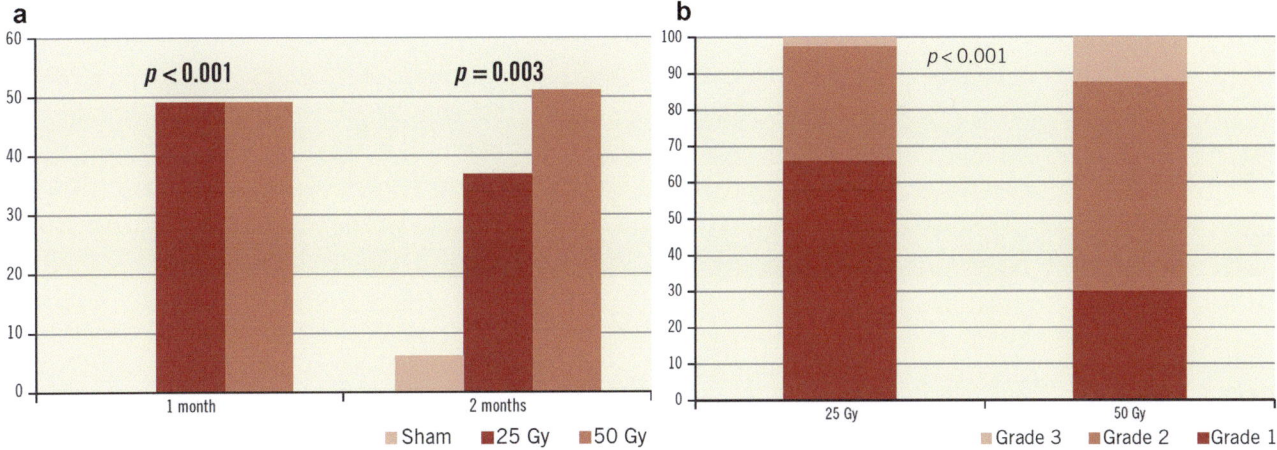

Fig. 12.5 Assessment of renal nerve injury and dose-response relationship. (**a**) Percentage of damaged renal nerves. (**b**) Renal nerve injury grade. A higher percentage of advanced nerve injury was seen among the 50 Gy group (Reprinted from Waksman et al. [13] with permission from Europa Digital & Publishing)

Conclusions

For over two decades, VBT has been safely used for the management of coronary artery in-stent restenosis. This method of cellular disruption and injury has recently crossed into the renal sympathetic denervation. It joins a rapidly growing field of RDN catheter systems currently under development, or already in clinical use, including RF ablation catheters, ultrasound energy, and local drug delivery-based systems. Ideally, any system implemented for RDN will need to maximize permanent nerve injury in a predictable pattern while minimizing damage to the local artery and surrounding structures, have a short procedure time, as well as minimize patient discomfort. The search for this system continues with VBT.

References

1. Krum H, Schlaich M, Whitbourn R, Sobotka PA, Sadowski J, Bartus K, et al. Catheter-based renal sympathetic denervation for resistant hypertension: a multicentre safety and proof-of-principle cohort study. Lancet. 2009;373:1275–81.
2. Esler MD, Krum H, Sobotka PA, Schlaich MP, Schmieder RE, Bohm M. Renal sympathetic denervation in patients with treatment-resistant hypertension (the symplicity HTN-2 Trial): a randomised controlled trial. Lancet. 2010;376:1903–9.
3. Templin C, Jaguszewski M, Ghadri JR, Sudano I, Gaehwiler R, Hellermann JP, et al. Vascular lesions induced by renal nerve ablation as assessed by optical coherence tomography: pre- and post-procedural comparison with the simplicity catheter system and the EnligHTN multi-electrode renal denervation catheter. Eur Heart J. 2013;34:2141–8.
4. Kinsella TJ, Sindelar WF, DeLuca AM, Pezeshkpour G, Smith R, Maher M, et al. Tolerance of peripheral nerve to intraoperative radiotherapy (IORT): clinical and experimental studies. Int J Radiat Oncol Biol Phys. 1985;11:1579–85.
5. LeCouteur RA, Gillette EL, Powers BE, Child G, McChesney SL, Ingram JT. Peripheral neuropathies following experimental intraoperative radiation therapy (IORT). Int J Radiat Oncol Biol Phys. 1989;17:583–90.
6. Sindelar WF, Hoekstra H, Restrepo C, Kinsella TJ. Pathological tissue changes following intraoperative radiotherapy. Am J Clin Oncol. 1986;9:504–9.
7. Park SH, Hwang SK. Outcomes of gamma knife radiosurgery for trigeminal neuralgia after a minimum 3-year follow-up. J Clin Neurosci. 2011;18:645–8.
8. Waksman R, Cheneau E, Ajani AE, White RL, Pinnow E, Torguson R, et al. Intracoronary radiation therapy improves the clinical and angiographic outcomes of diffuse in-stent restenotic lesions: results of the Washington Radiation for In-Stent Restenosis Trial for Long Lesions (Long WRIST) Studies. Circulation. 2003;107:1744–9.
9. Stoeteknuel-Friedli S, Do DD, von Briel C, Triller J, Mahler F, Baumgartner I. Endovascular brachytherapy for prevention of recurrent renal in-stent restenosis. J Endovasc Ther. 2002;9:350–3.
10. Jahraus CD, Meigooni AS. Vascular brachytherapy: a new approach to renal artery in-stent restenosis. J Invasive Cardiol. 2004;16:224–7.
11. Use of gamma radiation for treatment of renal artery in-stent restenosis. Cardiovasc Radiat Med. 2001;2:197–8.
12. Waksman R, Ajani AE, White RL, Chan R, Bass B, Pichard AD, et al. Five-year follow-up after intracoronary gamma radiation therapy for in-stent restenosis. Circulation. 2004;109:340–4.
13. Waksman R, Barbash IM, Chan R, Randolph P, Makuria AT, Virmani R. Beta radiation for renal nerve denervation: initial feasibility and safety. EuroIntervention. 2013;9:738–44.

Perivascular Renal Denervation (PVRD™): Chemical Renal Denervation with Micro-Doses of Ethanol Using the Peregrine™ Renal Denervation Device

Tim A. Fischell, Félix Vega, and Vartan E. Ghazarossian

Introduction

In the 1930s–1950s surgical renal sympathectomy was used to treat severe hypertension [1–3]. Despite a successful lowering of blood pressure (BP) observed with surgical denervation, this technique was abandoned due to a relatively high morbidity and mortality, and as a result of the development of more effective oral antihypertensive medications.

Recently, catheter-based renal sympathetic denervation has been performed using a point-by-point, mono-polar radiofrequency (RF) ablation catheter from within the renal artery [4–11]. This technique has been shown to disrupt renal sympathetic nerve activity [4–7], resulting in substantial and sustained blood pressure lowering in patients with severe and medically resistant hypertension [4–11].

The ability to lower blood pressure using a catheter-based ablative technique from within the renal artery has led to a proliferation of new technologies intended to expand and validate this observation, and to improve the ease-of-use, safety, and predictability of catheter-based renal sympathetic denervation [12–14].

Virtually all of these new denervation devices have focused upon "energy-based" denervation, utilizing predominantly RF or ultrasound catheters. These catheters are designed to deliver ablative thermal injury through the intima and medial layers of the renal artery, in order to target and destroy the sympathetic nerve fibers that traverse from the

T.A. Fischell, MD, FACC (✉)
Heart Institute at Borgess Medical Center, Kalamazoo, MI, USA

Ablative Solutions, Inc., Kalamazoo/Menlo Park, MI/CA, USA
e-mail: tafisc@gmail.com

V.E. Ghazarossian, PhD
Ablative Solutions, Inc., Kalamazoo/Menlo Park, MI/CA, USA
e-mail: Vartan@ablativesolutions.com

F. Vega, VMD
Preclinical Consultants, 53 Carmelita Street,
San Francisco, CA, USA
e-mail: PreclinicalConsultation@gmail.com

aorta, to the kidney within the adventitial and peri-adventitial space surrounding the renal arteries [4–12].

A number of these "next generation" RF and ultrasound transmural thermal- ablation catheters have been tested in patients and have validated the results from the original Simplicity Trials, with significant BP lowering seen after renal sympathetic (thermal) denervation [11–14].

Despite the moderate efficacy of both the first and next generation RF and ultrasound catheters, there are limitations, and potential safety concerns associated with the use of transmural thermal injury traversing the intimal and medial layers of the renal artery in order to create thermal injury to the sympathetic nerves that may run from 2 to 10 mm deep to the intimal surface [15–18]. In addition, the early generation RF devices appear to have a relatively modest effect upon BP when measured with ambulatory BP monitoring, as well as a relatively high "non-responder" rate.

Rationale for Chemical Renal Denervation with Ethanol

Given the potential limitations of RF and ultrasound, we have developed a novel micro-needle based drug delivery catheter (Peregrine™, Ablative Solutions, Inc. Menlo Park, CA). This device was developed in order to study the feasibility, safety and efficacy of chemical denervation using very small volumes of ethanol (EtOH), a known potent neurolytic agent. With this device (see Fig. 13.1) one can deliver micro-doses (150–600 µL) of EtOH precisely and locally to the adventitial and peri-adventitial space of the renal artery (termed PeriVascular Renal Denervation; PVRD™), with three simultaneously deployed micro-needles. This system has now been evaluated in pre-clinical testing and most recently, in an early human safety and feasibility clinical study, as a means to perform renal sympathetic denervation.

The key concepts and rationale for this methodology to create renal denervation are: (1) to deliver a very small volume of a highly potent neurolytic agent (EtOH) precisely

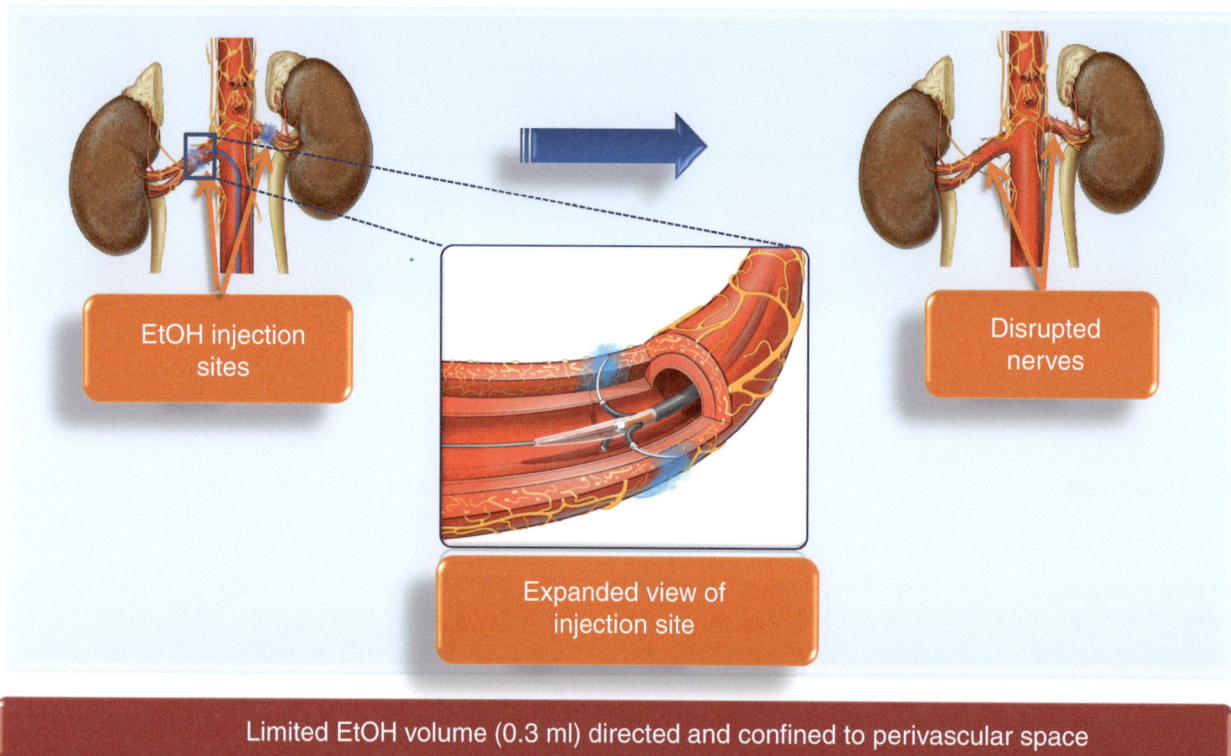

Fig. 13.1 Schematic drawings showing sequence of chemical denervation with EtOH. The *upper left panel* shows the anatomy of the mid-portion of the renal artery and shows no significant organs in the vicinity of the very localized EtOH delivery. The *middle panel* shows the device deployed with micro-dosing of EtOH targeted to the adventitial space (*blue halos* in *right panel*)

to the target area in the adventitia and the peri-adventitia; (2) to deliver the agent with such tiny (micro) needles such that even with full systemic heparin treatment there would be essentially no peri-arterial bleeding risk after the needle entry through the intima and media and into the adventitia, (3) to use an agent such as EtOH that is lipophilic and agrascopic, such that simultaneous injection from three needles placed in one step, at 120° needle separation radially around the renal artery would reproducibly create circumferential spread of the neurolytic agent, and confined to the adventitial space, and allow circumferential sympathetic nerve kill with minimal effects upon the intima and media of the renal artery (nerve kill without renal artery vessel wall injury); (4) to determine the needle depth and doses required to get "deep" sympathetic nerve kill (nerve injury out to 10–12 mm deep to intimal surface), which may be crucial in achieving reproducible and efficient sympathetic denervation; (5) to determine whether or not there is predictable and dose-dependent sympathetic denervation, as judged by the drop in renal parenchymal norepinephrine levels in a porcine model; (6) to determine the safety as judged by short-term (2 weeks) and longer term (3 month) histopathological and angiographic studies in a porcine model; (7) to determine whether or not this technology could be safely applied in clinical cases and finally; (8) to determine whether or not this procedure could have the potential to create renal denervation in humans without the pain that is associated with "thermal" renal denervation using either RF or ultrasound techniques.

Pre-clinical Testing

Extensive pre-clinical testing has now been completed in order to evaluate the safety and efficacy of chemical neurolysis, via adventitial injection of very small doses of dehydrated EtOH to as a means to perform sympathetic denervation, in a porcine model [19].

A novel, three needle-based delivery device, (Peregrine System™, Ablative Solutions, Inc., Menlo Park, CA) was introduced via the femoral artery into renal arteries of adult swine using fluoroscopic guidance. The drug injection catheter is an endovascular delivery catheter that contains three distal needles housed inside of individual guide tubes, which are contained within the catheter. The catheter has a steerable, radio-opaque 2 cm fixed, floppy guide-wire at its distal end to minimize renal artery trauma and allow steerability, when needed, into appropriate branch vessels (Figs. 13.1 and 13.2a–c).

The animal studies were conducted under the general principles of Good Laboratory Practice (GLP) regulations as set forth in 21 CFR 58. Animals were pre-medicated with 325 mg

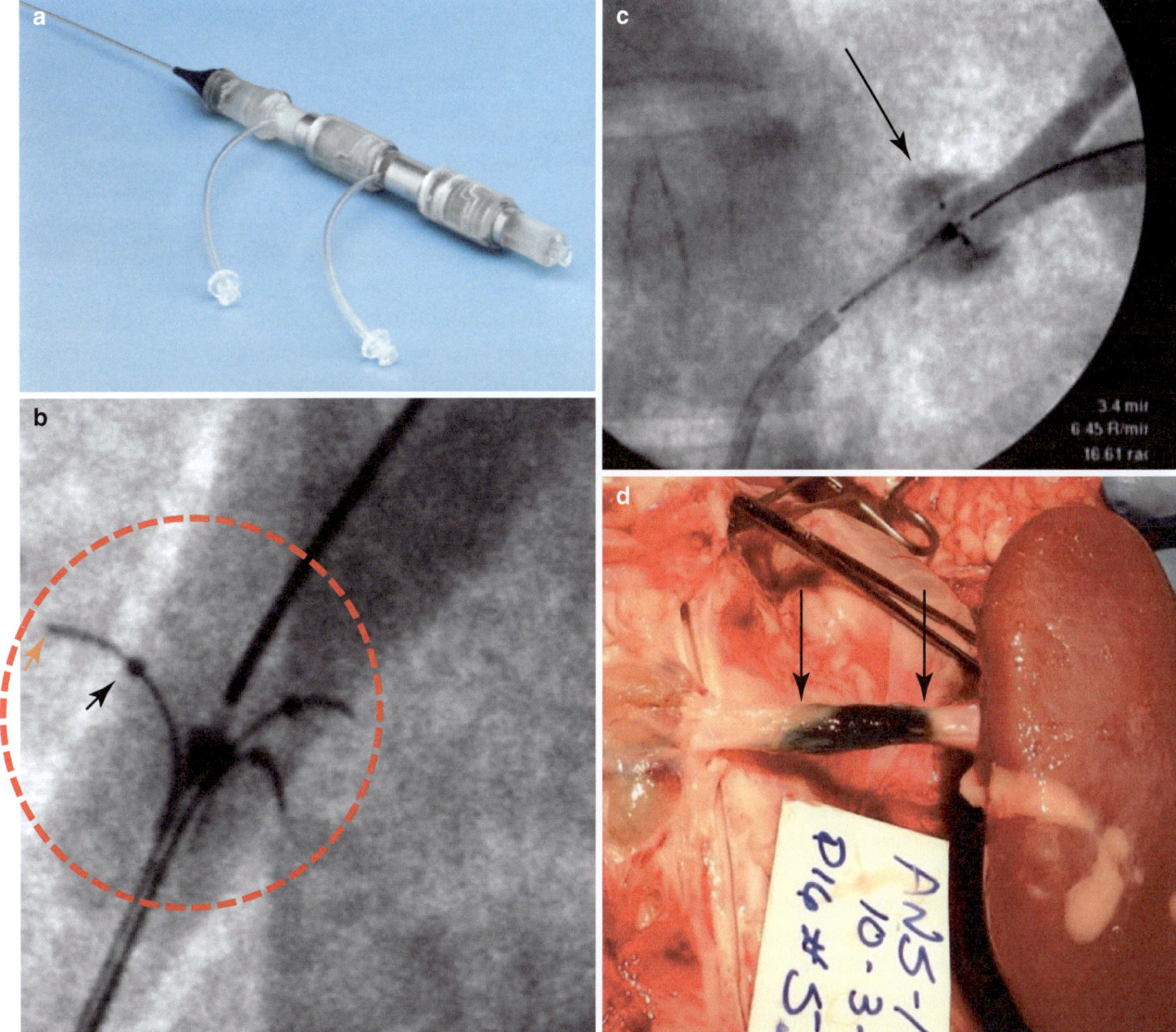

Fig. 13.2 Panel (**a**) shows the device handle that controls the tubes, needles and injection port. In (**b**), the device is deployed and centered in a porcine renal artery during contrast injection from the guiding catheter. *Black arrow* shows tip of guide tube against the intima and *orange arrow* shows tip of radio-opaque 0.008″ injection needle. Panel (**c**) show injection of ~0.2 ml of dilute contrast demonstrating injection 100 % limited to the adventitial space. The *black arrow* shows the appearance of a small volume of dilute contrast that is angiographically apparent in the adventitial and peri-adventitial layer of the renal artery after the purposeful injection of 0.30 ml of dilute contrast through the deployed Peregrine needles. In Panel (**d**) immediate necropsy is shown after injecting 0.15 ml EtOH combined with methylene blue to define the circumferential and very defined longitudinal (*black arrows*) spread of EtOH in the tunica adventitia

of aspirin and 75 mg of clopidogrel by mouth once daily for 2 days before the procedure. The animals were assigned to study groups at random, before the procedure began.

The animals were pre-medicated with intramuscular injection of telazol combined with atropine. When recumbent, animals were anesthetized with a mixture of isoflurane and oxygen delivered via facemask. When sufficiently anesthetized the animals were intubated and connected to a closed-circuit anesthesia system and maintained on isoflurane combined with oxygen. Blood was collected for evaluation of hematology (CBC) and serum chemistry. Urine was obtained via cystocentesis.

After the animals were prepared for sterile surgery, one femoral artery was accessed using the Seldinger technique, and a seven French introducer was placed. Intravenous heparin was given in all animals to achieve an ACT of >250 s. In all cases the right and left renal arteries of the pig were engaged using a seven French RDC guiding catheter. Prior to ethanol or saline injections, angiography of each renal artery was performed using iodixanol contrast diluted by 25 % with normal saline.

The Peregrine™ device was advanced into the left or right renal artery via the guiding catheter. Once the operational section of the device was positioned within the target site in the mid-portion of the renal artery, the three guide tubes are deployed spatially at 120°, one to another (see Figs. 13.1 and 13.2b). The tubes were simultaneously deployed up against the intimal surface (Figs. 13.1 and 13.2b), using the advancement mechanism in the control handle (Fig. 13.2a). These atraumatic tubes have radiopaque distal tip markers such that one can clearly define the position of the tubes, particularly when contrast is injected via the guiding catheter (Fig. 13.2b).

Once deployed, the three tubes serve to reproducibly "center" the device within the renal artery. The 0.008″ needles that reside within the distal tip of the tubes are advanced to a depth of 3.5 ± 0.25 mm deep to the intima (i.e., beyond the tip of the guide tube). This function is also performed via the specialized handle, which allows simultaneous advancement of the three injection needles. These tiny needles are made radiopaque, so that they can be easily seen under fluoroscopy. Although not part of the clinical protocol, in animals dilute contrast can be injected once the needles are positioned to confirm placement relatively deep in the adventitial space (Fig. 13.2c).

It should be noted that these needles are the equivalent of a ~30 gauge needle so that they can be safely advanced through the renal arterial wall without causing bleeding. Prior to conducting this study we confirmed that needles of this size could be repeatedly advanced through the wall of the renal artery of pigs that had been pre-treated with high doses of heparin (ACTs 300–600), with no detectable bleeding at the needle puncture sites. This is a key observation relevant to the safety of this approach.

Once the tubes and needles are deployed it is easy to confirm, fluoroscopically, that the needle tips are well outside the luminal space and ~2.5–3.0 mm deep to the media and the external elastic lamina in a normal porcine renal artery (Fig. 13.2b). This corresponds to an injection depth that approximates the border between the renal artery adventitia and peri-adventitia, and which corresponds to a depth to the middle of the renal sympathetic nerve field, as defined in pressure-fixed human histopathological studies by Virmani et al. [18].

The successful deployment of the tubes and needles was confirmed by angiography. EtOH or saline (sham) fluid was then administered, using a 1.0 ml luer-lock syringe attached to the proximal injection lumen at the handle of the catheter. This injection lumen is in fluid continuity with the distal end of all three needles. The injection is performed over 15–20 s.

Three volumes of EtOH were used in this study: 0.15 ml/artery (n = 3 pigs/6 arteries), 0.30 ml/artery (n = 3 pigs/6 arteries) and 0.60 ml/artery (n = 3 pigs/6 arteries). A procedural control group was also studied using the injection of 0.4 ml of saline/artery (n = 3). This was a "sham" arm to control for nonspecific effects that might be caused by mechanical injury from either the guide tubes or the needles, and/or any non-specific effects of fluid delivery. Once the treatment

agent was injected, the dead-space of the catheter was flushed with a very small volume of normal saline. After treatment of the first renal artery the device was removed from the animal, inspected and flushed. The contra-lateral renal artery was then engaged and the same fluid injection sequence was performed in the contralateral renal artery. After the treatment of the second renal artery, the animals were recovered and housed for restudy and sacrifice at 2 weeks post-intervention. The animals were treated with aspirin 162 mg/day for 7 days after intervention.

The circumferential spread of EtOH was evaluated in separate experiments by combining 0.125 ml of EtOH with 0.25 ml of methylene blue (stain). The volume of 0.15 ml was then injected under fluoroscopic guidance. Immediate necropsy was performed and demonstrated reproducible and circumferential spread of the 0.15 ml of the EtOH/methylene blue mixture (Fig. 13.2d). Histopathology was also used to evaluate circumferential spread of alcohol by having the pathologist evaluate and document the location (in terms of circumference) of any noted neuritis and neurolysis. The histopathological examination showed extensive and circumferential nerve injury at the 0.15, 0.30 and 0.60 ml EtOH injection volumes.

Safety and effectiveness of the device were evaluated. The efficacy of denervation was determined by measurement of renal parenchymal norepinephrine (NE) levels (analyzed by HPLC, with electrochemical detection), and using histopathologic evaluation of the peri-renal nerves at the end of the 2-week survival period (Fig. 13.3). Safety was evaluated by histopathologic evaluation of the renal artery and kidney as well as evaluation of clinical pathology. Blood and urine were collected in all animals treated with the device for evaluation of systemic and renal health at baseline and at the time of sacrifice.

The animals were survived for 14 ± 3 days after treatment. At the end of the study period the animals were anesthetized and angiography of the treated right and left renal arteries was obtained to evaluate vessel patency and to look for any luminal narrowing compared to baseline angiography. Four additional animals were studied with follow-up with angiography and pathology at 3 months after ethanol denervation using 300 µL of EtOH (Figs. 13.4 and 13.5).

After angiographic follow-up at 14 days and at 3 months, a necropsy was performed. The renal arteries and kidneys were harvested for histopathological evaluation. Gross pathology to examine the status of the renal arteries was performed to look for renal artery abnormalities such as aneurysms, perforations, dissections, hematoma, etc., as well as inspection of the surrounding tissues for any abnormalities. The renal arteries and kidneys were harvested, retaining the peri-adventitial tissue around the artery. The renal artery tissue was embedded in paraffin using standard techniques. Tissue was stained with H&E. Multiple sites

Fig. 13.3 Bar graph showing the dose-response effect of adventitial EtOH delivery upon renal parenchymal norepinephrine level at 14 ± 3 days. There is a marked and dose-dependent reduction of NE levels versus both naive control animals and sham control animals injected with saline. Mean NE reduction was 54 % with 0.15 ml; 78 % with 0.30 ml and 88 % using 0.60 ml/artery. Standard deviation (SD) for each data set as shown. P values as shown

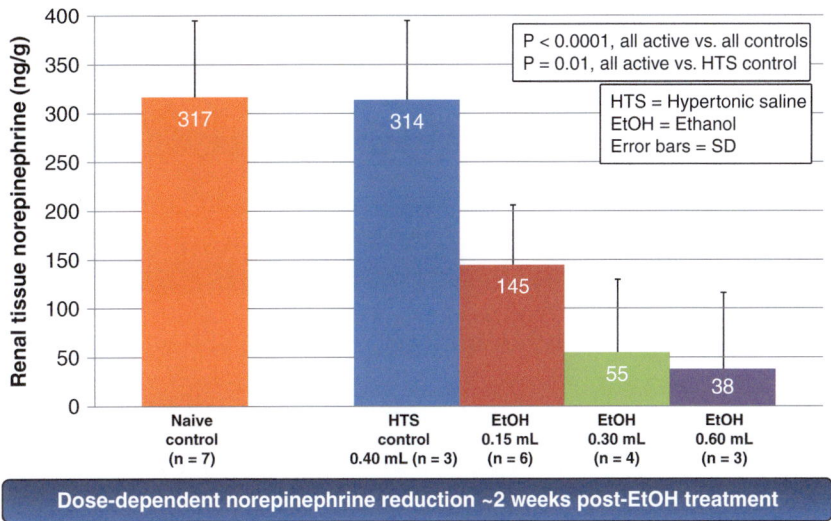

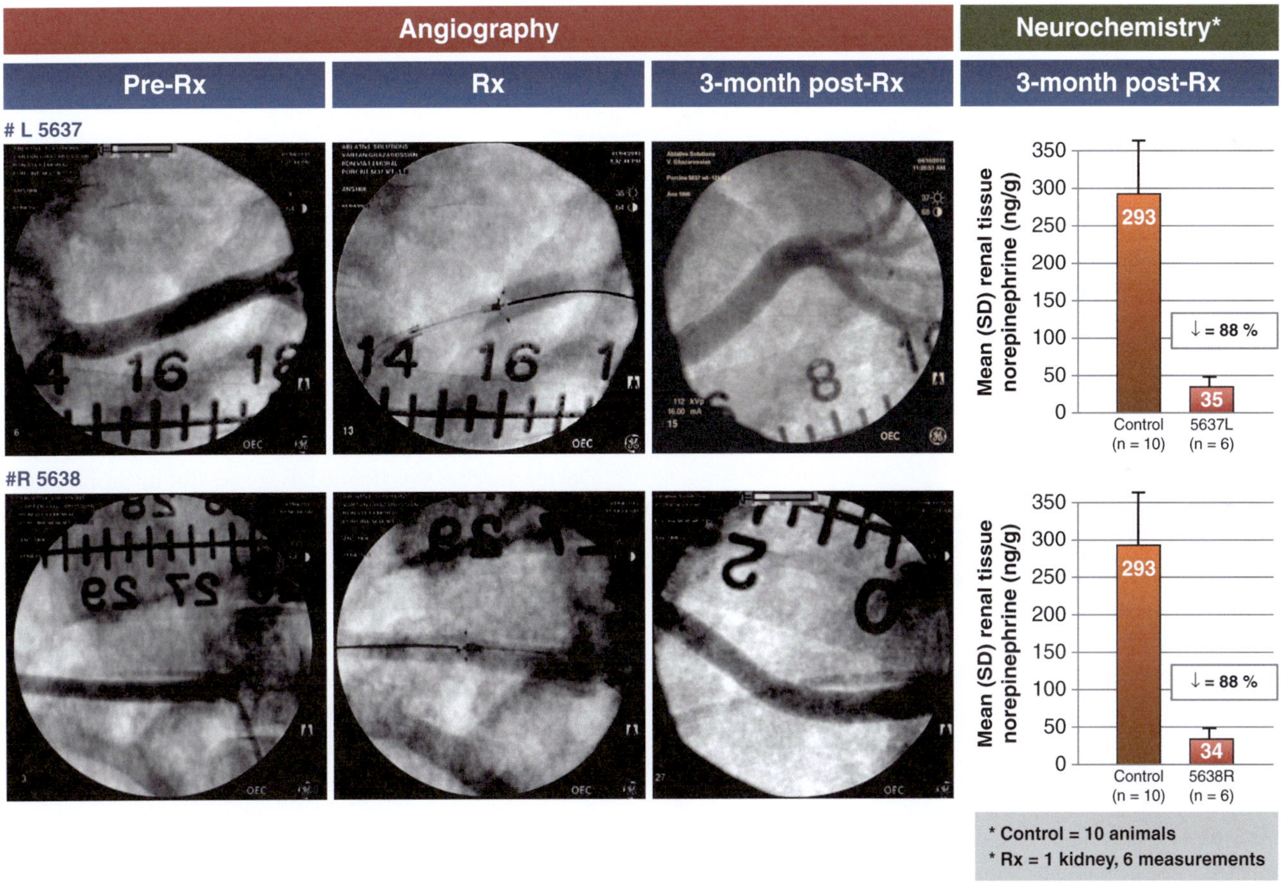

Fig. 13.4 Angiographic pictures and norepinephrine data from two pigs (*upper* and *lower panel* sets) at 3 month follow-up after 0.30 ml injection of EtOH in adventitial space by Peregrine™ device. *Left panels* show renal angiogram prior to treatment. Middle angiogram shows Peregrine™ device deployed during EtOH delivery and right angiographic panels show 3-month results with no evidence of any stenosis. In both of these kidneys there was an 88 % drop in renal parenchymal norepinephrine relative to untreated control kidneys (*far right panels*)

from each renal artery segment were labeled and sent for (blinded) microscopic evaluation by a board certified veterinary pathologist.

In all kidneys, four samples were obtained from random locations at each of the proximal, mid and distal regions of each kidney for a total of 12 samples/kidney. The tissue

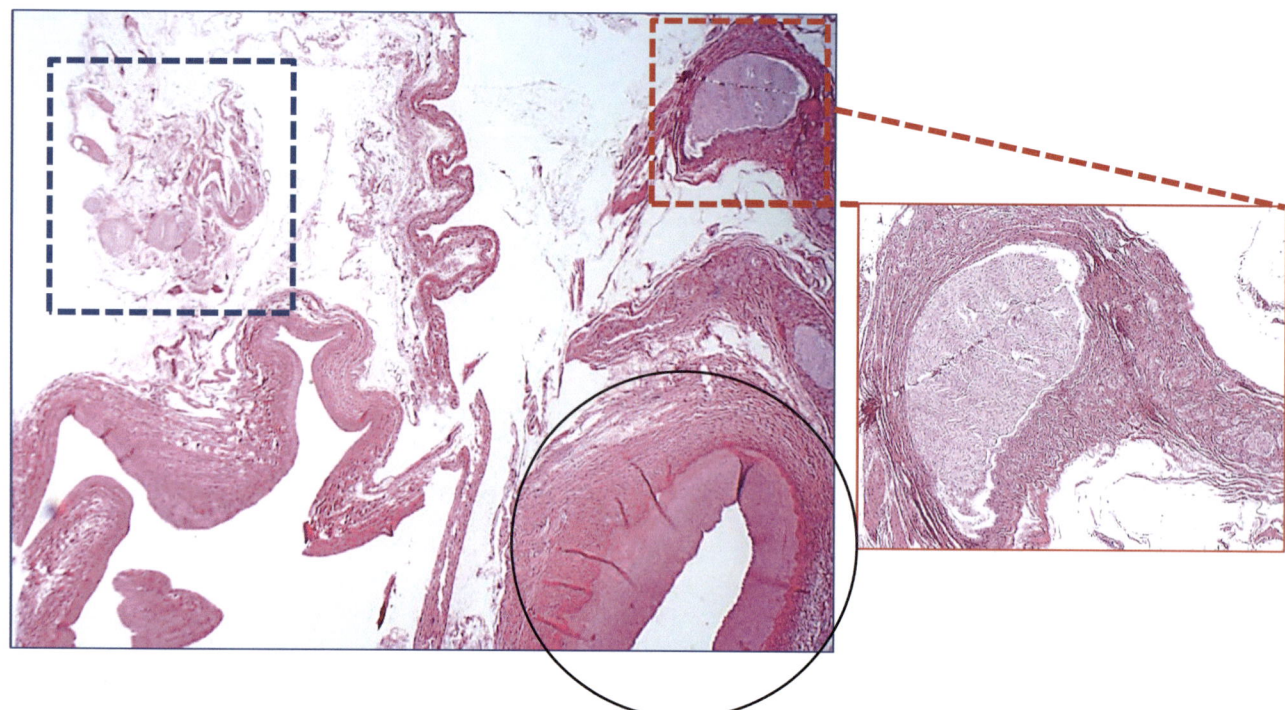

Fig. 13.5 Histopathology (H & E) of renal denervation at 30 days with 0.30 ml EtOH injection. The renal artery (intima and media) appears intact without evidence of injury or inflammation (*black circle*). The reaction to the EtOH appears quite limited to the adventitial layers.

There is severe damage to the deep renal nerve bundles with vacuolization, nerve fiber disruption, and fibrosis of the perineural structures at a depth of 4–14 mm deep to the intima (*blue hatched and red hatched boxes* and magnified view from *red* box)

samples were weighed, placed in cryovials and flash frozen by immersion into dry ice. The frozen samples were then stored at −70 °C. They were sent in dry ice to an independent laboratory for (blinded) measurement of renal parenchymal norepinephrine levels.

Renal norepinephrine concentrations in the treated animals from this study were also compared to values from naïve control animals of the same age and species (n = 7) with renal tissue sampling performed in an identical fashion to the treated animals.

The safety of ethanol injection was also assessed in a separate nephrotoxicology study (n = 4). After deep engagement of the renal arteries 0.6 ml of EtOH was injected directly in both the right and left renal arteries (1.2 ml total EtOH/animal), over 20–30 s to replicate the timing of injection into the adventitial space when therapeutic EtOH neurolysis was performed. These animals had serial measurement of serum BUN, creatinine, electrolytes and body weight at days 1, 7 and at 30 days after the injection. Histopathological evaluation of the renal parenchyma was performed in all such treated kidneys at 30 days to look for any evidence of renal injury.

Additional, longer-term safety evaluation was obtained with angiographic follow-up at 90 days, in four additional animals (n = 8 arteries) treated with 300 μl (0.30 ml) EtOH. These studies were performed to look for any evidence of late renal artery stenosis (Fig. 13.4).

For statistical analysis, between-group comparisons were made using a Wilcoxon rank-sum test, performed in R (Version 2.14.1, Vienna, Austria). Data are shown in graphs as mean ± SD. A p value of <0.05 was considered significant.

Device success was defined as successful injection of the designated fluid without serious adverse events. The device was used successfully in all 16 animals and 32 renal arteries. Procedure time, measured from the advancement of the device into the renal artery, followed by deployment of needles, injection, and withdrawal back into the guiding catheter averaged approximately 90 s for each renal artery (range – 55–140 s). A small hematoma at the femoral access site was recorded in one animal. There was no other study-related morbidity or mortality.

At 2-weeks after ethanol-mediated renal denervation measurements of renal tissue NE showed an essentially linear dose response ($R^2 = 0.95$) between the EtOH volume delivered and the reduction of the renal parenchymal NE level (Fig. 13.3). The mean renal NE reductions were 54, 78 and 88 % at doses of 0.15 ml/artery, 0.30 ml/artery and 0.60 ml/artery, respectively (p < 0.0001 vs. combined controls; Fig. 13.3). The other statistical comparisons are shown in Fig. 13.3 and demonstrate a statistically significant reduction (p < 0.05) in renal parenchymal NE at all three doses, vs. sham controls.

Angiographic follow-up of all 24 treated vessels at 14 ± 3 days showed no evidence of renal artery narrowing at

EtOH doses of 0.15, 0.30 or 0.60 ml/artery. There were no other abnormalities noted, including no aneurysmal changes or thrombus. Angiography at the 90-day time point in four additional animals (eight arteries) treated with 0.3 ml EtOH, demonstrated no detectable renal artery narrowing (Fig. 13.4).

Histological examination revealed marked, and deep, circumferential renal nerve injury at depths of 1.5–12 mm from the intimal surface (Fig. 13.5). There was no discernible nerve injury in the saline, sham control injected animals. Nerve injury in the EtOH treated vessels was characterized by vacuolization, loss of internal architecture, and the development peri-neural fibrosis (Fig. 13.5). There was no evidence of device-related or EtOH-induced injury to the intimal layer of treated vessels. There were no thrombi. There was no evidence of any significant EtOH-induced injury to the intimal or medial layers of the renal arteries at the 0.30 ml dose at 3 month follow-up (Fig. 13.5). There was no discernible injury to tissue deep to the peri-adventitial plane.

There were no adverse nephrotoxic or systemic effects seen. The pigs' serum creatinine, BUN and electrolytes remained unchanged over the study period. Finally, direct injection of EtOH into the renal artery, at 200 % the likely therapeutic dose (i.e., 0.6 ml vs. 0.30 ml), resulted in no detectable renal toxicity as measured by creatinine, BUN, or electrolytes measured at 1, 3, 7 and 30 days after EtOH injection (all p's=NS). There were no discernible renal pathological effects seen on sectioning of the renal parenchyma at the 30-day follow-up.

First in Man Feasibility

The first in man early safety and feasibility study was started in September 2013. Bilateral renal angiography was performed in nine patients with severe refractory hypertension. Heparin was administered to achieve an ACT of >250 in all patients. Following anticoagulation unilateral denervation using 300 μL of EtOH was performed successfully in the first five patients. Unilateral intervention was done in these first five patients, as per protocol, to make certain that this technique was safe, prior to attempting bilateral denervation in one setting.

These patients were re-studied at 1 month after their first intervention. Angiography demonstrated no injury, stenosis or thrombus in any of the five treated vessels. After re-study of the initial target vessel, bilateral denervation was completed by denervation, as per protocol with 300 μL (0.3 ml) in the contralateral renal artery. Four additional patients were treated with bilateral denervation following this first "staged" cohort.

The procedure is very simple technically and also much faster than first or even second generation energy-based "burning" catheters. The mean time from device advancement into the target renal artery, to device withdrawal and final angiography was ~3 min (range 1.5–4 min). There were no complications, and device success was achieved in 9/9 cases and in 19/19 vessels (one patient treated who had dual renal/accessory renal arteries). There were no observations of vasospasm, thrombus, dissection or perforation in any of the 19 renal arteries treated. Interestingly, in two of the nine patients radiofrequency renal denervation would have been contraindicated (one patient with a short (12 mm) main renal artery length; one patient with dual renal arteries to the left kidney).

Perhaps most importantly, the ethanol denervation procedure was essentially painless. In 6/9 patients there was 0/10 pain throughout the procedure. In three patients there was a very transient (~60 s of discomfort, rated as 3–4/10). Only modest conscious sedation was used. In all cases the patients were essentially awake and actively conversant during the EtOH injection. In the three patients who had any discomfort, the pain was rated as 0/10 at 1–2 min after the EtOH injection. Lab tests, including BUN and CR were unchanged at 24 h after the procedure. Further follow-up is pending. Early data suggests a significant drop in both systolic and diastolic BP at 4 weeks after unilateral denervation (n=5). These data need to be confirmed in a larger cohort.

Discussion

In these studies we have demonstrated the apparent safety, and predictability, as well as a dose-dependent efficacy of low dose ethanol injection via micro-needles into the perivascular space to achieve circumferential sympathetic nerve ablation (PeriVascular Renal Denervation, or PVRD™), with minimal injury to the normal renal artery intimal and medial layers, in a porcine model. The ability to target and deliver a neurolytic agent to a deep peri-adventitial space may allow more complete renal denervation than might be easily, or safely obtained using energy-based systems from within the renal artery.

Renal denervation may prove to be a valuable intervention to treat severe hypertension as well as a number of other conditions that may be driven by sympathetic imbalance, or "overdrive." Denervation of the renal artery has been shown to be effective in the treatment of refractory and drug-resistant hypertension [4–7], and possibly in the treatment of congestive heart failure [20], central obstructive sleep apnea [21, 22], left ventricular hypertrophy [23], metabolic syndrome [24, 25], chronic kidney disease [26, 27] and in patients with atrial and/or ventricular arrhythmias [28, 29]. There is a need to develop and evaluate the safest and most effective methods to perform renal denervation.

The drug-delivery catheter used in this study is a novel endovascular delivery device that contains three distal needles housed inside of individual guide tubes, which are contained within the catheter. The catheter is used under fluoroscopic guidance by a single-operator using standard endovascular techniques to access the vessel of choice and perform injection into the adventitial and peri-adventitial space of that vessel. The radio-opaque micro-needles are deployed with minimal trauma to the normal renal arterial wall and to target delivery in the adventitial and peri-adventitial space. There is no obstruction of renal blood flow during the deployment of this device. The device was very simple to use, with catheter positioning and denervation being performed in less than 2 min from the time that the catheter entered the renal artery via the guiding catheter in virtually all cases. There were no device-related complications.

The known neurolytic agent, Dehydrated Alcohol Injection, USP (ethanol – EtOH, 98 %), was chosen for the evaluation of the drug-delivery catheter used in this study [30–34]. Ethanol is indicated and FDA approved for therapeutic neurolysis, and produces injury to tissue cells by dehydration and by precipitation of protoplasm. At very low doses, ethanol is known to produce neuritis and nerve degeneration (neurolysis). Deliberate injury to nerves by the targeted injection of ethanol results in more or less enduring block of sensory, motor and autonomic function [29–33].

As seen in this study, the dose of ethanol that is effective to create nearly complete renal sympathetic neurolysis involves a dose that is so small that it will produce no apparent systemic effects. Even when double the expected therapeutic dose of 0.3 ml EtOH was purposefully injected directly into the renal artery, we could not detect any signs of renal toxicity. Even at the highest dose used in this study (0.60 ml), contains less alcohol than a single alcoholic drink.

The porcine renal denervation model has been well characterized, and does appear to predict the efficacy in the treatment of refractory hypertension in human subjects. In this study it was possible to verify, and quantify denervation of the kidneys by measurement of the renal parenchymal levels of the neurohormone, norepinephrine (NE). We further validated the neurohormonal effects of ethanol-mediated denervation by using careful, and blinded histological examination of both treated and sham controlled arteries.

The histopathology demonstrated profound and circumferential renal sympathetic nerve damage, with nearly complete sparing of the normal intimal and medial architecture of the renal artery, using doses of 0.15–0.60 ml of EtOH/ artery. Evaluation at this time point indicates normal arterial healing, although evaluation at longer time points is needed to more fully evaluate safety.

At ethanol doses of 0.30 and 0.60 ml there was essentially complete denervation, as judged by the 78 % and 88 % reduction in renal parenchymal norepinephrine levels, respectively. These reductions observed with 0.30 and 0.60 ml EtOH are substantially equivalent to the reduction seen with surgical denervation in a porcine model.

Despite the reasonable efficacy of both the first and next generation RF and ultrasound catheters [3–7], there are a number of potential limitations, and safety concerns associated with the use of transmural thermal injury using either RF or ultrasound, traversing the intimal and medial layers of the renal artery. In order to create thermal injury to the sympathetic nerves that may run from 2 to 10 mm deep to the intimal surface [15–18], there will be collateral damage to the intimal and medial layers of the renal artery wall. The ability to predictably damage the renal sympathetic nerves in a dose-dependent fashion, using very low volumes of EtOH delivered in the adventitial space may have a number of potential advantages over energy-based systems.

The concerns and limitations of transmural, thermal-injury catheters, that could potentially be overcome with chemical neurolysis, include: (1) potential failure to adequately denervate deeper nerve fibers due to the heat sink as the thermal injury traverses the renal artery wall, resulting in "non-responders" and/or an inadequate BP lowering response (See Fig. 13.6) [4, 6, 7, 9], (2) failure to create circumferential nerve ablation such that many nerves pass uninjured to the kidney, resulting in suboptimal efficacy [4, 6, 7, 34], (3) intense pain related to thermal ablation requiring high doses of benzodiazepines in combination with very high doses of narcotic analgesia, with attendant respiratory depressive effects and the risk of prolonging hospitalization [4–10], (4) the risk of luminal thrombus formation on the endoluminal surface at sites of thermal "burn" injury, with the subsequent risk of downstream thrombo-embolization and potential for renal injury [15], (5) large volumes of contrast use injected directly into the renal arteries bilaterally during repeated positioning of a unipolar electrode RF system, with the potential risk of contrast induced renal injury, (6) long case duration with high levels of radiation exposure to the patient and the operator [4–11], (7) the expense of purchasing and maintaining complex capital equipment required to perform RF and/or ultrasonic ablation, and finally, (8) the risk of provoking neointimal hyperplasia and/or negative remodeling from transmural thermal arterial injury, which may result in subsequent renal artery stenosis and recurrent hypertension [16, 17].

In addition, a recent study by Meier and colleagues, they have found that ~45–50 % of patients with refractory hypertension have renal anatomy that is not suitable for energy-based "burning" denervation systems. The large majority of these cases could, in theory, be treated with the current Peregrine™ chemical denervation catheter, since this device can treat 3.5–7 mm diameter arteries, only requires a 2–3 mm landing zone for the operational piece of the catheter, and can perform denervation in ~1.5–2.0 min per artery.

Although the limitations of thermal ablation for renal denervation are real, and the very early clinical use of the Peregrine™ device appears promising, it remains to be

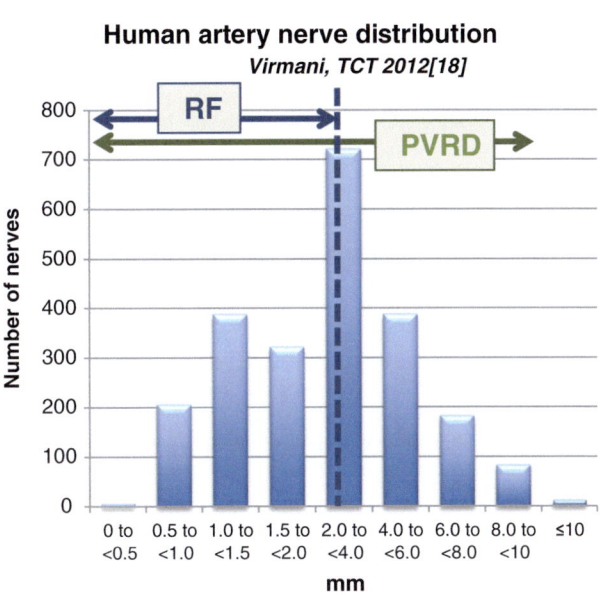

Human artery nerve distribution
Virmani, TCT 2012[18]

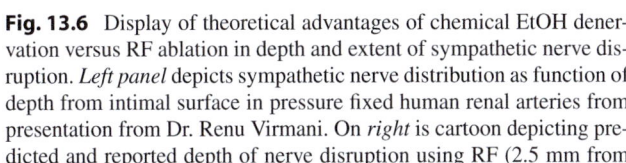

Fig. 13.6 Display of theoretical advantages of chemical EtOH denervation versus RF ablation in depth and extent of sympathetic nerve disruption. *Left panel* depicts sympathetic nerve distribution as function of depth from intimal surface in pressure fixed human renal arteries from presentation from Dr. Renu Virmani. On *right* is cartoon depicting predicted and reported depth of nerve disruption using RF (2.5 mm from intima; *blue circle*) vs. EtOH when delivered as 0.30 ml into adventitia using the Peregrine™ device (*green circle*; 10–14 mm depth from intima). Overall it is estimated that the cross-sectional area of nerve disruption is potentially six to seven times greater with chemical neurolysis using EtOH as compared to RF delivered from the intimal surface

determined how effectively chemical denervation with EtOH, and the use of this novel drug delivery catheter might overcome each of these drawbacks.

Limitations

There, of course, remain a number of unanswered questions regarding the long-term safety and efficacy of ethanol mediated renal denervation. It should be appreciated that renal parenchymal norepinephrine is only a surrogate marker for efficacy in patients. The exact correlation between drops in renal parenchymal norepinephrine levels and antihypertensive efficacy in humans has not been definitively correlated.

Although these data from the porcine model and the first in human experience are encouraging, the true safety and efficacy of ethanol mediated perivascular renal denervation will need to be validated in long-term clinical trials.

Summary

In summary, we report the first use of adventitial and peri-adventitial, local delivery of very low doses of dehydrated EtOH to perform successful renal sympathetic denervation in a porcine model. Circumferential and deep peri-adventitial

delivery of very low doses of EtOH has the potential to be a simple, safe, predictable and appealing alternative to energy-based systems to achieve substantial, and dose-dependent renal denervation, with minimal injury to the normal renal arterial wall. Ongoing clinical trials demonstrate that this device and method can be used safely in patients and with essentially no pain during renal denervation. Further clinical evaluation and longer term follow-up will be required to determine the role of alcohol renal denervation using the Peregrine™ system in treating patients with refractory hypertension.

Acknowledgments We wish to acknowledge the expert technical contributions of Jeff A. Burke, Phil C. Burke, Andy E. Denison, and Chris S. Hayden from REV-1 Engineering.

Disclosures, Conflict of Interest TAF and VEG are principles, employees and co-founders of Ablative Solutions and have equity positions in the company. FV has is a paid consultant working with Ablative Solutions, Inc.

References

1. Harris SH. Renal sympathectomy: its scope and limitations. R Soc Med. 1935;28:1497–510.
2. Smithwick RH, Thompson JE. Splanchnicectomy for essential hypertension; results in 1,266 cases. J Am Med Assoc. 1953;152:1501–4.

3. Schlaich MP, Sobotka PA, Krum H, Whitbourn R, Walton A, Esler MD. Renal denervation as a therapeutic approach for hypertension: novel implications for an old concept. Hypertension. 2009;54(6):1195–201.

4. Krum H, Schlaich M, Whitbourn R, Sobotka PA, Sadowski J, Bartus K, et al. Catheter-based renal sympathetic denervation for resistant hypertension: a multicentre safety and proof-of-principle cohort study. Lancet. 2009;373:1275–81.

5. Investigators, SH-1. Catheter-based renal sympathetic denervation for resistant hypertension: durability of blood pressure reduction out to 24 months. Hypertension. 2011;57:911–7.

6. Symplicity HTN-2 Investigators, Esler MD, Krum H, Sobotka PA, Schlaich MP, Schmieder RE, Esler MD, Krum H, Sobotka PA, Schlaich MP, Schmieder RE, et al. Renal sympathetic denervation in patients with treatment-resistant hypertension (the Symplicity HTN-2 trial): a randomised controlled trial. Lancet. 2010;376:1903–9.

7. Esler MD, Krum H, Schlaich M, Schmieder RE, Bohm M, Sobotka PA, et al. Renal sympathetic denervation for treatment of drug-resistant hypertension: one-year results from the Symplicity HTN-2 randomized, controlled trial. Circulation. 2012;126:2976–82.

8. Kandzari DE, Bhatt DL, Sobotka PA, O'Neill WW, Esler M, Flack JM, et al. Catheter-based renal denervation for resistant hypertension: rationale and design of the SYMPLICITY HTN-3 trial. Clin Cardiol. 2012;35:528–35.

9. Mahfoud F, Cremers B, Janker J, Link B, Vonend O, Ukena C. Renal hemodynamics and renal function after catheter-based renal sympathetic denervation in patients with resistant hypertension. Hypertension. 2012;60:419–24.

10. Krum H, Schlaich M, Sobotka P, Scheffers I, Kroon AA, de Leeuw PW. Device-based antihypertensive therapy: therapeutic modulation of the autonomic nervous system. Circulation. 2011;123:209–15.

11. Lambert GW, Hering D, Esler MD, Marusic P, Lambert EA, Tanamas SK. Health-related quality of life after renal denervation in patients with treatment-resistant hypertension. Hypertension. 2012;60:1479–84.

12. Ormiston JA, Watson T, van Pelt N, Stewart R, Haworth P, Stewart JT. First-in-human use of the OneShot™ renal denervation system from Covidien. EuroInterv. 2013;8:1090–4.

13. Schlaich MP, Hering D, Sobotka PA, Krum H, Esler MD. Renal denervation in human hypertension: mechanisms, current findings, and future prospects. Curr Hypertens Rep. 2012;14:247–53.

14. Schlaich MP, Krum H, Sobotka PA, Esler MD. Renal denervation and hypertension. Am J Hypertens. 2011;24:635–42.

15. Cook S, Goy J, Togni M. Optical coherence tomography findings in renal denervation. Eur Heart J. 2012;10:1093.

16. Kaltenbach B, Id D, Franke JC, Sievert H, Hennersdorf M, Maier J, Bertog S. Renal artery stenosis after renal sympathetic denervation. J Am Coll Cardiol. 2012;60(25):2694–5.

17. Vonend O, Antoch G, Rump LC, Blondin D. Secondary rise in blood pressure after renal denervation. Lancet. 2012;380:778.

18. Virmani R. Perirenal nerve distribution, density and quantification: implications for the evaluation of device safety and efficacy. Presentation at TCT Conference, 2012, TCT 2012. p. 1–32 http://www.tctmd.com/show.aspx?id=114463.

19. Fischell TA, Vega F, Raju N, Johnson ET, Kent DJ, Ragland RR, Almany ST, Fischell DR, Ghazzorossian VE. Ethanol-mediated perivascular renal denervation: preclincal validation of safety and efficacy in a porcine model. EuroInterv. 2013;9:140–7.

20. Sobotka PA, Krum H, Bohm M, Francis DP, Schlaich MP. The role of renal denervation in the treatment of heart failure. Curr Cardiol Rep. 2012;14:285–92.

21. Linz D, Mahfoud F, Schotten U, Ukena C, Neuberger H-R, Wirth K, et al. Renal sympathetic denervation suppresses postapneic blood pressure rises and atrial fibrillation in a model for sleep apnea. Hypertension. 2012;60:172–8.

22. Witkowski A, Prejbisz A, Florczak E, Kadziela J, Sliwinski P, Bielen P, et al. Effects of renal sympathetic denervation on blood pressure, sleep apnea course, and glycemic control in patients with resistant hypertension and sleep apnea. Hypertension. 2011;58: 559–65.

23. Brandt MC, Mahfoud F, Reda S, Schirmer SH, Erdmann E, Bohm M, et al. Renal sympathetic denervation reduces left ventricular hypertrophy and improves cardiac function in patients with resistant hypertension. J Am Coll Cardiol. 2012;59:901–9.

24. Schlaich MP, Hering D, Sobotka P, Krum H, Lambert GW, Lambert E. Effects of renal denervation on sympathetic activation, blood pressure, and glucose metabolism in patients with resistant hypertension. Front Physiol. 2012;3:10.

25. Mahfoud F, Schlaich M, Kindermann I, Ukena C, Cremers B, Brandt MC. Effect of renal sympathetic denervation on glucose metabolism in patients with resistant hypertension: a pilot study. Circulation. 2011;123:1940–6.

26. Schlaich MP, Bart B, Hering D, Walton A, Marusic P, Mahfoud F. Feasibility of catheter-based renal nerve ablation and effects on sympathetic nerve activity and blood pressure in patients with end-stage renal disease. Int J Cardiol. 2013;168(3):2214–20.

27. Hering D, Mahfoud F, Walton AS, Krum H, Lambert GW, Lambert EA. Renal denervation in moderate to severe CKD. J Am Soc Nephrol. 2012;23:1250–7.

28. Linz D, Mahfoud F, Schotten U, Ukena C, Hohl M, Neuberger HR. Renal sympathetic denervation provides ventricular rate control but does not prevent atrial electrical remodeling during atrial fibrillation. Hypertension. 2013;61:225–31.

29. Ukena C, Bauer A, Mahfoud F, Schreieck J, Neuberger HR, Eick C. Renal sympathetic denervation for treatment of electrical storm: first-in-man experience. Clin Res Cardiol. 2012;101:63–7.

30. Moller JE, Helweg-Larsen J, Jacobsen E. Histopathological lesions in the sciatic nerve of the rat following perineural application of phenol and alcohol solutions. Dan Med Bull. 1969;16:116–9.

31. Streitparth F, Walter A, Stolzenburg N, Heckmann L, Breinl J, Rinnenthal JL. MR-guided periarterial ethanol injection for renal sympathetic denervation: a feasibility study in pigs. Cardiovasc Intervent Radiol. 2013. doi:10.1007/s00270-013-0570-x.

32. Wali FA, Suer AH, Hayter A, Tugwell AC. The effect of ethanol on spontaneous contractions and on the contraction produced by peri-arterial nerve stimulation and by acetylcholine in the rat isolated ileum. Gen Pharmacol. 1987;18:631–5.

33. Kocabas H, Salli A, Demir AH, Ozerbil OM. Comparison of phenol and alcohol neurolysis of tibial nerve motor branches to the gastrocnemius muscle for treatment of spastic foot after stroke: a randomized controlled pilot study. Eur J Phys Rehab Med. 2010; 46:5–10.

34. Wilkes D, Ganceres N, Doulatram G, Solanki D. Alcohol neurolysis of the sciatic and femoral nerves to improve pressure ulcer healing. Pain Pract. 2009;9:145–9.

Vincristine Local Delivery for Renal Artery Denervation

Konstantinos Toutouzas, Andreas Synetos, and Christodoulos Stefanadis

The contribution of renal sympathetic nerve activity to the development and progression of resistant hypertension, has been convincingly demonstrated in both preclinical and human experiments. Preclinical experiments in hypertension models of hypertension [5, 6, 14], have successfully used renal denervation as both an experimental tool and a therapeutic strategy, but even earlier, in the absence of appropriate drugs to pharmacologically reduce blood pressure in severely hypertensive patients, therapeutic splanchnicectomy and even radical surgical sympathectomy were used since the 1930s. These surgical techniques have been abandoned due to their severe side effects. Recent studies have further investigated the close relationship between kidneys and brain, and gave light to some important parameters of this transaction. Low frequency stimulation of the sympathetic system resulted in renin excretion only, intermediate frequency stimulation results on decreased urinary sodium excretion and high frequency stimulation, results on direct renal artery vasoconstriction, decrease in renal blood flow and decrease glomerular filtration rate [2, 5, 10].

Nowadays, recently-developed endovascular catheter technology enabled selective denervation of the human kidney, with radiofrequency energy delivered to the renal artery wall, targeting the renal nerves located in the adventitia of the renal arteries. Early clinical results demonstrated the efficacy of this technique in producing renal denervation and significant reductions in blood pressure over a 18 month period [9, 10, 15]. During the last years, the use of different systems of renal sympathetic denervations, has raised several questions regarding the safety and more recently, the efficacy of the method. One of the major disadvantages of the method is that is painful, so that the patient has to be treated with painkillers or have a slight sedation during the process. More importantly, there is no evidence regarding the long term efficacy of the method, since it is well known that renal sympathetic efferent nerves in kidney and heart transplant models can regenerate. In some cases, the use of ablation catheters has been associated with other complications such as transient intraprocedural bradycardia, post-procedural hypotension, urinary tract infection, Paresthesias and renal artery stenosis [9, 10, 13, 15]. However the most important concern regarding this method, emerged over the past few months, when the SYMPLICITY HTN-3 study, the most rigorous renal denervation clinical trial conducted to date, and the first of its kind to include a sham-control group, failed to meet its primary goal [20]. The goal was to enroll patients who had severe drug-resistant hypertension – office values of 160 mmHg or higher on at least two occasions while on at least three drugs at maximum tolerated doses, including a diuretic. However, about two out of three patients initially involved in the SYMPLICITY HTN-3 trial never made it to randomization because their blood pressure medication wasn't optimum, while optimization of that regimen knocked out a number of people from the actual trial itself.

All the previously mentioned concerns, gave rise to new ideas and new alternatives that shared the same target: The renal sympathetic system. These new approaches include ultrasonic ablation, barodenervation and chemical denervation [17, 24–27].

Chemical denervation refers to an alternate approach to induce renal sympathetic nerve injury through the delivery of neurotoxins. Previously used agents such as guanethidine, had some initial good results. Guanethidine exerts its action after local delivery with the use of the Bullfrog microinfusion catheter that is designed to inject therapeutic agents directly through the arterial wall and into the perivascular tissues. Systemic guanethidine administration is known to have reversible interference with the transmission of neural pathways, while local its administration induces autonomic denervation directly and through an immune-mediated pathway [18]. In an experimental study, perivascular renal artery

K. Toutouzas, MD, FESC, FACC (✉) • A. Synetos, MD, FESC
C. Stefanadis, MD, FESC, FACC
First Department of Cardiology, Athens Medical School, Hippokration Hospital, Vas. Sofias 114, Athens, Greece
e-mail: Ktoutouz@gmail.com; synetos@yahoo.com; chstefan@med.uoa.gr

R.R. Heuser et al. (eds.), *Renal Denervation: A New Approach to Treatment of Resistant Hypertension*,
DOI 10.1007/978-1-4471-5223-1_14, © Springer-Verlag London 2015

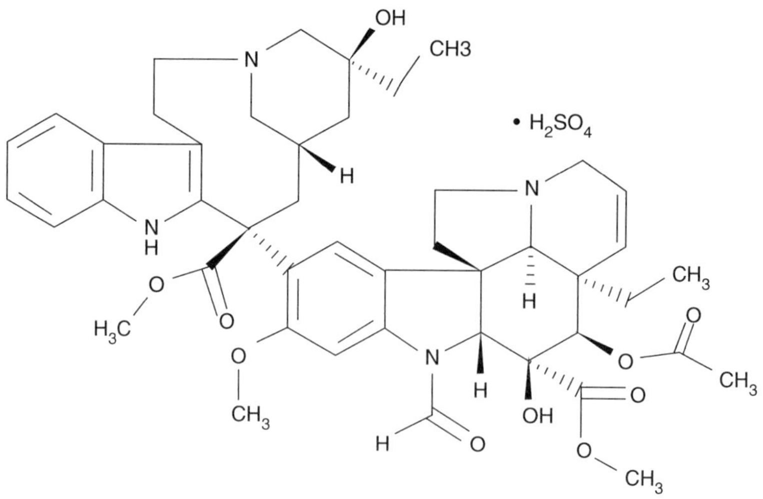

Fig. 14.1 Chemical structure of vincristine

delivery of salicylic acid, hypertonic saline and paclitaxel, were capable of performing renal denervation that was assessed by depletion of renal noradrenaline [4]. In this chapter we will concentrate on the renal sympathetic system denervation that is performed by local administration of vincristine.

Vincristine

Vincristine is a vinca alkaloid from the Catharanthus roseus (Madagascar periwinkle). It is a mitotic inhibitor, and is used in cancer chemotherapy. Vincristine is created by the coupling of indole alkaloids vindoline and catharanthine in the vinca plant (Fig. 14.1). Vincristine is widely used in the treatment of lymphoblastic leukemias, malignant lymphomas, multiple myelomas, and a number of other malignancies [11]. Moreover, vincristine has potent irreversible neurotoxicity by causing giant axonal swellings and secondary demyelination of the paranodal type mainly in the proximal portions of the peripheral nerves outside the spinal canal [1, 7, 8, 19, 21]. Although reduction in its total dosage and injection schedule, resulted in decreasing considerably, the incidence of severe neurotoxic effects, the induced of polyneuropathy is still reported in an unpredictable number of cancer patients. Vincristine is unique among the chemotherapeutic agent that is predictably and uniformly neurotoxic to all who receive it [16]. In therapeutic doses, it produces dose-related neuropathy, very early in the course of treatment [22], and its clinical antineoplastic efficacy is limited by the development of a mixed sensorimotor neuropathy [23]. Vincristine neurotoxicity is not only dose but also duration dependent as there is a progressive increase in the clinical and electrophysiological evidence of toxicity with continuing treatment [3, 22]. The symptoms usually start in the hands and/or feet and creeps up the arms and legs. An

estimated 30–40 % of cancer patients treated with chemotherapy experiences these symptoms, a condition called chemotherapy-induced peripheral neuropathy.

Peripheral neuropathy can be defined as a derangement in structure and function of peripheral motor, sensory, and autonomic neurons causing peripheral neuropathic symptoms and signs. Vincristine induced neuropathy tend to occur early during therapy, whereas cisplatin-induced neuropathy tends to develop only after a certain cumulative dose level. In a study that assessed the natural course of vincristine-induced peripheral neuropathy in patients with lymphoma receiving vincristine in two different dose intensities, it was noticed that neuropathic changes were observed in both dose intensity groups, but the higher dose intensity group reported significantly more symptoms during therapy, whereas neurologic signs were significantly more prominent after a cumulative dose of 12 mg vincristine. Furthermore, offtherapy worsening of symptoms (24 %) and signs (30 %) occurred [30].

The way of action of vincristine on the peripheral nerves (demyelination) was depicted in many experimental studies. In a study that assessed vincristine neurotoxicity in experimental animals from clinical, electrophysiological, and histological points of view, 65 rats were used as a control group and 31 rats were divided into two groups and given vincristine in two different regimens: the fixed-dose group (0.2 mg/kg) and the increasing-dose group (0.1 mg/kg, by an increment of 0.05 mg/kg/week). Vincristine was given intraperitoneally once weekly for 5 consecutive weeks. Progressively with the treatment, an increasing number of rats showing signs of neurological deficits were observed. During the first 5 weeks of this study, electrophysiological testing showed a nonsignificant difference in the conduction velocities of sciatic and tail nerves between the control and the treated groups, whereas a significant decrease in the amplitude of the sensory nerve action potential and compound muscle

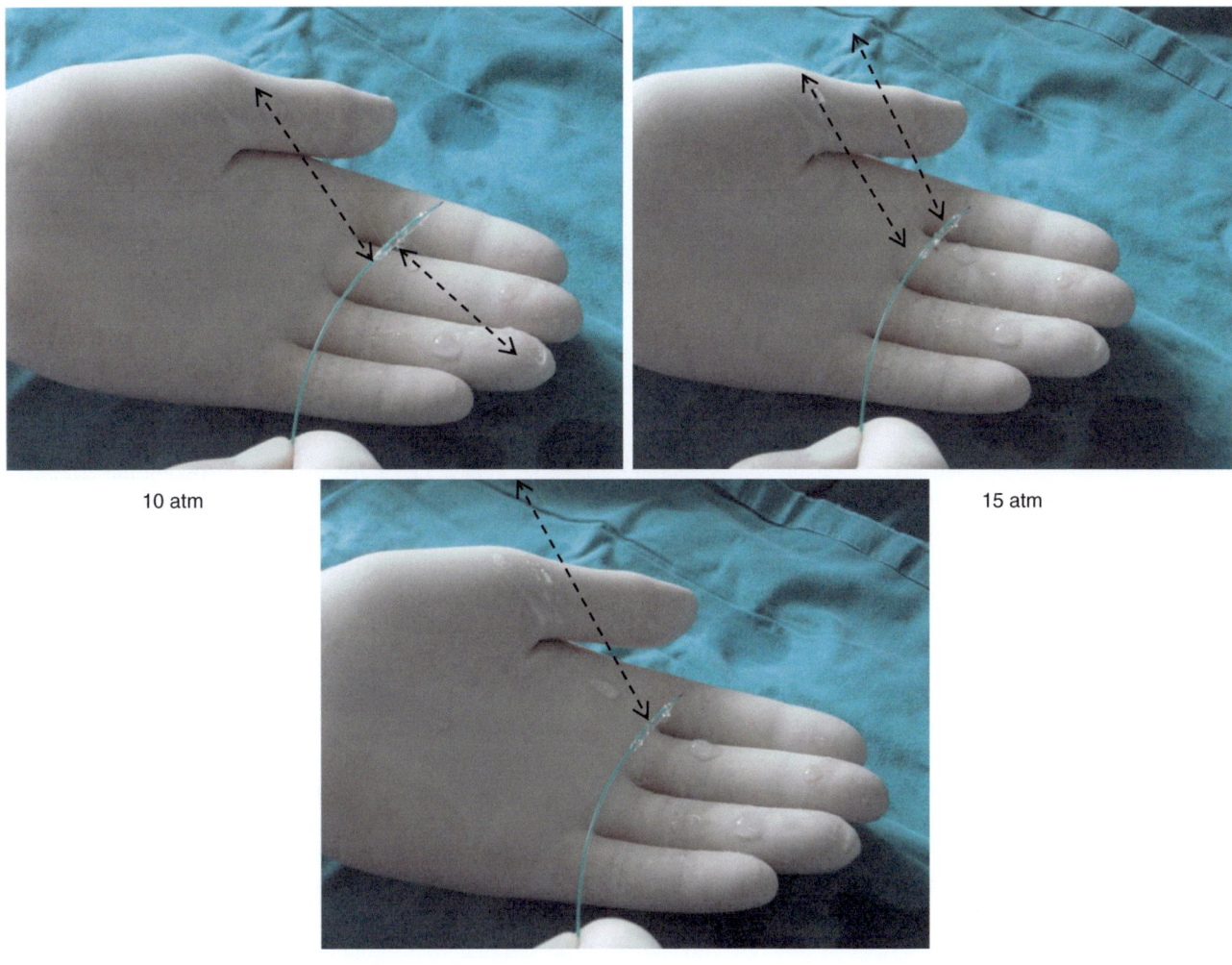

10 atm

15 atm

20 atm

Fig. 14.2 The first catheter used for the local delivery of vincristine. Itdelivers vincristine to the media layer of the renal artery with a random flow rate

action potential of the tested nerves was recorded. The reduction in the amplitude of the action potential was associated with histological changes characterized by axonal degeneration with relative demyelination [12].

This important side effect of vincristine, created the hypothesis that this agent can cause irreversible demyelination and therefore denervation of the renal sympathetic system when applied locally in the media layer of the renal artery. This hypothesis has been tested both in experimental models and in humans.

Experimental Models

The first attempt that proved that local delivery of vincristine in a safe concentration is safe and effective and can cause chemical denervation of the sympathetic nervous system of the renal artery was performed in 2011. A dedicated catheter

for the local delivery of vincristine in the media layer or the renal artery was created in the laboratory of the First Department of Cardiology of the University of Athens. This catheter consisted of a modified conventional non-compliant balloon angioplasty catheter. Six sideholes of 25 μm diameter were created circumferentially across the balloon in fixed intervals of 60°. The catheter was checked in vitro so that different balloon inflation pressures could create different pressures of vincristine delivery (Fig. 14.2). The experimental model chosen for this protocol were 14 juvenile Landrace swine (3–5 months old, weight 28 ± 0.5 kg). In order to visualize under fluoroscopy the process, a mixture of vincristine was diluted to a final concentration of 25 mg/l in a mixture consisting of 20 ml of sterile 0.9 % NaCl solution and 20 ml of contrast. The mixture used for the placebo procedure, contained 20 ml of sterile 0.9 % NaCl solution and 20 ml of contrast, without the addition of vincristine. The protocol of the procedure was the following: The experiment was performed with the animals under general anesthesia, with continuous monitoring of the vital signs. The trachea was intubated with a 6.5–7.0 mm cuffed tracheal tube and ventilation was performed via a mechanical respirator. General anesthesia was maintained via 1–2 % isoflurane and oxygen. After the insertion of a 6 Fr introducer sheath though the right femoral artery, an initial (reference) angiogram was performed in both renal arteries using a 6 Fr Judkins Right four guiding catheter in order to evaluate the preprocedural anatomy of the arteries and define the desired segment of the renal artery for chemical denervation. The femoral catheter was used to obtain blood samples and to monitor systolic arterial pressure, diastolic arterial pressure mean arterial pressure and heart rate before, immediately after and 28 days after the procedure. The systolic arterial pressure, diastolic arterial pressure, mean arterial pressure and the heart rate, derived from pulsatile arterial pressure, were recorded continuously during the procedure. After the canulation of the renal artery with the JR4 guiding catheter, a guidewire was advanced to the distal segment of the renal artery and the modified balloon catheter was advanced in the main branch of the renal arteries. In order for the modified catheter to produce enough pressure to the media layer of the renal artery, and to cause small dissections so that the agent can pass through the media layer and reach the sympathetic nervous system of the renal artery, the diameter of the balloon for both treated and control segments was selected on a 1:1 ratio according to the diameter of the target vessel. The noncompliant balloon was then inflated at 20 atm to cover the target segment, using the mixture containing vincristine, allowing for delivery of vincristine into the vascular wall. The inflation was interrupted when a total of 4 ml of the mixture, that contained 0.1 mg of vincristine was delivered. The procedure was then repeated in the contralateral renal artery using the placebo mixture for inflation. All angiograms before and after the procedure were recorded on video and blood samples were drawn before, immediately after and 28 days after the procedure in order to determine serum creatinine levels. After the completion of the initial procedures, in all animals delivery of vincristine and placebo mixtures was successful and uncomplicated, with no acute or short-term complications related to the intervention. Moreover the safety for the renal function was proved by the fact that serum creatinine was 1.37 ± 0.12 mg/dl before the procedure, 1.41 ± 0.09 mg/dl after the procedure, and 1.36 ± 0.24 mg/dl 28 days after the procedure (p = NS for all comparisons) [24, 27].

After 28 days all animals were alive for euthanasia and it was previously shown their kidney function was normal. A final renal artery angiography before euthanasia showed that all vincristine and placebo treated renal arteries were angiographically patent at the end of the procedure, without evidence of thrombus formation, abrupt occlusion of the arterial segments or aneurysmal dilatation of the target segments at the post-procedural angiography. Moreover systolic blood pressure showed a significant drop between baseline and follow up at 28 days (132 ± 34.05 versus 125 ± 32.19 mmHg, p=0.024), although this was beyond the scope of this study.

After euthanasia, both the vincristine and the placebo treated renal arteries were prepared for histology and immunohistology, with neuron specific enolase in order to visualize the sympathetic nerve fibers. It should be noted that during the harvest of the renal arteries, all renal arteries of both groups were patent, with no signs of thrombus. Each renal artery was dissected into 8 equal segments of 2 mm, and the sections of the vincristine treated arteries were compared to the sections of the renal arteries treated with the control mixture. The mean number of intact nerves in all sections was significantly lower in the group of vincristine, (8.6 ± 3.4 versus 11.7 ± 3.1, p<0.01), showing the effectiveness of renal sympathetic denervation by the local delivery of vincristine [24, 27].

This was actually the first attempt to deliver locally to the renal artery a pharmaceutical agent, although this was performed previously in the coronary arteries, there was not any attempt to perform this on the renal arteries, This first attempt to produce renal artery denervation in an experimental model by vincristine, had the disadvantage that the flow rate of vincristine administration was not checked in vitro, a limitation that however was similar for both groups treated with vincristine or the placebo and therefore had no effect on the conclusions. However this method with the catheter-based chemical renal denervation and had the advantage that vincristine was not only delivered to nerves in the deeper layers of the vascular wall through the injured intima, but it could also exert a direct toxic effect on the sympathetic nerve axons in proximity with the tubular epithelial cells, resulting in an enhancement of its antihypertensive effect. Despite this possible beneficial effect, the spill out of vincristine towards the parenchymal renal tissue de novo raises some issues of safety, although these they were not observed in this preliminary study.

In order to overcome these limitations of the channeled dedicated catheter that delivers vincristine with an uncontrolled flow rate, a new double balloon delivery catheters was tested in vitro and in the same experimental model.

This new catheter was designed and manufactured by Rontis AG Switzerland, and consists of an over the wire triple lumen catheter with two non compliant balloons at its distal tip. It has two differences compared to the previously used channeled dedicated catheter. Firstly it strongly engages the balloon catheter (when the balloon is inflated) in the renal artery allowing all the pharmaceutical mixture to be delivered in the media layer of the renal artery and not spilled out by the circulation, and secondly, it delivers the pharmaceutical agent with a constant flow rate. The outer balloon is channeled and allows the delivery of the drug to the tissues, and the inner balloon, is used for the fixation of the catheter

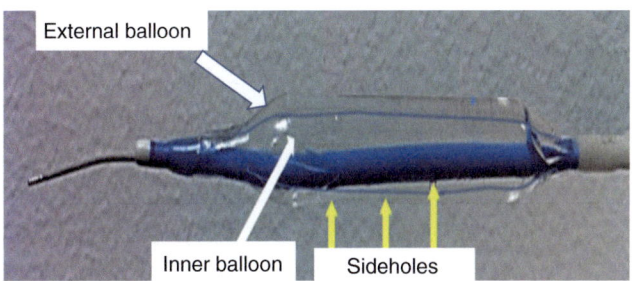

Fig. 14.3 The double balloon delivery catheter for the local delivery of vincristine with constant flow rate

on the arterial wall and the obstruction of the renal artery so that the whole vincristine will be delivered to the arterial wall and not washed out by the blood flow. The third lumen allows the use of a guidewire for the advancement of the catheter. The outer balloon design similarly to the previous catheter consisted of six sideholes of 25 μm diameter, in fixed intervals of 60°. The injected mixture reached the arterial wall by diffusion or as a result of applied hydrostatic pressure. High-pressure inflation of the outer balloon catheter, using normal saline resulted in producing a jet of the solution from the sideholes in jets (Fig. 14.3).

This catheter was checked in vitro in various pressures for both the inner and the outer balloon, in order to assess the optimal inflation pressures in order to achieve a constant flow rate. After calculating the viscosity of the vincristine mixture that was 6.9 cP, the optimal pressures to achieve a constant flow rate of 10.11 cc/min was 2 Atm for the inner balloon and 6 Atm for the outer balloon [26].

Thereafter, the initial experiment with the local delivery of vincristine in the renal arteries was repeated with the use of the new double balloon catheter. Similarly 16 juvenile Landrace swine (3–5 months old, weight 27±0.5 kg) were used to study the effect of vincristine, and the whole procedure was repeated, via a 7F Judkins right catheter that was advanced though a 7F femoral sheath, and this was due to the increased profile of the new catheter. Both vincristine and the control mixtures remained the same. The assessment of the effectiveness of denervation was performed by immunohistology with the use of neuron specific enolase.

The whole process was completed for animals with safety, and the delivery of vincristine and placebo mixtures was successful and uncomplicated with no acute or short-term complications related to the intervention. Serum creatinine was 1.32±0.15 mg/dl before the procedure, 1.35±0.12 mg/dl after the procedure, and 1.34±0.19 mg/dl 28 days after the procedure. (p=NS for all comparisons), and this was indicative of the safety of the local delivery of vincristine regarding the renal function. On the final angiography, just before euthanasia, all vincristine- and placebo-treated renal arteries were angiographically patent at the end of the procedure. On immunohistology similarly to the original findings, the mean

number of intact nerves in all sections was significantly lower in the group of vincristine (1.48±0.37 versus 4.56±0.99, p<0.001), proving the effectiveness of local delivery of vincristine for the demyelinating and therefore denervating the renal arteries. In this study, the lack of direct measurement of the vincristine that was delivered to the media of the renal arteries, is compensated by three indirect signs. In the angiography during the inflation of the balloons for the delivery of vincristine, it was evident that contrast was entrapped within the arterial wall after high-pressure inflation of the dedicated delivery system. Secondly, in the in vitro study, it was evident that the balloon inflation was correlated with the jet length and thus the force applied to the arterial wall, and finally, histology and immunohistology was convincing that the total and the mean number of nerve fibers of the renal arteries treated with vincristine, were significantly lower to the nerve fibers of the control group that were treated with a mixture not containing vincristine [26].

The direct comparison of the two methods for the local delivery delivery of vincristine, a head to head comparison of the two catheters (the one with a constant flow rate of delivery and the other with a random flow rate delivery) was performed in an experimental model that used ten juvenile Landrace swine (3–5 months old, weight 29.9±1.6 kg), that underwent renal artery denervation by vincristine by both catheters. After the introduction of a sheath into the right or left femoral artery and the advancement of a guidewire into the distal part of the right renal artery, the first delivery balloon catheter (4–5 mm in diameter, 12–15 mm in length) that delivers vincristine with a random flow rate was advanced in the proximal part of the renal artery. Then the balloon was inflated and the vincristine mixture was delivered locally to the media of the renal artery. Similarly the process was repeated in the contralateral renal artery, with the use of the double balloon catheter that delivers vincristine to the media with a constant flow rate.

At 28 days after the initial procedure and just before euthanasia, all animals were alive indicating the safety of both methods. The effectiveness of denervation was assessed again by immunohistochemistry, and actually the sections of the renal artery treated with vincristine via the constant flow rate delivery catheter had lower expression of enolase positive cells (sympathetic nerve fibers) compared to the sections treated with vincristine delivered by random flow rate (1.70±0.41 versus 1.48±0.37 p=0.04) [28].

This findings support the known knowledge that the biological effect of any chemical agent on vascular endothelium, such as intima hyperplasia, or dissection and denervation, does not depend only on the drug potency, but also on the properties of the local delivery (flow rate). The transport and the binding properties of the chemical agent are important for the maintenance of adequate concentrations in the media of the vascular wall, and this is more important for hydrophobic drugs such as vincristine, that are relatively insoluble in the aqueous phase and bind to hydrophobic sites. Therefore the constant flow rate of the local delivery ensures the proper transport and the optimal concentration of the vincristine into the small dissections of the intima and the media layer of the renal artery [4].

First in Man Application of Renal Denervation by Vincristine

The First in Man application of renal denervation with vincristine was performed to a 74-year-old male patient that was referred due to uncontrolled arterial hypertension. He had an office blood pressure of 174/104 mmHg under treatment with valsartan 320 mg, amlodipine 10 mg and HCTZ 25 mg as a fixed combination and bisoprolol 10 mg. The diagnosis of resistant hypertension was confirmed by the results of ambulatory blood pressure monitoring that showed that the daytime average systolic blood pressure was 146 mmHg and average diastolic blood pressure was 85 mmHg. Moreover the patient was non-dipper, as there was no significant reduction in both systolic and diastolic blood pressures during the night.

Chemical renal denervation with vincristine was performed under local anesthesia via an eight French introducing sheath that was inserted into the right femoral artery. After the insertion and advancement of an eight French guiding catheter (Renal long, Boston Scientific, Natick, MA, USA) in the ostium of the left renal artery, and the performance of an initial angiogram of the renal artery, a guidewire was advanced to the distal segment of the renal artery and a single balloon delivery balloon-catheter (5 mm in diameter, 15 mm in length) described, was advanced into the main branch of the renal artery. The dedicated balloon was inflated at 20 atm, using a mixture containing vincristine and contrast and the inflation was interrupted when a total of 4 ml of the mixture (containing 0.1 mg of vincristine) was delivered. The same procedure was performed for chemical denervation of the right renal artery. After the completion of the procedure the patient was transferred to ICU unit and was discharged the following day, with no signs of renal damage. Follow up, was scheduled at 4 weeks. The office blood pressure was 132/80 mmHg, and the ambulatory blood pressure confirmed the control of blood pressure. The average SBP/DBP was 123/72 mmHg, the day time blood pressure was 124/73 mmHg and the night blood pressure was 124/73 mmHg [29].

All the previous data suggest the safety and efficacy of vincristine induced renal denervation both in experimental models and in humans. Although data from large scaled randomized studies are absent, the decrease of the number of sympathetic nerve fibers located in the media layer of the renal arteries, that was present in all experimental studies, and the treatment of the resistant hypertension in the first in

man application of the method, strongly suggest that this method can give solutions in patients with uncontrolled hypertension. An important limitation of the method is the midterm follow up of the studies, so the long term duration of its demyelinating effect, that it was reported in clinical studies in patients treated for cancer, needs to be verified in larger studied long term follow up [7].

References

1. Arndt C, Tefft M, Gehan E, Anderson J, Jenson M, Link M, Donaldson S, Breneman J, Wiener E, Webber B, Maurer H. A feasibility, toxicity, and early response study of etoposide, ifosfamide, and vincristine for the treatment of children with rhabdomyosarcoma: a report from the Intergroup Rhabdomyosarcoma Study (IRS) IV pilot study. J Pediatr Hematol Oncol. 1997;19(2):124–9.
2. Barajas L, Muller J. The innervation of the juxtaglomerular apparatus and surrounding tubules: a quantitative analysis by serial section electron microscopy. J Ultrastruct Res. 1973;43(1):107–32.
3. Carbone PP, Bono V, Frei 3rd E, Brindley CO. Clinical studies with vincristine. Blood. 1963;21:640–7.
4. Consigny PM, Davalian D, Donn R, Hu J, Rieser M, Stolarik D. Chemical renal denervation in the rat. Cardiovasc Intervent Radiol. 2013;37(1):218–23.
5. DiBona GF. The sympathetic nervous system and hypertension: recent developments. Hypertension. 2004;43(2):147–50.
6. Doumas M, Papademetriou V, Douma S, Faselis C, Tsioufis K, Gkaliagkousi E, Petidis K, Zamboulis C. Benefits from treatment and control of patients with resistant hypertension. Int J Hypertens. 2010;2011:318549.
7. Earl HM, Connolly S, Latoufis C, Eagle K, Ash CM, Fowler C, Souhami RL. Long-term neurotoxicity of chemotherapy in adolescents and young adults treated for bone and soft tissue sarcomas. Sarcoma. 1998;2:97–105.
8. Egbelakin A, Ferguson MJ, MacGill EA, Lehmann AS, Topletz AR, Quinney SK, Li L, McCammack KC, Hall SD, Renbarger JL. Increased risk of vincristine neurotoxicity associated with low CYP3A5 expression genotype in children with acute lymphoblastic leukemia. Pediatr Blood Cancer. 2011;56(3):361–7.
9. Esler MD, Krum H, Sobotka PA, Schlaich MP, Schmieder RE, Bohm M. Renal sympathetic denervation in patients with treatment-resistant hypertension (The Symplicity HTN-2 Trial): a randomised controlled trial. Lancet. 2011;9756:1903–9.
10. Gewirtz JR, Bisognano JD. Catheter-based renal sympathetic denervation: a targeted approach to resistant hypertension. Cardiol J. 2011;1:97–102.
11. Holland JF, Scharlau C, Gailani S, Krant MJ, Olson KB, Horton J, Shnider BI, Lynch JJ, Owens A, Carbone PP, Colsky J, Grob D, Miller SP, Hall TC. Vincristine treatment of advanced cancer: a cooperative study of 392 cases. Cancer Res. 1973;33(6):1258–64.
12. Ja'afer FM, Hamdan FB, Mohammed FH. Vincristine-induced neuropathy in rat: electrophysiological and histological study. Exp Brain Res. 2006;173(2):334–45.
13. Kaltenbach B, Id D, Franke JC, Sievert H, Hennersdorf M, Maier J, Bertog SC. Renal artery stenosis after renal sympathetic denervation. J Am Coll Cardiol. 2012;60(25):2694–5.
14. Kato T, Kassab S, Wilkins Jr FC, Kirchner KA, Granger JP. Decreased sensitivity to renal interstitial hydrostatic pressure in Dahl salt-sensitive rats. Hypertension. 1994;23(6 Pt 2):1082–6.
15. Krum H, Schlaich M, Whitbourn R, Sobotka PA, Sadowski J, Bartus K, Kapelak B, Walton A, Sievert H, Thambar S, Abraham WT, Esler M. Catheter-based renal sympathetic denervation for

resistant hypertension: a multicentre safety and proof-of-principle cohort study. Lancet. 2009;9671:1275–81.

16. LeQuesne. Neuropathy due to drugs; diseases of the peripheral nervous system. Peripheral neuropathy. 2nd ed. Philadelphia: WB Saunders Co; 1984. p. 2173–4.

17. Mabin T, Sapoval M, Cabane V, Stemmett J, Iyer M. First experience with endovascular ultrasound renal denervation for the treatment of resistant hypertension. Eur Interv. 2012; 8(1):57–61.

18. Manning PT, Powers CW, Schmidt RE, Johnson Jr EM. Guanethidine-induced destruction of peripheral sympathetic neurons occurs by an immune-mediated mechanism. J Neurosci. 1983;3(4):714–24.

19. Mantadakis E, Amoiridis G, Kondi A, Kalmanti M. Possible increase of the neurotoxicity of vincristine by the concurrent use of posaconazole in a young adult with leukemia. J Pediatr Hematol Oncol. 2007;29(2):130.

20. Medtronic pr (2014) http://newsroom.medtronic.com/phoenix. zhtml?c=251324&p=irol-newsArticle&ID=1889335&highlight=.

21. Moore AS, Norris R, Price G, Nguyen T, Ni M, George R, van Breda K, Duley J, Charles B, Pinkerton RV. Vincristine pharmacodynamics and pharmacogenetics in children with cancer: a limited-sampling, population modelling approach. J Paediatr Child Health.

22. Pal PK. Clinical and electrophysiological studies in vincristine induced neuropathy. Electromyogr Clin Neurophysiol. 1999;39(6):323–30.

23. Rosenthal S, Kaufman S. Vincristine neurotoxicity. Ann Intern Med. 1974;80(6):733–7.

24. Stefanadis C. Renal denervation in resistant hypertension: radiofrequency ablation and chemical denervation. Hellenic J Cardiol. 2011;52(6):481–2.

25. Stefanadis C, Synetos A, Toutouzas K, Tsioufis C, Drakopoulou M, Tsiamis E, Agrogiannis G, Patsouris E, Tousoulis D. Barodenervation of the sympathetic nervous system of the renal artery. A new concept. Int J Cardiol. 2013;168(4):4443–4.

26. Stefanadis C, Synetos A, Toutouzas K, Tsioufis C, Drakopoulou M, Tsiamis E, Agrogiannis G, Patsouris E, Tousoulis D. New double balloon delivery catheter for chemical denervation of the renal artery with vincristine. Int J Cardiol. 2013;168(4):4346–8.

27. Stefanadis C, Toutouzas K, Synetos A, Tsioufis C, Karanasos A, Agrogiannis G, Stefanis L, Patsouris E, Tousoulis D. Chemical denervation of the renal artery by vincristine in swine. A new catheter based technique. Int J Cardiol. 2013;167(2):421–5.

28. Stefanadis C, Toutouzas K, Synetos A, Tsioufis C, Karanasos A, Agrogiannis G, Stefanis L, Patsouris E, Tousoulis D. Effectiveness of the denervation of the renal sympathetic nervous system by vincristine, by a constant flow rate delivery catheter. Int J Cardiol Subm. 2014.

29. Stefanadis C, Toutouzas K, Vlachopoulos C, Tsioufis C, Synetos A, Pietri P, Tousoulis D, Tsiamis E. Chemical denervation of the renal artery with vincristine for the treatment of resistant arterial hypertension: first-in-man application. Hellenic J Cardiol. 2013;54(4):318–21.

30. Verstappen CC, Koeppen S, Heimans JJ, Huijgens PC, Scheulen ME, Strumberg D, Kiburg B, Postma TJ. Dose-related vincristine-induced peripheral neuropathy with unexpected off-therapy worsening. Neurology. 2005;64(6):1076–7.

NephroBlate™ Renal Denervation System: Urologic-Nephrologic Based Approach to Resistant Hypertension

Richard R. Heuser, Terrence J. Buelna, Adam Gold,
Rahul R. Rao, William G. Van Alstine, Randy I. Cooper,
and Mihir Desai

Introduction

Hypertension affects more than a quarter of adults in developed countries. In the USA, it was estimated to affect 65–70 million people in 2012 [1–4]. Hypertension is the leading treatable cardiovascular risk factor directly responsible for seven million deaths worldwide. There are over one billion (1.2 billion) hypertensive patients worldwide and by 2025, it is thought that we will have 1.5 billion patients with hypertension [1, 3, 5, 6]. Up to 20 % of the hypertensive population have resistant hypertension [1–3] which is defined as uncontrolled systolic blood pressure despite therapy with equal or greater than three antihypertensive agents from at least three different classes including a diuretic. Resistant hypertension often occurs in disorders where there is an enhanced sympathetic drive such as obesity, obstructive sleep apnea and chronic kidney disease [7, 8]. Resistant hypertensive patients show a strikingly greater

R.R. Heuser, MD, FACC, FACP, FESC, FSCAI (✉)
Department of Cardiology, St Lukes Medical Center,
555 N 18th St, Suite 300, Phoenix, AZ 85006, USA
e-mail: rheuser@phoenixheartcenter.com

T.J. Buelna • A. Gold, MSME • R.R. Rao, PE, BSc
Verve Medical Inc, 13660 N. 94th Drive, Suite D, Peoria,
AZ 85381, USA
e-mail: Terry@buelna.com; adam@verve-medical.com;
rahul@verve-medical.com

W.G. Van Alstine, DVM, PhD, DACVP
Department of Veterinary Medicine, Purdue University,
1625 Waterstone Drive, Lafayette, IN 47909, USA
e-mail: billvanDVM@gmail.com

R.I. Cooper, MD
Department of Nephrology, Southwest Vascular Center/Southwest
Kidney Institute, 1100 East University Drive, STE 100, Tempe,
AZ 85281, USA
e-mail: rcooper@swkidney.com

M. Desai, MD
Department of Urology, University of Southern California, USC
Institute of Urology, Los Angeles, CA, USA
e-mail: adityadesai2003@gmail.com

cardiovascular morbidity and mortality than controlled hypertensive patients [9].

The role of the renal sympathetic nerves in the pathogenesis of reno-vascular hypertension is paramount; excessive activation of the sympathetic system contributes to the development and perpetuation of hypertension. Afferent and efferent sympathetic nerves are thought to play a critical role. Efferent nerves (pre- and post ganglionic) signal sympathetic inflow to the kidneys and stimulates renin release activating the Renin-Angiotensin-Aldosterone (RAS) system, which in turn increases tubular reabsorption of sodium and causes extra-cellular volume expansion. The vaso-constriction caused by activation of the RAS pathway further increases the secretion of renin which perpetuates the process leading to hypertension. Afferent sympathetic nerves signaling out of the kidney to the renal artery plexus, celiac plexus, and sympathetic trunk, into the central nervous system, modulate central sympathetic tone and contribute to maintaining the neurogenic elevation of blood pressure [10, 11]. It is felt that up-regulation of the sympathetic nervous system is particularly important in resistant hypertension [12].

Sympathetic renal denervation's impact on reduction of hypertension has been recognized for many decades from the surgical literature. Most recently renal denervation (RDN) has been shown in unblinded studies (SYMPLICITY HTN-1 and 2) to be effective in reducing blood pressure in 85 % of patients with resistant hypertension with follow up to 3 years [13, 14]. Some patients have been excluded from arterial based device trials for multiple reasons, abnormal renal artery anatomy, renal aneurysms, renal stents, or severe kidney disease. Renal arteries are not always easily cannulated. Anatomical abnormalities such as acute angles of the take off of the renal artery, short renal artery, or no-common renal artery trunk, might make it impossible to perform arterial based RDN. Furthermore, there is variability in renal artery diameter; it may vary between 2 and 8 mm. Because of these issues, not all vessels can be treated with the currently available devices. One of the devices, the Medtronic-Ardian renal denervation device studied in the SYMPLICITY trial,

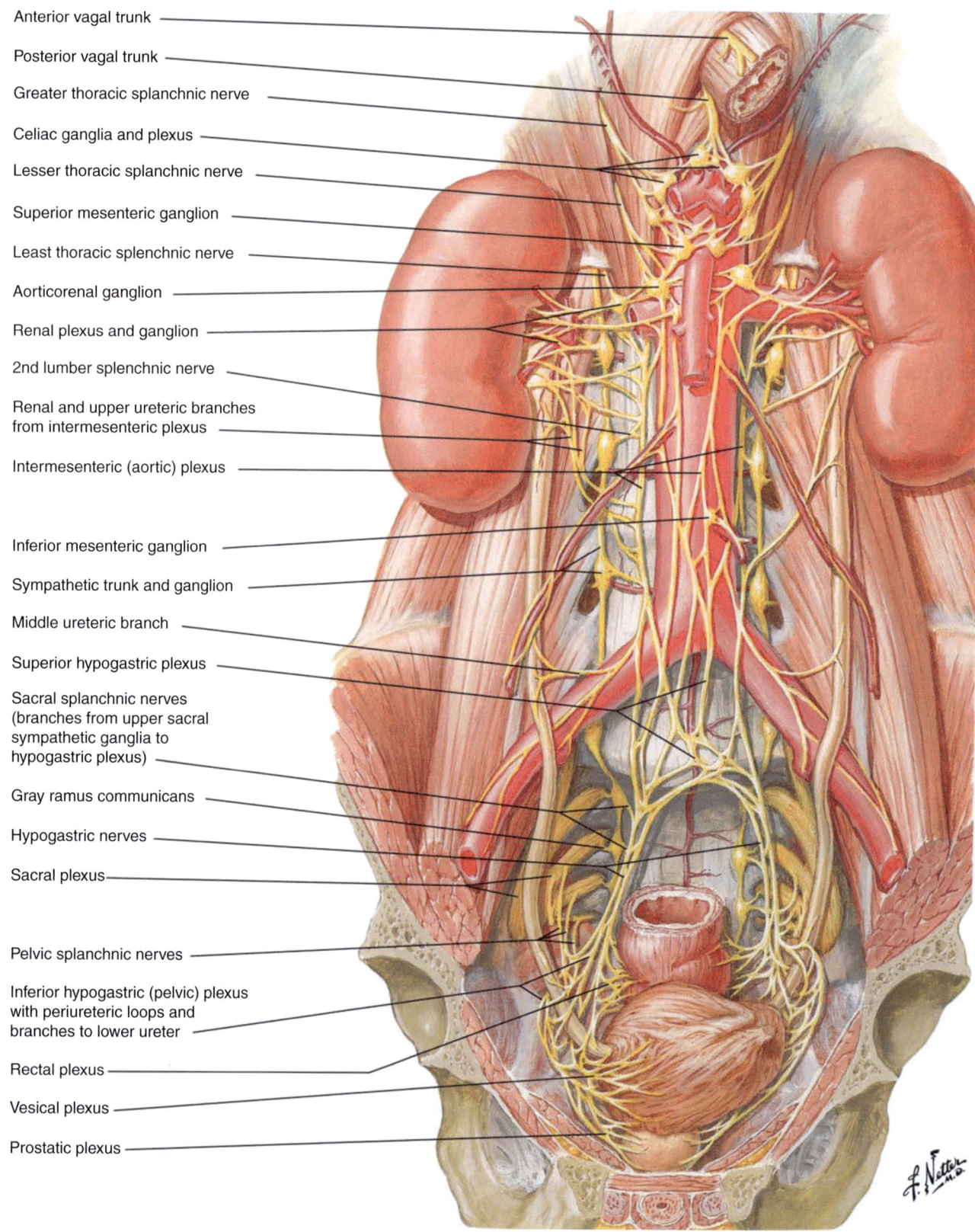

Anterior vagal trunk

Posterior vagal trunk

Greater thoracic splanchnic nerve

Celiac ganglia and plexus

Lesser thoracic splanchnic nerve

Superior mesenteric ganglion

Least thoracic splanchnic nerve

Aorticorenal ganglion

Renal plexus and ganglion

2nd lumber splenchnic nerve

Renal and upper ureteric branches
from intermesenteric plexus

Intermesenteric (aortic) plexus

Inferior mesenteric ganglion

Sympathetic trunk and ganglion

Middle ureteric branch

Superior hypogastric plexus

Sacral splanchnic nerves
(branches from upper sacral
sympathetic ganglia to
hypogastric plexus)

Gray ramus communicans

Hypogastric nerves

Sacral plexus

Pelvic splanchnic nerves

Inferior hypogastric (pelvic) plexus
with periureteric loops and
branches to lower ureter

Rectal plexus

Vesical plexus

Prostatic plexus

Fig. 15.1 Illustration of renal enervation. The netter collection of medical illustrations, volume 6, kidneys, ureters, and urinary bladder, page 27 (With permission from Elsevier, Health Sciences Division)

currently requires a procedural time greater than 45 min which can result in increased exposure to contrast and radiation. RDN procedural outcomes may not be known until at least 15 days of follow up, and more recent studies suggest as many as 20–30 % of patients are non-responders [14]. It is not clear if this non response is due to a lack of destruction of sufficient efferent or afferent nerve fibers, or other factors. Intra-arterial renal denervation is believed to primarily affect

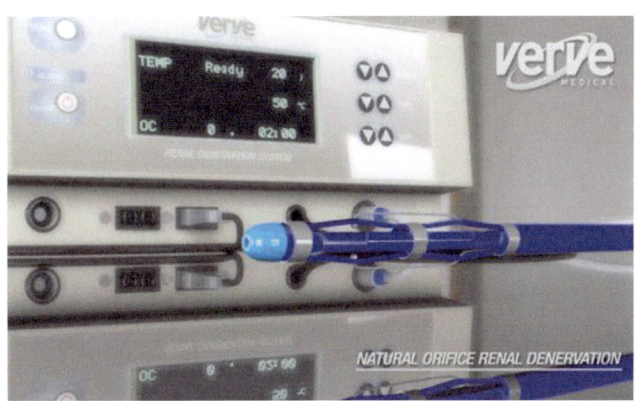

Fig. 15.2 The radiofrequency generator used for the Verve Medical device (Reprinted from Heuser et al. [17] with permission from Europa Digital and Publishing)

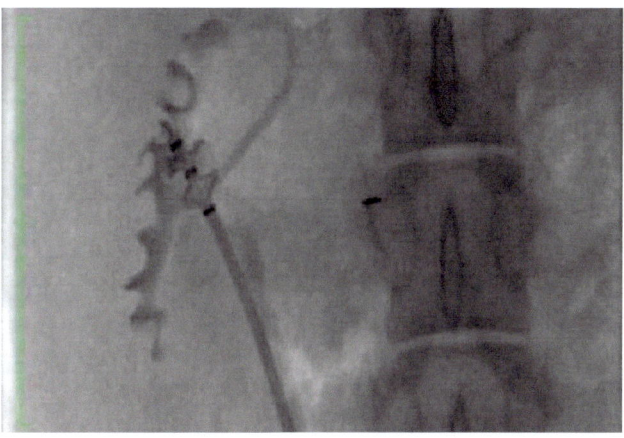

Fig. 15.4 Fluoroscopic image of the device in a swine's renal pelvis (Reprinted from Heuser et al. [17] with permission from Europa Digital and Publishing)

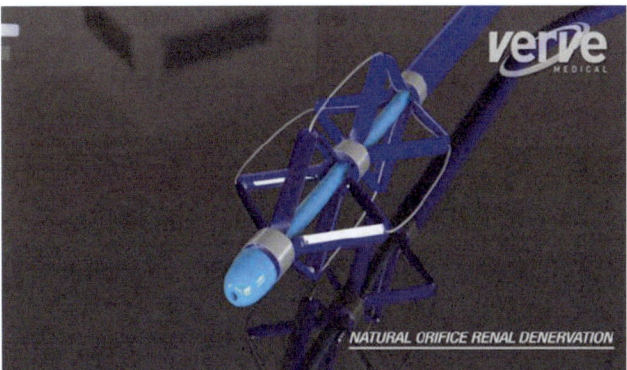

Fig. 15.3 The monopolar radiofrequency electrode catheter for delivery to the renal pelvis (Reprinted from Heuser et al. [17] with permission from Europa Digital and Publishing)

efferent nerves. There are other sources of enervation to the kidneys other than nerves that parallel the renal arteries (Fig. 15.1). There seems to be increased concentration of afferent sympathetic nerve fibers in the hilum of the kidney adjacent to the renal pelvis.

Verve Medical has developed NephroBlate™, a proprietary RF catheter system which can be introduced transurethrally to the renal pelvis, exploiting the proximity of the renal nerves to the renal pelvis with standard urologic techniques [15] (Figs. 15.2 and 15.3). It has been shown in the pelvic location, both efferent and afferent nerves are located and intertwined within the multiple layers of the renal pelvic wall [16]. This procedure is not restricted by anatomic variances of the artery and does not necessitate utilization of intra-arterial contrast. If contrast is administered, it will be delivered in a retrograde manner and not systemically (Fig. 15.4). The procedure can be performed in patients with bleeding diathesis without treatment with antiplatelets agents or heparin.

The Verve Medical system consists of a monopolar radiofrequency electrode catheter and a low power 50 W custom radiofrequency generator which monitors and regulates power, temperature, time and impedance. A standard 0.035 guidewire is delivered into the renal pelvis under direct

vision through the working channel of a cystoscope. The 9f catheter is then threaded over a standard 0.035 guidwire into the renal pelvis, distal to the UPJ and proximal to the calyces. The electrode array is located at the distal end of the catheter and radially expands to contact and dilate the renal pelvis. Low power, <10 W, monopolar energy is delivered from the generator through the electrodes into the renal pelvic wall for 4–6 min ablating the residing afferent and efferent nerves (Figs. 15.2, 15.3 and 15.4).

Methods and Results

Sixteen female domestic swine weighing 60–65 kg underwent bilateral renal denervation via ureteral access. Sixteen other similar animals were used for control. In each of the groups, three animals were euthanized immediately after delivery of RF energy; five animals at 7 days, six animals at 14 days and two animals at 30 days. Renal cortical tissue was harvested and Norepinephrine (NE) levels were measured using HPLC in all groups of animals. Histopathology of the treated zone was performed to confirm nerve damage.

Animals were fasted overnight then sedated with Ketamine, intubated, and maintained on Isoflurane anesthesia throughout the procedure. No anticoagulant was administered. A ventral midline laparotomy was performed to expose the urinary bladder. A 5 cm incision was made in the ventral aspect of the bladder to access the ureteral orifice. The Verve Medical device was passed retrograde over a 0.035″ guidewire from the bladder to the renal pelvis and RF ablation was performed. Treatment time/temperature algorithms were established with a range from 1 to 12 min and temperatures from 55 to 90 °C. The procedure was repeated in the contralateral kidney. In two animals, RF energy was not applied to the contralateral kidney (sham procedure). The device was not passed into the contralateral kidney. The urinary bladder and laparotomy were closed and the animals were allowed to recover from anesthesia. Bilateral pyelogram, ureterogram,

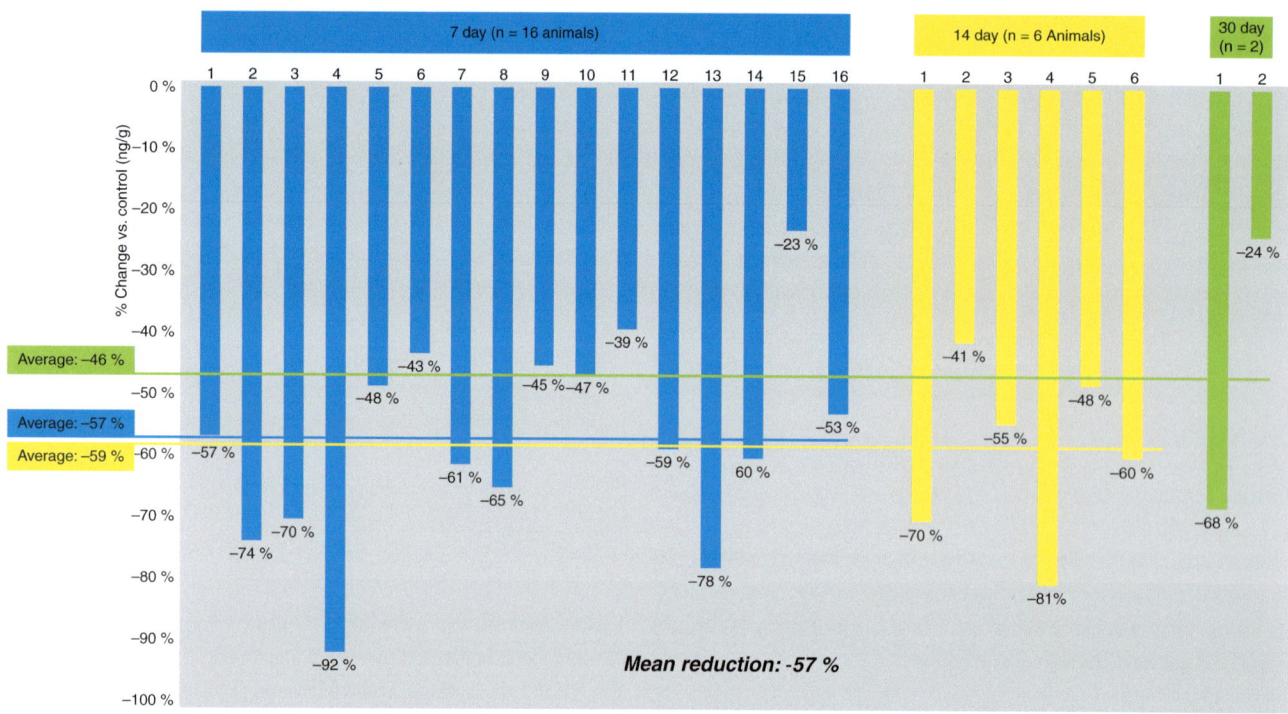

Fig. 15.5 Reduction from baseline of norepinephrine in the swine model post-intrapelvic RF ablation. Note that the data are per kidney (Reprinted from Heuser et al. [17] with permission from Europa Digital and Publishing)

and renal angiography were performed to insure no procedural related injury to the renal pelvis, ureters or the renal arteries. Immediately following euthanasia renal cortical tissue was harvested for determination of tissue norepinephrine concentration by High Performance Liquid Chromatography (HPLC) (Fig. 15.5). The kidneys were then perfusion fixed for histopathologic analysis (Fig. 15.6). In all animals there was a reduction of NE levels compared to control samples. Mean reduction of norepinephrine levels was 57 %, compared to control (Fig. 15.5). Histopathology confirmed nerve ablation in the treated zone with no parenchymal or vascular thermal injury.

With these results, we developed a protocol to treat a small number of patients (n=3, four kidneys) undergoing elective nephrectomy at Muljibhai Patel Urological Hospital in Nadiad, India. After submission to the hospital institutional review board and after patient informed consent we treated three patients with chronic kidney disease (two with nephrolithasis, one with end stage kidney disease from polycystic kidney disease (PKD)). The patients were treated on the side which was planned for elective nephrectomy. One patient (PKD) was pre-renal transplant and had both kidneys were treated. The RDN treatment was done under general anesthesia. One week after transurethral RDN treatment (Fig. 15.7a, b), the previously planned nephrectomy was performed. The procedure time was between 9 and 15 min. The procedures were well tolerated and no adverse effects were

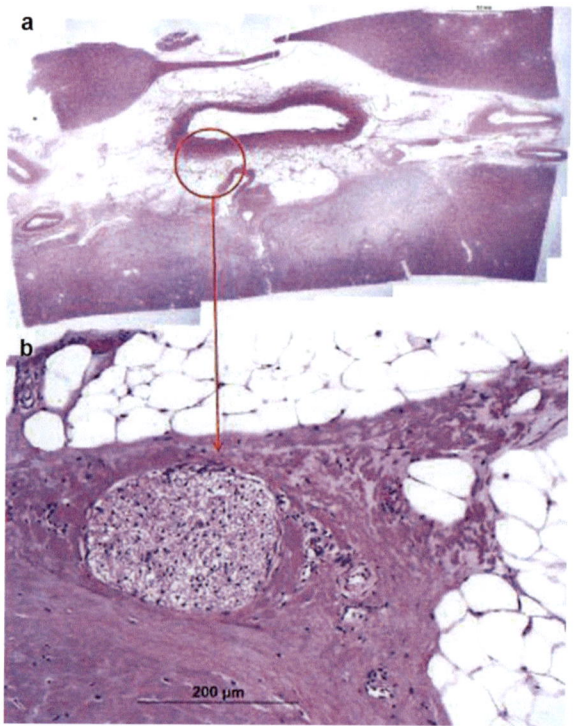

Fig. 15.6 (**a**) Image shows the relation to the surrounding renal pelvis tissue. Not all nuclei are damaged. (**b**) High power showing severe nerve injury with necrosis of endoneural cells and perineural thermal injury. Not all nuclei are damaged (From Heuser et al. [17] with permission from Europa Digital and Publishing)

Fig. 15.7 (**a**) Verve's NephroBlate™ (From Verve Medical with their permission) (**b**) NephroBlate™ Catheter – Fluoroscopic View – with wings extended

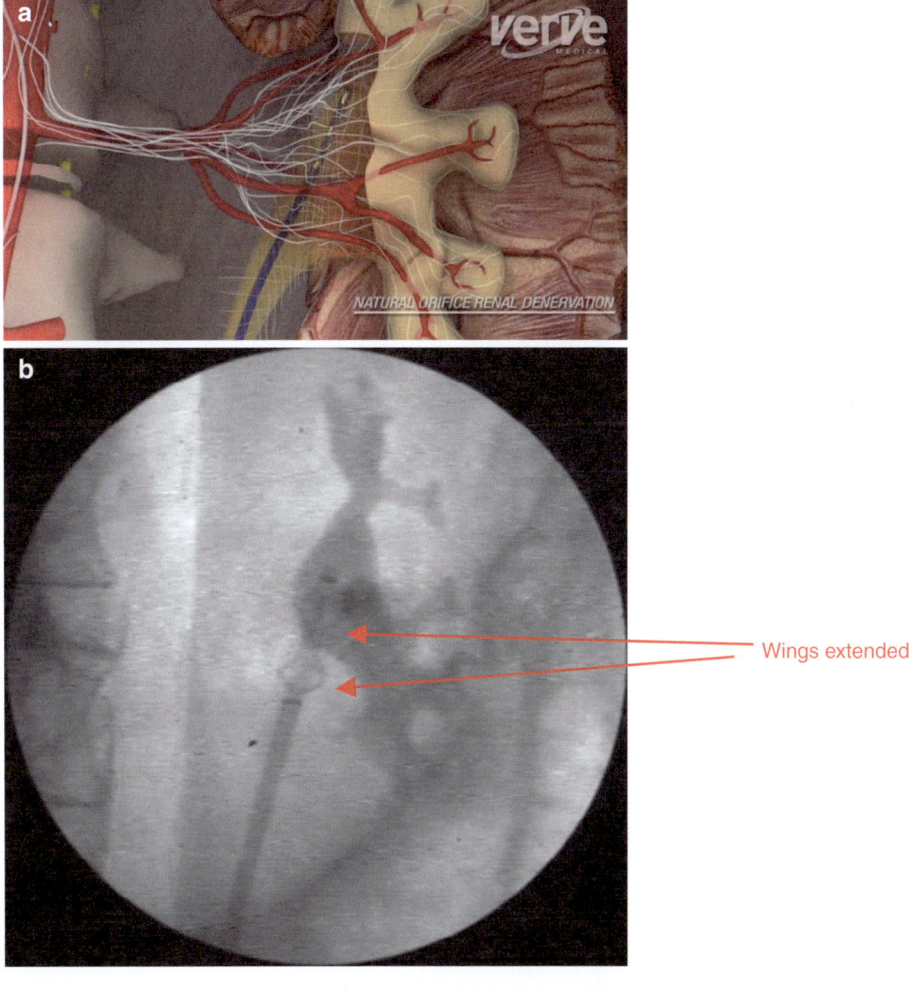

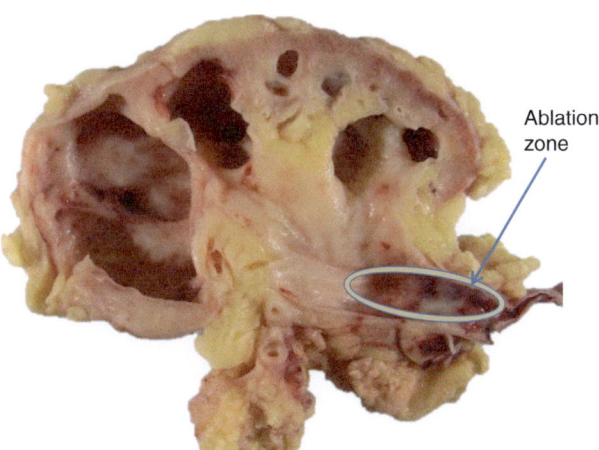

Fig. 15.8 Explanted human kidney 7 days post treatment (From Verve Medical with their permission)

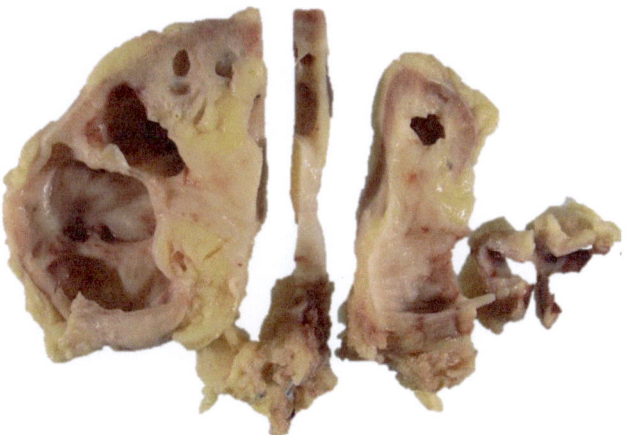

Fig. 15.9 Tissue sectioning for pathology (From Verve Medical with their permission)

recorded. The histopathological results on the treated kidney in all cases showed a significant destruction of the peri-pelvic nerves from the renal pelvic space to the serosa (1.75 mm) (Figs. 15.8, 15.9, 15.10, 15.11, 15.12, 15.13, 15.14 and

15.15). With a virtual elimination of the afferent and efferent nerves in the treated area and no change to the nerves in the control (untreated) segments in the histopathologic specimens, we proceeded with our clinical studies on resistant hypertensive patients.

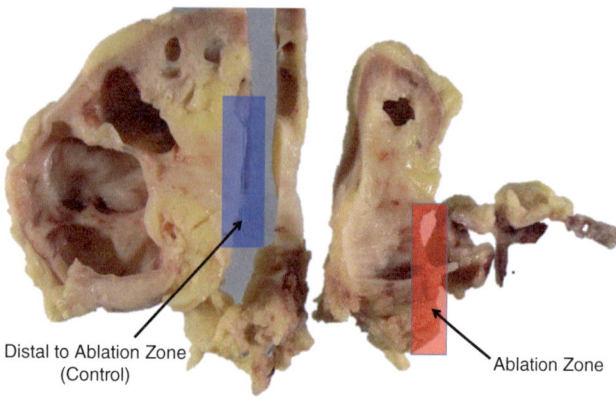

Histopathology Sampling Zones

Fig. 15.10 Histopathology sampling zones (From Verve Medical with their permission)

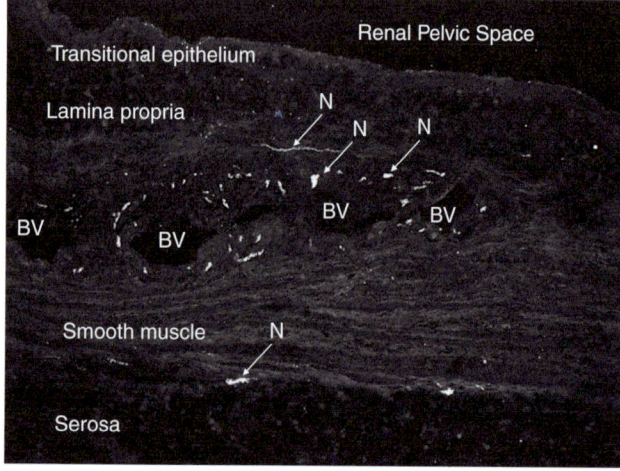

Fig. 15.11 Pelvis wall – distal to ablation zone (Control) (From Verve Medical with their permission)

With the above data, we proceeded with our clinical trial after Ethics Committee approval. Four patients were treated via trans-urethral approach under general anesthesia. The catheter was introduced via 9FR sheath. The RF energy was applied for 6 min, 70° Centigrade, 5 W. The operating room (OR) time ranged from 16 to 25 min. All patients had Double-J Stent placed post procedure as a precaution, and were removed 2 weeks later. The patients characteristics pre-procedure:

- Systolic BP Ave 172 mmHg
- eGFR Ave 82.4* ml/min/1.7
- Creatinine Ave 1.03* ml/dL
- (*Average not including the end-stage renal disease ESRD patient). If the ESRD patient data is included, the average systolic BP is the same (172 mmHg, GFR 65.02 ml/min/1.73 m^2, and Serum Creatinine is 1.80 mg/dL).

The inclusion criteria included: Office systolic blood pressure (SBP) ≥160 mmHg (SBP ≥ 150 mmHg with Type II diabetes mellitus), on >2 antihypertensive agents, with at least one agent being a diuretic. The procedures were performed in India. Practically speaking, few patients in our demographic territory could afford any more than two antihypertensive agents. As in the diseased kidney study, the procedure was done under general anesthesia. In either study, no patients received aspirin, heparin or any antiplatelet agents. Within minutes of treatment of the first kidney, a blood pressure response was noted and following the procedure, none of the patients had significant pain post procedure, bleeding, or urologic complications such as perforation or stricture formation or obstruction. There was a mean drop in systolic blood pressure of 44 mmHg (Systole: 20.55; Diastole: 13.58), with no significant change in renal function (Fig. 15.16 and Table 15.1).

Fig. 15.12 Pelvis wall – distal to ablation zone (Landscape) (From Verve Medical with their permission)

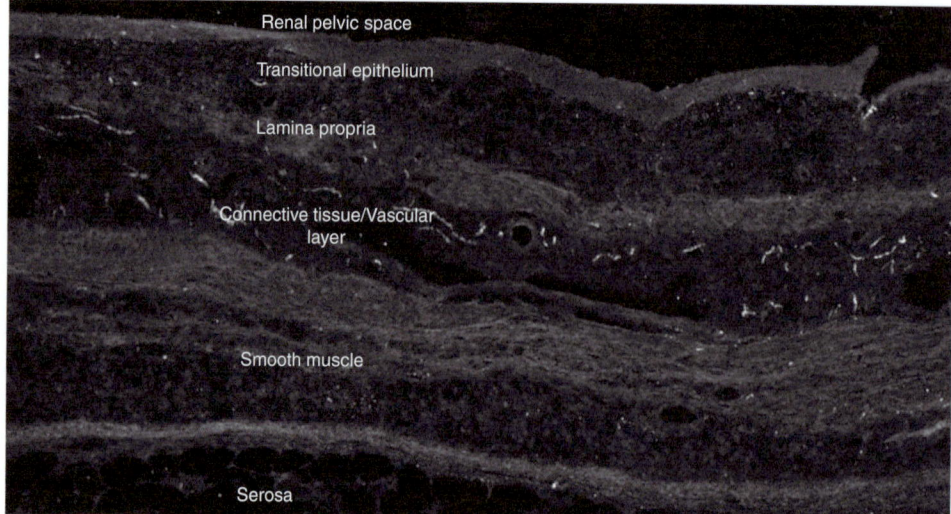

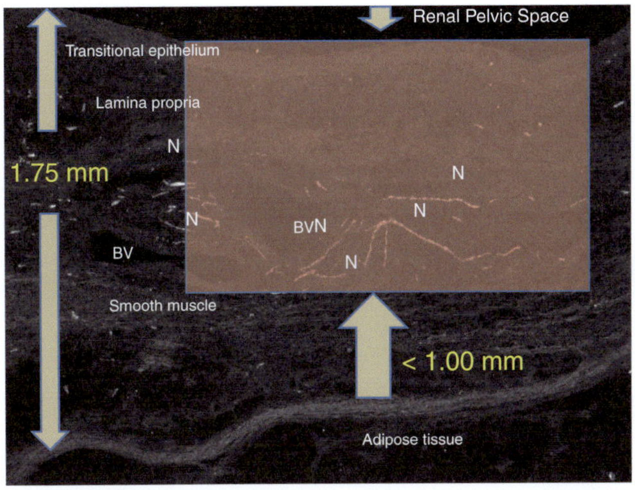

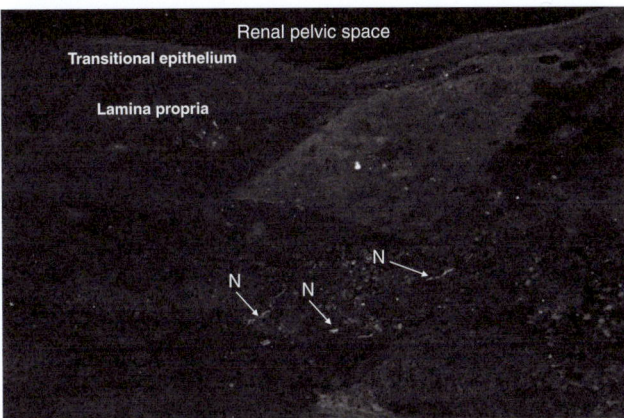

Fig. 15.13 Treatment depth (From Verve Medical with their permission)

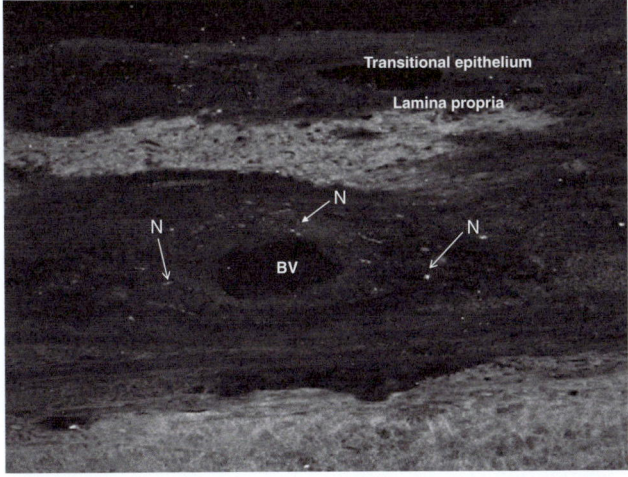

Fig. 15.14 Pelvis wall – ablation zone (From Verve Medical with their permission)

Fig. 15.15 Pelvis wall – ablation zone (From Verve Medical with their permission)

Discussion

In general terms, renal sympathetic efferent nerve activity is involved in renal excretion, sodium retention, reduced renal blood flow and peripheral and cardiovascular effects. Renal sympathetic afferent nerves affect central nervous drive; therefore, the inhibition of renal afferent nerves is a potential target for RH and carries the promise that control may result in a subsequent decline in associated cardiovascular morbidity/mortality. Targeted afferent ablation could not only reduce blood pressure, but could ameliorate organ specific damage caused by chronic sympathetic over activity.

When one considers renal disease, the concept of renal denervation is an intriguing theoretical approach. There is increased sympathetic activity with progressive deterioration of renal function [17]. There is microneurographic evidence of increased sympathetic activity in chronic renal disease [18–21].

Recent studies have shown that chronic kidney disease occurs in over one-half of the individuals born in the United States in their lifetime [22]. Studies of arterial RDN approaches to these patients have not only occurred, but have been effective. One series in patients with end stage renal disease, however, revealed that 25 % of patients attempted to be treated with the arterial approach with RDN could not be treated because of severe arterial disease [23]. This could be a real niche for a non-vascular device such as the Verve device.

Clearly, this is a small clinical sample of patients with resistant hypertension. Further human trials will need to confirm the efficacy and safety of the NephroBlate™ renal denervation system. The device may allow treatment of patients with arterial anatomic abnormalities. For instance, only 55 % of patients have a single hilar renal artery [24]. Limitations of the current vascular approaches for RDN include the possibility of renal artery anomalies, inappropriate vessel size or vessel origination from the aorta, previous stents, aneurysms, bifurcated renal arteries or renal insufficiency. With the vascular approach, complications are rare, but do occur (2.6 %) [25]. Because of where the vascular RDN applies the RF energy, we suspect that the efferent nerves are preferentially ablated. It is thought that the efferent nerves can anatomically regrow after renal denervation. Furthermore, it is believed that the afferent sympathetic nerves have a greater impact on the activation of the RAS pathway [26–28]. There seems to be a preferentially increased concentration of the afferent nerves adjacent to the renal pelvis.

Some unique potential problems with the arterial approach have been described by new imaging techniques. Optical coherence tomography was performed pre and post renal nerve ablation in 32 renal arteries in patients with treatment resistant hypertension [28]. Vasospasm occurred more often after RDN than before (0 % vs. 42 % p<0.001) [28]. A decrease in renal artery diameter after RDN was documented with the EnligHTN™ device (4.69±0.73 vs. 4.21±0.88 mm p<0.0012). This was also seen with the Medtronic-Ardian

Fig. 15.16 Reduction in blood pressure; 1 month results. Four drug resistant patients on ≥2 drugs (From Verve Medical with their permission)

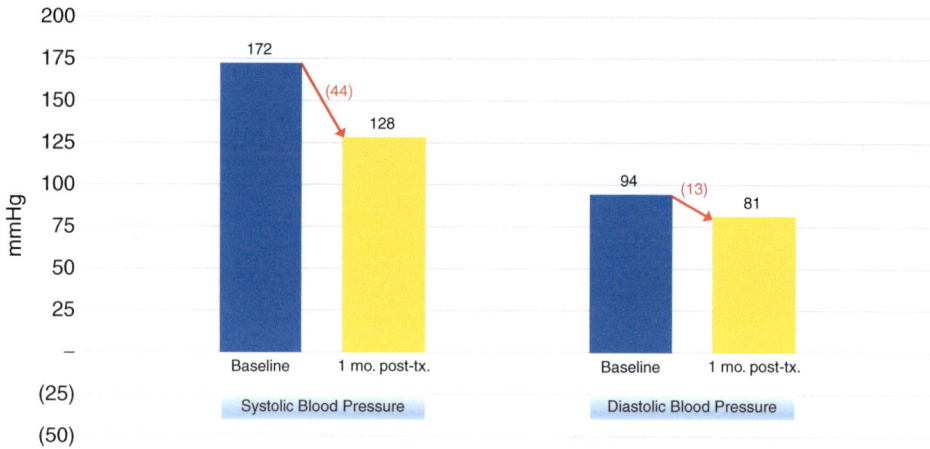

Table 15.1 Kidney function: 1 month follow up. Consistent results; minimal change (From Verve Medical with their permission)

GFR (ml/min/1.73 m²)			Serum creatinine (mg/dL)		
Pre	Post	% Change	Pre	Post	% Change
65.02	61.13	6.0 %	1.80	1.79	−0.8 %

SYMPLICITY device (15.04±0.66 vs. 4.55±0.88 mm p<0.001). Intimal edema was noted in 96 % of cases after RNA. Thrombus formation occurred 67 % vs. 18 % p<0.001 (after vs. before). Whether this is clinically relevant is unknown, but we definitely need to consider antiplatelet therapy with the arterial approaches [26].

Treatment of patients who have renal insufficiency that preclude contrast utilization during the procedure and treatment of patients with previously placed renal stents could be unique advantages of the NephroBlate™ renal denervation system. It is enticing to consider applications in patients who otherwise are not candidates for renal denervation the current available technology at this time. In a general hypertensive population, patients do not achieve blood pressure control in 28–53.1 % of cases [1] and future applications could be in patients with mild hypertension only, heart failure medication intolerant patients, diabetic patients, patients with sleep apnea or even patients with metabolic syndrome. In contrast to other devices, the NephroBlate™ device does not require the operator to reposition the ablation catheter to multiple sites for treatment. It is possible that only a single ablative treatment in each renal pelvis is needed. The device is delivered using standard urologic techniques and the procedure could be performed with cystoscopy and ultrasound in an outpatient or possibly an office setting.

It is conceivable that the treatment of efferent and afferent nerves which are in close proximity to the NephroBlate™ catheter may require less energy delivery with lower temperatures than current RF, Ultrasound, or other energy based systems. It is also possible the monopolar RF catheter may also reduce procedure time compared to arterial delivery

systems. Because the NephroBlate™ catheter ablates the nerves within the pelvis which are predominantly afferent nerves [16], there may be a more direct effect on the sympathetic nervous system in patients with pelvic directed RDN.

Possible unique applications of the non-vascular approach in a resistant hypertensive patient would include the following clinical scenarios:

- Patients with existing disease or anatomic anomalies
- Patients who have failed arterial approaches
- Patients with severe chronic kidney disease who are more prone to contrast nephropathy
- Patients who might need physiologic "nephrectomy"
- Renal transplant patients with severe high blood pressure (treatment the existing non- functioning kidney)
- Patients with antiplatelet intolerance or bleeding disorders

Nonresponders from the Symplicity Trial have averaged about 15 %, but in some other studies the number has been as high as 50 % [29]. Those with the most severe hypertension seem to be the biggest responders. Most studies have had only short follow up; in fact, less than 70 % of studies published have had at least 6 month follow up. Although in some studies, efficacy has been shown to be up to 36 months, the size and durability of the antihypertensive effect, long term safety and hard cardiovascular and renal endpoints still need to be verified before denervation is established as an approved technique. Currently, the overall duration of the procedure and associated discomfort and pain requiring sedation is an issue and bradycardia can occur in 13 % of the cases [30, 31]. Inconsistency and unpredictably is further aggravated by the absence of actual renal enervation direct measurements as the procedure offers no acute endpoint on the treatment outcome during the intervention [31].

It has been suggested that over the next two decades up to 50 % of the adult population will be diagnosed with hypertension [1]. We do need other approaches to treat these patients. New devices, however, need to be safe, effective and durable. Patients with renal anomalies; stents, aneurysms, multiple arteries, difficult access patients need therapy. Patients who have renal insufficiency should be able to be treated without risk of contrast nephrotoxicity. We should be able to treat patients who have not responded to arterial treatments. A certain percentage of patients have aspirin intolerance or allergy may also need treatment for resistant hypertension [32]. Patients with bleeding disorders would be unlikely candidates for RDN using the arterial approach. Clopidogrel allergy occurs in 1–1.6 % of patients [33, 34]. With the possibility that RDN will be more widely utilized in the future, it would be important not to exclude these patients. In our clinical experience, the blood pressure response was immediate and maintained at 3 month follow up. Further studies will need to be conducted to see if this continues, and if it does and since the procedures were performed under general anesthesia, a sham control would probably not be necessary to confirm success since with anesthesia the placebo affect is minimized if not eliminated. A serious limitation in all the other devices is the lack of immediate feedback of success is eliminated. Ideally, this should be able to be performed as an outpatient procedure. The procedure should be done fairly quickly with minimal pain to the patient.

Limitations

This may not be an interventional cardiology procedure. It may be performed by urologists since cystoscopy must be utilized for access. The catheter is a 9F system which is a normal French size for urologists who perform catheter procedures routinely utilizing an 0.035″ wire. Perhaps the urologist will perform the procedure in concert with an interventional nephrologist, interventional radiologist or interventional cardiologist in the future. Some clinical limitations of this new technique have to be described. Patients with nephrolithiasis, pelvic ureteral junction (PUJ) obstruction, previous renal surgery and other obstructive/reflex uropathies, ascending urinary tract infections and patients with indwelling catheters probably would not be considered candidates for this approach.

Conclusion

Although numerous articles show renal interruption of the renal afferent nerves will attenuate systemic tone lowering blood pressure, most studies have primarily included treatment of efferent systems. In contrast to the zwidespread distribution of efferent sympathetic nerve fibers in the kidneys the majority of the afferent renal sensory nerves are located in the renal pelvic area [16].

As many as 44 % of patients in the Symplicity HTN-1 and 2 trials were excluded because of clinical and anatomic study entry requirements [28]. Even with improvements in arterial devices, anatomic exclusions still occur

(in 23 % with the Stylus device) [35]. If Verve Medical's clinical experience confirms efficacy and safety, this approach may be one way to treat patients who cannot be treated with the standard percutaneous arterial devices. It also may have a unique application in patients with resistant hypertension and renal insufficiency because of the lack of utilization of systemic contrast.

References

1. Kearney PM, Reynolds K, Muntner P, Whelton PK, He J. Global burden of hypertension: analysis of worldwide data. Lancet. 2005;365:217–23.
2. Lloyd-Jones D, Adams RJ, Brown TM, Carnethon M, Dai S, De Simone G, Ferguson TB, Ford E, Furie K, Gillespie C, Go A, Greenlund K, Haase N, Hailpern S, Ho PM, Howard V, Kissela B, Kittner S, Lackland D, Lisabeth L, Marelli A, McDermott MM, Meigs J, Mozaffarian D, Mussolino M, Nichol G, Roger VL, Rosamond W, Sacco R, Sorlie P, Roger VL, Thom T, Wasserthiel-Smoller S, Wong ND, Wylie-Rosett J. Heart disease and stroke statistics – 2010 update: a report from the American Heart Association. Circulation. 2010;121:E46E215.
3. Wolf-Maier K, Cooper RS, Banegas JR, Giampaoli S, Hense HW, Joffres M, Kastarinen M, Poulter N, Primatesta P, Rodríguez-Artalejo F, Stegmayr B, Thamm M, Tuomilehto J, Vanuzzo D, Vescio F. Hypertension prevalence and blood pressure levels in 6 European countries, Canada, and the United States. JAMA. 2003;289:2363–9.
4. Sekikawa A, Hayakawa T. Prevalence of hypertension, its awareness and control in adult population in Japan. J Hum Hypertens. 2004;18:911–2.
5. Lewington S, Clarke R, Qzilbash N, Peto R, Collins R. Age-specific relevance of usual blood pressure to vascular mortality: a meta-analysis of individual data for one million adults in 61 prospective studies. Lancet. 2002;360:1903–13.
6. Writing group members, Lloyd-Jones D, Adams RJ, Brown TM, Carnethon M, Dai S, De Simone G, Ferguson ATB, Ford E, Furie K, Gellespie C, Go A, Greenlund K, Haase N, Hailpern S, Ho PM, Howard V, Kissela B, Kittner S, Lackland D, Lisabeth L, Marelli A, McDermott MM, Meigs J, Mozaffarian D, Mussolino M, Nichol G, Roger VL, Rosamond W, Sacco R, Sorlie P, Roger VL, Thom T, Wasserthiel-Smoller S, Wong ND, Wylie-Rosett J. American Heart Association Statistics Committee and Stroke Subcommittee. Heart disease and stroke statistics – 2010 update: a report from the American Heart Association. Circulation. 2010;121:948–54.
7. Grassi G. Assessment of sympathetic cardiovascular drive in human hypertension: achievements and perspectives. Hypertension. 2009;54(4):690–7.
8. Pedrosa RP, Drager LF, Gonzaga CC, et al. Obstructive sleep apnea: the most common secondary cause of hypertension associated with resistant hypertension. Hypertension. 2011;58(5):811–7.
9. Pierdomenico SD, Lapenna D, Bucci A, Di Thommaso R, Di Mascio R, Manente BM, Caldarella MP, Neri M, Cuccurullo F, Mezzetti A. Cardiovascular outcome in treated hypertensive patients with responder, masked, false resistant and true resistant hypertension. Am J Hypertens. 2005;18:1422–8.
10. DiBona GF, Kopp UC. Neural control of renal function. Physiol Rev. 1997;77(1):75–197.
11. Gu YM, Asayama K, Liu YP, Staessen JA. Renal denervation: time to open Pandora's box. Swiss Med Wkly. 2012;142:213638.
12. Tsioufis C, Kordalis A, Fiessas D, et al. Pathophysiology of resistant hypertension: role of the sympathetic nervous system. Int J Hypertens. 2011;2011:642416.

13. Schlaich MP, Sobotka PA, Krum H, Whitbourn R, Walton A, Esler MD. Renal denervation as a therapeutic approach for hypertension: novel implications for an old concept. Hypertension. 2009;54:1195–201.

14. Henry Krum, for the Symplicity I Investigators. Radiofrequency energy provides safe and durable blood pressure reduction: complete 3 year results from the Symplicity HTN-1. ESC, May 2013.

15. Heuser RR, Buelna TJ, Berci WL, Hubbard BS. A novel non-vascular system to treat resistant hypertension. EuroIntervention. 2013;9:135–8.

16. Kopp UC. Neural control of renal function. Colloquium series on integrated systems physiology: from molecule to function. In: Granger D, Granger J, editors. Morgan & Claypool Publishers; 2011.

17. Sampaio F, Uflacker R. Renal anatomy applied to urology, endourology and interventional radiology. 1st ed. Chapter 7; NY: Thieme Medical Publishing; 1993. p. 49.

18. Polimeni A, Curcio A, Indolfi C. Renal sympathetic denervation for treating resistant hypertension. Circ J. 2013;77(4):857–63. Epub 2013 Mar 19.

19. Templin C, Jaguszewski M, Ghadri JR, Sudano I, Gaehwiler R, Hellermann JP, Schoenenberger-Berzins R, Landmesser U, Erne P, Noll G, Luscher TF. Vascular lesions induced by renal nerve ablation as assessed by optical coherence tomography: pre- and post-procedural comparison with the Symplicity(R) catheter system and the EnligHTN™ multi-electrode renal denervation catheter. Eur Heart J. 2013;34:2141–8.

20. Hausberg M, Kosch M, Harmelink P, Barenbrock M, Hohage H, Kisters K, Dietl KH, Rahn KH. Sympathetic nerve activity in end-stage renal disease. Circulation. 2002;106:1974–9.

21. Klein I, Ligtenberg G, Liamoey P, Koomans HA, Blanestijn PJ. Sympathetic activity is increased in polycystic kidney disease and is associated with hypertension. JASN. 2001;12:2427–33.

22. Charnow JA. Lifetime CKD risk high in the U.S. Renal & Urology News. 10 Sept 2013.

23. Schlaich MP, Bart B, Hering D, Walton A, Marusic P, Mahfoud F, Bohm M, Lambert EA, Krum H, Sobotka PA, Schmieder RE, Ika-Sari C, Eikelis N, Straznicky N, Lambert GW, Esler M. Feasibility of catheter-based renal nerve ablation and effects on sympathetic nerve activity and blood pressure in patients with end-stage renal disease. EuroPCR. 2013.

24. Converse Jr RL, Jacobbsen TN, Toto RD, Jost CMT, Consentino F, Foud-Tarazi F, Victor RG. Sympathetic overactivity in patients with chronic renal failure. N Engl J Med. 1992;327:1912–8.

25. Ligtenberg G, Blankestijn PJ, Oey PL, Klein I, Dijkhorst-Oei LT, Boomsma F, Wieneke GH, van Huffelen AC, Koomans HA. Reduction of sympathetic hyperactivity by Enalapril in patients with chronic renal failure. N Engl J Med. 1999;340:1321–8.

26. Campese VM, Kogosov E, Koss M. Renal afferent denervation prevents the progression of renal disease in the renal ablation model of chronic renal failure in the rat. Am J Kidney Dis. 1995;26:861–5.

27. Kopp UC, Cicha MZ, Smith LA, Mulder J, Hökfelt T. Renal sympathetic nerve activity modulates afferent renal nerve activity by pge2-dependent activation of α1-and α2-adrenoceptors on renal sensory nerve fibers. Am J Physiol Regul Integr Comp Physiol. 2007;293:R1561–72.

28. Johansson M, Elam M, Rundquist B, Eisenhofer G, Herlitz H, Lambert G, Friberg P. Increased sympathetic nerve activity in renovascular hypertension. Circulation. 1999;99:2537–42.

29. Kaltenbach B, Franke J, Bertog SC, Steinberg DH, Hofmann I, Sievert H. renal sympathetic denervation as second-line therapy in mild resistant hypertension: a pilot study. Catheter Cardiovasc Interv. 2013;81:335–9.

30. Esler MD, Krum H, Schlaich M, Schmieder RE, Böhm M, Sobotka PA. Symplicity HTN-2 Investigators. Renal sympathetic denervation for treatment of drug-resistant hypertension: one-year results from the Symplicity HTN-2 randomized, controlled trial. Circulation. 2012;126:2976–82.

31. Krum H, Schlaich M, Sobotka P, Murray E, Felix M, Michael B, Mark Dunlap M, Rocha-Singh K, Katholi R. TCT 12 long-term follow-up of catheter-based renal denervation for resistant hypertension confirms durable blood pressure reduction. J Am Coll Cardiol. 2012;60:B3.

32. Ramanuja S, Breall J, Kalaria V. Approach to "aspirin allergy" in cardiovascular patients. Circulation. 2004;110:e1–4.

33. Lokhandwala J, Best PJ, Henry Y, Berger PB. Allergic reactions to clopidogrel and cross-reactivity to other agents. Curr Allergy Asthma Rep. 2011;11(1):52.

34. Cheema AN, Mohammad A, Hong T, Jakubovic HR, Parmar GS, Sharieff W, Garvey MB, Kutryk MJ, Fam NP, Graham JJ, Chisolm RJ. Characterization of clopidogrel hypersensitivity reactions and management with oral steroids without clopidogrel discontinuation. J Am Coll Cardiol. 2011;58(14):1445.

35. Mahfoud F, on behalf of Professor Robert Whitbourn. Simulataneous multi-electrode renal denervation treatment for resistant hypertension: results from a First-in-Man Feasibility study. Presented at ESC, May 2013.

Mark H. Wholey, Emily Stein, Michael Evans, and K.T. Venkateswara Rao

Introduction

Renal denervation through catheter-based ablation of renal nerves appears to be a promising therapy to treat resistant hypertension. Currently, there are several approaches in development to achieve ablation. These include energy-based approaches using radiofrequency (RF), ultrasound (intravascular and extra-vascular), beta-radiation and cryo-ablation [1–8]. All energy-based approaches are untargeted and have the potential to damage the vascular wall and surrounding tissue. Moreover, OCT findings have shown that RF probes damage the endothelial layer and cause thrombus formation on the intraluminal side [9]. Late stenosis in renal arteries have also been reported in a limited number of cases with RF ablation [10, 11]. In addition, energy-based approaches are not suitable for treating stented areas of the renal arteries [12].

M.H. Wholey, MD (✉)
UPMC Shadyside, Pittsburgh Vascular Institute,
5230 Centre Avenue, Pittsburgh, PA 15232, USA

Northwind Medical, 6254 Grand Oak Way,
San Jose, CA 95135, USA
e-mail: wholeymh@upmc.edu

E. Stein, PhD
963 Helen Ave., San Leandro, CA 94577, USA

Northwind Medical, 6254 Grand Oak Way,
San Jose, CA 95135, USA
e-mail: emilyste@gmail.com

M. Evans, BS
145 Tasso St., Palo Alto, CA 94301, USA

Northwind Medical, 6254 Grand Oak Way,
San Jose, CA 95135, USA
e-mail: Michael6501@gmail.com

K.T. Venkateswara Rao, PhD
Northwind Medical, 6254 Grand Oak Way,
San Jose, CA 95135, USA
e-mail: kt@northwindmed.com

Implant-based approaches have also been suggested. These include baroreceptor activation therapies to modulate the nerves at the carotid sinus [13]. Electrical generator implants, designed to sense local blood pressure and send electrical signals to modulate baroreceptor activity, are under investigation. Implants mechanically stimulate the carotid sinus and act on the baroreceptors. Lastly, implants that reduce vascular resistance by making an arterio-venous (A-V) fistula in the iliac arteries [14] have also been clinically tested in patients with resistant hypertension.

Agent-based therapies to treat resistant hypertension are also in development. These include catheter-mediated administration of non-targeted agents to ablate the renal artery tissue including ethanol and vinchristine and the adrenergic agent, guanethidine [15–17].

We believe that implant-based approaches to treat hypertension are not cost effective and that simpler and neuronal site-specific therapies can be developed based on targeted pharmacologic intervention. One such approach is to specifically induce renal nerve cell death using targeted delivery of one or more neurotropic agents using a catheter-based approach. Focal injection of a small volume of neurotropic agent delivered by microneedle catheters into the wall of the renal arteries has been shown to induce target-specific nerve cell deactivation in situ. In this paper, we describe the approach and present results from pre-clinical experiments conducted and discuss preliminary results from first-in-human studies.

The main objective of these studies was to demonstrate the feasibility of agent-based renal deactivation therapy to treat hypertension using Northwind agent formulations. Specific objectives were to evaluate the: (i) feasibility of delivering therapeutic amount of neurotropic agent into the vessel wall of renal arteries using microneedles, (ii) safety of the neurotropic agent, evaluated in terms of off-target cytotoxicity within the renal arterial wall and surrounding tissues, (iii) efficacy of neurotropic agent, evaluated in terms of the ability to induce nerve block and nerve cell death, and (iv) efficacy of agent to reduce blood pressure, as measured by a reduction in norepinephrine levels in blood and kidney tissue, at acute (14-day) and chronic (90-day) time points. In addition, the dose response of the neurotropic agent and its durability was also examined.

Background

Evidence supporting the role of the peripheral nervous system (PNS) in hypertension has been demonstrated in numerous clinical procedures involving phenol ablative and surgical ablation methods over past decades. The PNS serves as a feedback loop to transmit environmental or tissue-specific stress and damage signals as electrochemical feedback messages to the central nervous system (CNS) to trigger various 'flight-or-fight' responses. As a component of the sympathetic nervous system, the PNS plays a role in the regulation of blood pressure and heart rate. The identity and understanding of neurotransmitters such as neuropeptide Y, natriuretic peptides, neuronal nitric oxide synthase and others and their involvement in cardiovascular autonomic control build upon our understanding of the classical neurotransmitters involved in the regulation of heart rate and blood pressure, acetylcholine (AC) and the catecholamine, norepinephrine (NE) [18, 19]. In cardiac tissue, acetylcholine has an inhibitory effect and lowers heart rate while NE has a stimulatory effect on heart rate [18]. Clinically, NE is used as a vasopressive drug and is administered to patients with hypotension and shock to increase blood pressure [20]. In models of induced hypertension, intermittent increases in intra-renal adrenergic neurotransmitter levels have been sufficient to elicit chronic hypertension [21]. Further, elevated NE levels are correlated with clinical hypertension and its reduction has been shown to correlate with a drop in ambulatory blood pressure [22]. Elevated circulating catecholamine levels and PNS hyperactivity are hallmark symptoms in many patients with essential hypertension [22, 23]. We hypothesize that interruption of the electrochemical signaling of PNS neurons in tissue-specific neuronal bundles will inhibit local sympathetic neurotransmitter release and thus interrupt regional chemoelectrical signaling relay back to the CNS and result in a change in vascular tone. Furthermore, we hypothesize that sustained inhibition of neuronal signaling can induce intracellular stress responses that lead to apoptosis, a quieter cell death as opposed to more inflammatory types of cell death such as chemical and energy ablation. We have selected a number of pharmacologic agents known to bind cell surface receptors on neurons. A brief summary of our pre-clinical findings is provided below.

Experimental Methods

Various FDA approved agents were identified for having PK/PD and hydrophobicity profiles amenable for nerve-specific deactivation in the renal artery. Selected agents were screened in human neuronal cell cultures at established concentrations (ED_{50}, ED_{100}, LD_{50}) and their ability to induce a sustained drop in metabolic activity (using the MTT assay; Life Technologies), induction of apoptosis by monitoring Caspase-3 activation (Cell Signaling Technologies), and overall cytotoxicity (trypan blue staining) was evaluated in time-course experiments. The lead compound NW2013 was identified as having optimal kinetics and potency in vitro. NW2013, along with a few other efficacious agents and formulations thereof were then evaluated in vivo using the Sprague-Dawley rat sciatic nerve block model.

Studies in the Rat Sciatic Nerve-Block Model

Sprague-Dawley rats (250–300 g) were randomly assigned into treatment and control groups and were transiently anesthetized by ketamine. Following anesthetization, the sciatic notch was accessed by palpitation and 200 uL of NW2013, other proprietary pharmacologic agents, or the chemical agent ethanol were administered by a single intra-muscular injection using a 27-gauge needle near the sciatic notch. A single injection of phosphate-buffered saline in the right leg served as the negative control. The β-adrenergic receptor antagonist, guanethidine, served as positive control.

Animals were survived to 3 and 30 days and were assessed on a weekly basis for clinical manifestations of neuropathy. Clinical and analytical assessments included the ability of the sciatic nerve bundle to conduct signals at 5 Hz (results in a leg twitch) or 20 Hz (results in leg tetanus), sensory proprioception (slight pinch of the foot pad), motor nerve function (ability for animal to walk and step up), over-all leg function (ability to apply body pressure while walking). Animals were euthanized on day 3 and day 30 and immunohistochemical evaluation of the sciatic nerve bundles and surrounding tissue was performed.

Renal Nerve Deactivation Studies in the Porcine Model

Juvenile Yorkshire domestic swine (30–40 kg) were housed and quarantined for 7 days prior to the procedure. Animals were anesthetized and blood samples were collected before surgery. The target renal artery with surrounding tissue was

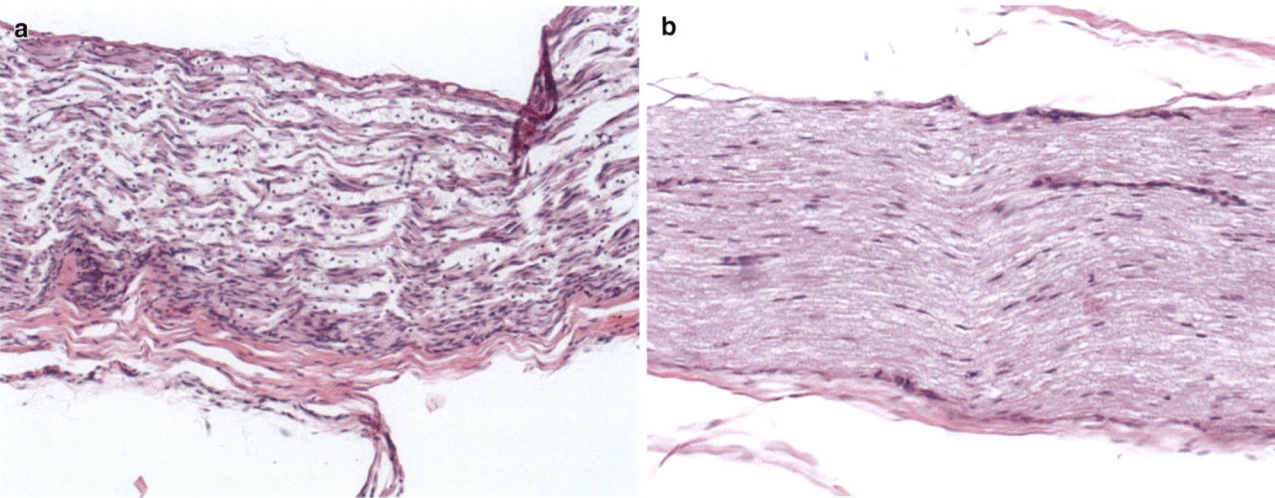

Fig. 16.1 Longitudinal sections of the 30 day endpoint histology of the sciatic nerve bundles from animals injected with (**a**) NW2013 and (**b**) normal saline

surgically accessed using laparotomy without disturbing the fascia (fatty layer) covering the artery. Two sites along the length of the artery were selected for injection with the respective orientation marked by placing 4-0 prolene sutures around the artery.

The animals were catheterized using standard endovascular techniques to access renal arteries and angiographic images were obtained prior to NW2013 administration. A microsyringe, equipped with a 33-gauge needle was used to inject the agent or saline (control) into the artery wall. Four (4) injections per renal artery were performed. Two injections were done in a single plane per site, roughly 180° apart. Two different doses of NW 2013 were injected. Angiograms were performed after agent injection into the vessels and the animal was closed surgically.

Animals were then survived for 14 and 90 days. Angiograms of both renal arteries were taken at 14 and 90 days prior to sacrifice. Blood collection and urine samples were collected on days 0, 7, 10, 14 and 90. At 14-day and 90-day sacrifice time points, animals were anesthetized and kidneys were accessed surgically using laparotomy. Kidney tissue samples from the renal cortex were collected, flash frozen, weighed and sent for norepinephrine measurement using HPLC mass spectrometry techniques.

After harvesting the renal tissue, the animals were euthanized. Aortas and renal arteries were perfused with formalin, harvested, and fixed. Following fixing, each kidney was sectioned at approximately 2 mm increments from the aorta to the kidney hilus. Sections were stained with hematoxylin and eosin (H&E); selected sections were then stained using immunohistochemical methods for Caspase 3, Neurofilament protein (NFP) and Tyrosine hydroxylase (TH).

Results

Rat Sciatic Nerve Model

All animals were successfully treated and survived their end points. All Northwind pharmacologic agents and combinatorial formulations outperformed the positive control (guanethidine) in nerve block efficacy (Fig. 16.4). A three-agent combinatorial formulation was identified as having superior effectiveness to all other single pharmacologic agents tested and to the chemoablative agent, ethanol, in blocking nerve conductance. There were no observed long term effects on motor or sensory function in Northwind pharmacologic agents. Surprisingly, ethanol-treated animals were found to be hypersensitive to touch and pain in the ethanol treated limb.

Histological examination of the hind-limb injected with NW2013 showed signs of edema and axonal degeneration on day 3. On day 30, in the animals treated with NW2013 the nerve bundles contained nerve axons showing signs of loss of perineurium and structural integrity as well as axonal degeneration (Fig. 16.1). An absence of inflammatory foci surrounding the degenerative nerve bundles was also noted. In contrast, the overall structure of the nerve bundle appears intact with individual neurons having an ordered appearance in the saline control samples.

Overall, agent NW2013 was determined to be safe, was demonstrated to be superior in blocking sensory nerve function and sciatic nerve electrical conductance, as well as to induce apoptosis/Caspase-3 activation (per immunohistochemical staining of tissue sections). No toxicity was observed to the surrounding tissue.

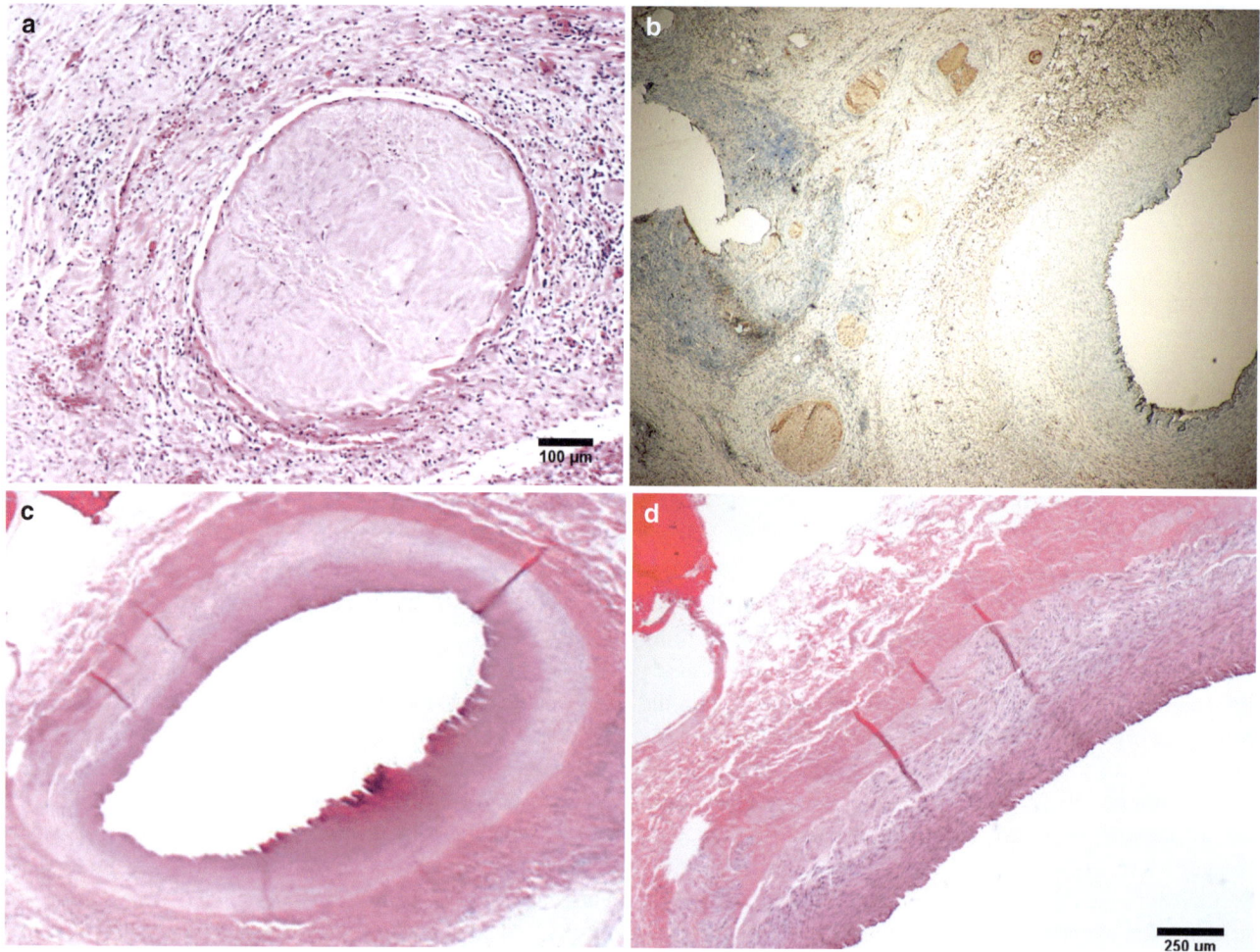

Fig. 16.2 Histology sections at 14-days after administering low dose NW2013 into the renal artery wall: (**a**) H&E stain and (**b**) Caspase-3 stain of nerve bundles; (**c**) vessel wall at low and (**d**) high magnifications

Renal Nerve Deactivation in the Porcine Model

All animals were successfully treated and survived to their endpoints. No complications, related to bleeding complications, perforations or other, were noted. Vessel spasm was noted both prior to and after agent injection in all animals. Nitroglycerine was injected in the first animal to reduce spasm. However, since the vessel spasm did not resolve after administering nitro, no nitro was used in subsequent treatments. Angiography after treatment confirmed good blood flow into both renal arteries.

Follow up angiograms at 14 and 90 days from all animals showed patent renal arteries with good blood to the kidneys. At 90-days, small degree of narrowing was noted with high-dose of NW2013. All animals were surgically exposed, kidney tissue was harvested and the animals were euthanized. Renal arteries and vital organs were harvested and fixed using standard techniques.

Porcine Histology at 14-Days

Sub-acute histologic changes were observed in NW2013 treated renal arteries. The renal nerves appear to be selectively affected in the treated vessel without any effect on the vascular tissue in the low-dose treatment group. The nerves showed the absence of nuclei and cellular structure, and were Caspase-3 positive, indicative of neuronal apoptosis (Fig. 16.2a, b). There were a few nerves that showed focal damage and others that showed total absence of nuclei. These neuronal changes were interpreted as neurodegenerative changes following treatment with NW2013. The saline-treated (control) renal nerves failed to show any degenerative changes indicative of site-specific action of the pharmacologic agent. The neurodegenerative changes were extensive and dose dependent. The high dose treatment resulted in greater neurodegenerative changes marked by total absence of nuclei within the nerve bundles; the surrounding tissue also showed fat necrosis and some

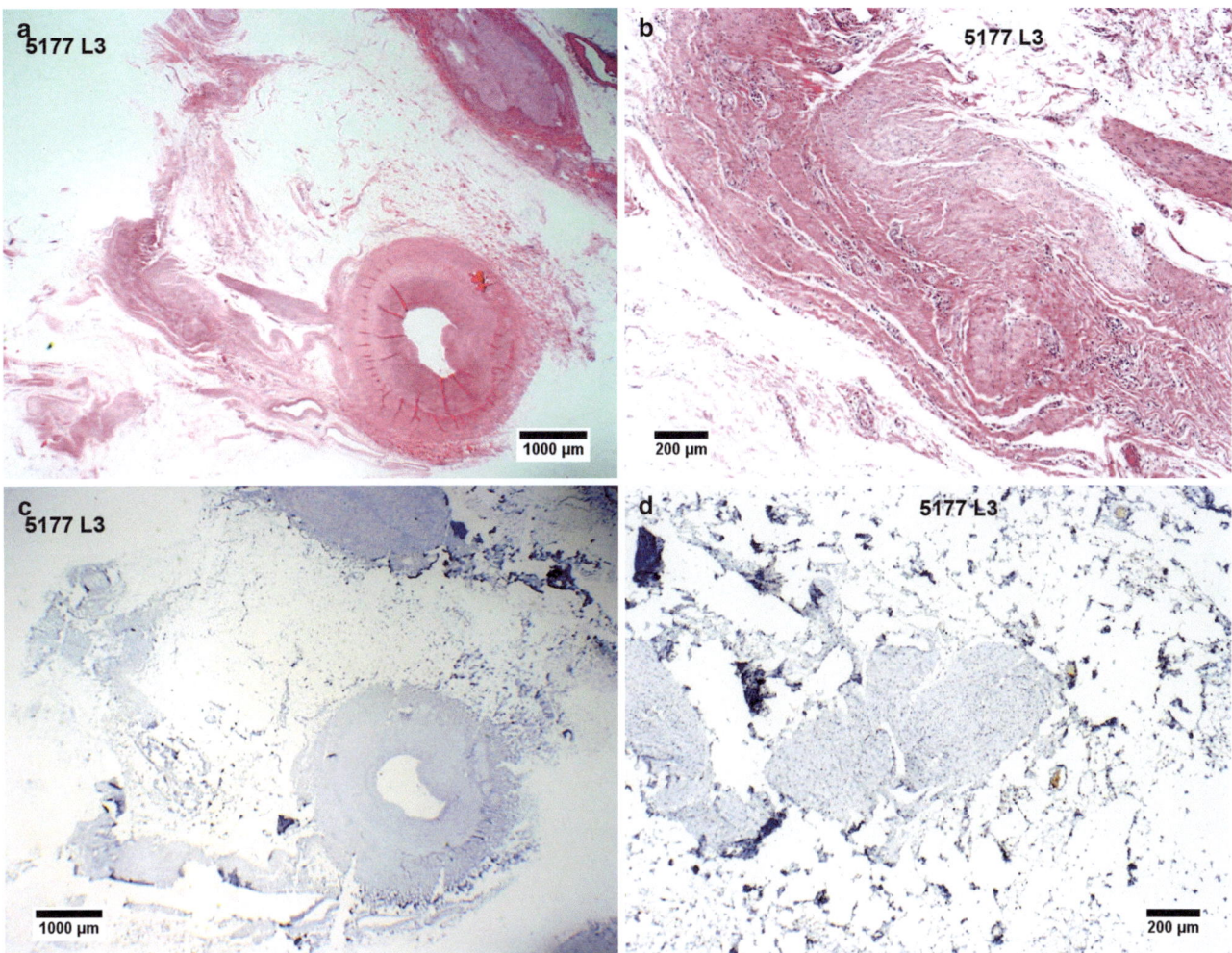

Fig. 16.3 Histology at 90-days after administering low dose NW2013 into the renal artery wall: (**a**, **b**) H&E stain and (**c**, **d**) Caspase-3 stain at (**a**, **c**) low and (**b**, **d**) high magnifications

arteriolar damage. In both groups the renal arteries were normal in appearance without any significant medial, intimal or adventitial injury (Fig. 16.2c, d).

Porcine Histology at 90-Days

Chronic changes after local administration of NW2013 showed extensive perineural fibrosis and modest inflammation (Fig. 16.3). At low concentrations, some nerves showed vacuolar degeneration as well as mild immune cell recruitment within the nerve bundles. The Caspase-3 stains were negative at the late time points, suggesting the completion of neuronal apoptosis. The renal arteries were normal in appearance without any medial, intimal or significant adventitial injury. At high dose, the arteries had moderate to severe necrosis and degenerative changes characterized by atrophied

nerve fibers with regions of more significant immune cells infiltrate including the presence of macrophages, eosinophils, lymphocytes and multinucleated giant cells.

Immunohistochemistry

Immunostaining against Neuro-filament protein (NFP) showed varying degrees of expression indicating structural axonal damage/loss in injured fascicles (Fig. 16.4). Immunostaining against Tyrosine hydroxylase (TH) was variable where a functional loss was detected, even in the absence of recognizable axonal change. There were no unexpected deleterious findings in the chronic phase of induced injury in the adjacent examined organs. The surrounding lymph nodes showed non-specific reactive lymphoid hyperplasia.

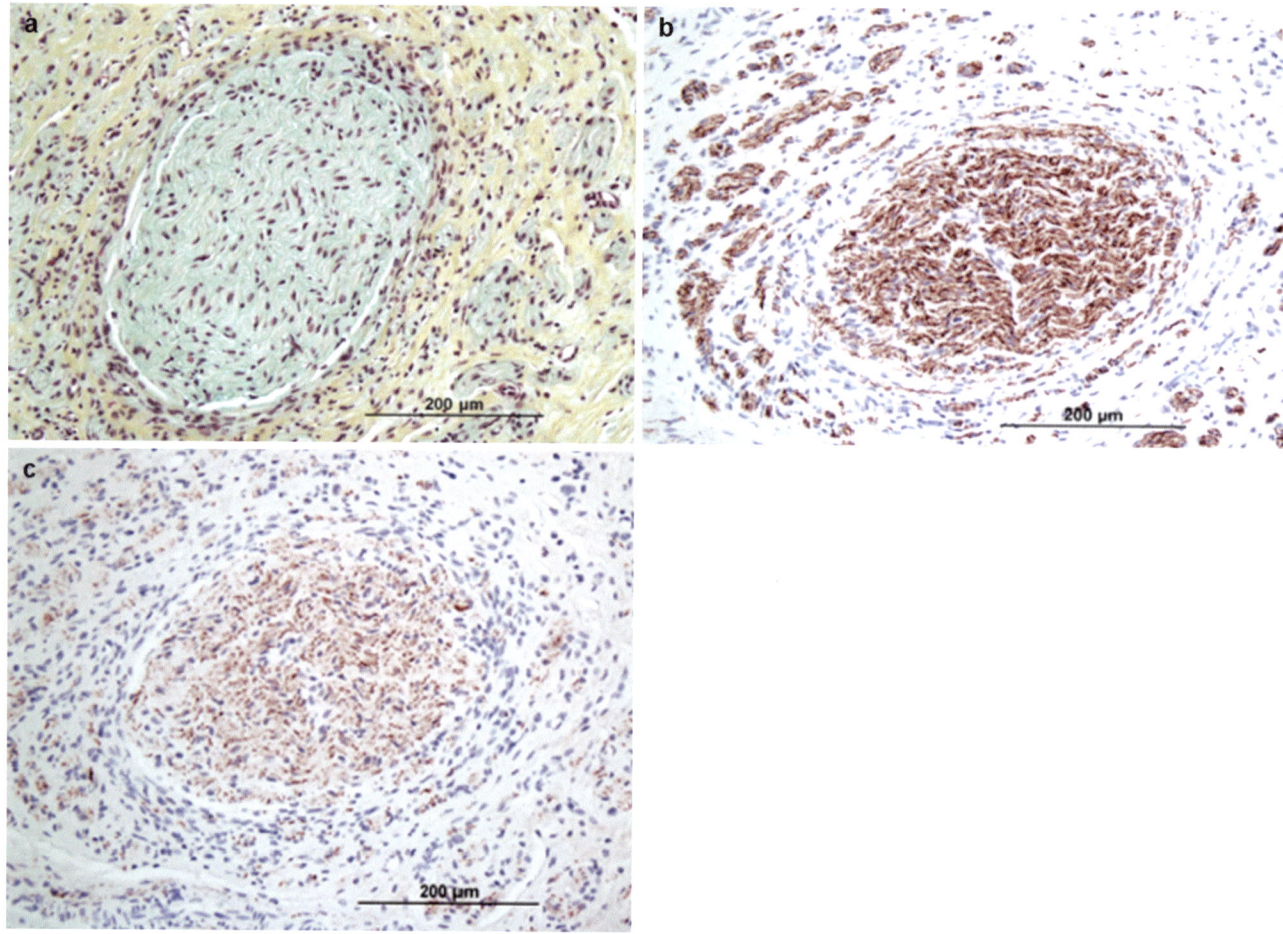

Fig. 16.4 Histology sections of renal nerve fascicle, at 90-days after administering low dose NW2013 into renal artery wall. (**a**) Movat stain, (**b**) Neurofilament protein (NFP) immunostain showing focal staining of fascicles, and (**c**) tyrosine hydroxylase (TH) showing no staining of fascicles

In summary, it may be concluded that the nerve fascicle pathology characterized by neurodegenerative histology, immune cell recruitment and perineural inflammation with fibrosis was consistent with post-injury healing in the NW2013-treated tissue. In addition, the observed differences in select neuronal markers suggest both structural injury and functional loss of nerves in bundles in a treatment-specific manner. All observed changes were restricted to the NW2013 treatment cohort and was demonstrably localized to the tissue surrounding the site of administration.

Norepinephrine Results

Results on kidney tissue norepinephrine (NE) levels in the renal cortex are shown in Fig. 16.5 at the 90-day time points. It is noted that local administration of neurotropic agents into the vessel wall caused a decrease in NE levels compared to controls in a dose-dependent manner.

Discussion

Results from the above studies clearly demonstrate that local administration of neurotropic pharmacologic agents in particular NW2013, into renal artery walls can abrogate nerve function and induce local neurodegenerative changes in a manner that is safe to surrounding tissue. All animals survived to the designated end point, and renal arteries remained fully patent without local toxicity or deleterious effects, especially at the low dose. No significant damage was noted to the vessel wall. The neurotropic pharmacologic agents acted with specificity and selectively inducted degenerative changes exclusive to the neurons surrounding the renal artery. At 14-days after NW2013 administration, nerves in the nerve bundles lacked structure and nuclei, and showed signs of significant apoptosis, as confirmed by Caspase-3 immunostaining. At 90-days, the apoptotic process was complete and the neurons were replaced by fibrous connective tissue. Axonal degeneration was observed in some nerve

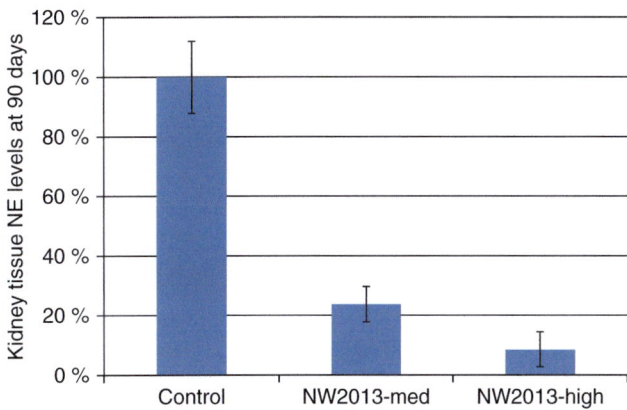

Fig. 16.5 Kidney tissue norepinephrine (NE) levels at 90 days after local administration of NW2013 compared to controls (error bars denote one standard deviation)

bundle regions. In other bundle regions, axons remained visible but they were non-functional, as evidenced by NFP staining. Correspondingly, NW2013 treatment resulted in reduced kidney tissue-specific norepinephrine levels consistent with selective damage to neurons. NE results are equivalent to those reported in preclinical studies conducted using energy-based ablative methods.

Agent NW2013 had the optimal (most safe and effective) response at low concentrations, both at 14 and 90 days and demonstrated effective dose-response. At high concentrations, the agent was not soluble and drug particulates caused localized tissue damage characterized by necrosis. Although a higher reduction in tissue NE levels was observed at a higher dose, the lack of observed side effects in the low dose NW2013 treatment cohort favor the use of NW2013 at lower concentrations.

In summary, preclinical studies have successfully demonstrated that targeted and selective nerve deactivation and degeneration can be achieved through the local administration of neurotropic pharmacologic agents in a safe and effective manner. It is recommended that further studies be conducted to evaluate the feasibility of delivering these neurotropic pharmacologic agents percutaneously using a catheter or other minimally-invasive methods to achieve similar sympathetic neuromodulatory effects.

Early Clinical Experience

A First-In-Human safety study was initiated at The Center of Vascular and Heart Diseases of Georgia (Tbilisi, Georgia) with Dr. Konstantine Kipiani as Principal Investigator. The study protocol was consistent with European Society of Cardiology (ESC) and American College of Cardiology (ACC) guidelines for treating patients suffering from resistant hypertension by renal denervation [24, 25], and approved by the Ethics Committee and Institutional Review Board. After careful screening, patients were enrolled after they met the following key inclusion criteria:

- Office systolic blood pressure ≥ 160 mmHg;
- Stable use of ≥3 antihypertensive drugs, concurrently at maximum tolerated doses, for a minimum of 14 days prior to enrollment, of which one is a diuretic;
- No change in medication 1 month prior to enrollment;
- CT angiogram was obtained prior to treatment.

After patient preparation, the femoral artery was accessed using standard endovascular methods and an abdominal aortogram was obtained to define the vasculature of the abdominal aorta including renal arteries and to determine the presence of any supplementary renal arteries. A 7F sheath with a renal distal curve was used to selectively enter the ostium of the renal artery. Once the 7F sheath was in position, contrast media was injected to image the renal circulation including hilar branches as well as second and third order vessels extending to the renal cortex.

Procedural steps are shown in Fig. 16.6. The delivery system was advanced over an 0.014″ guidewire, through the sheath, and positioned in the renal artery proximal to the bifurcation to ventral and dorsal divisions. The integrated balloon-needle system was then inflated to advance the microneedle into the peri-adventitial region. This was verified by injecting contrast proximal to the balloon and checking for vessel occlusion. Following injection of the agent, the balloon was deflated and the needle was retracted. The delivery catheter was then positioned 10 mm distal to the ostium and the procedure was repeated at the second site. The post procedure angiogram demonstrated no intimal disruption with a normal appearing renal artery without any occlusion, clot, dissection or spasm, as noted in Fig. 16.6d. These steps were repeated on the contralateral kidney. When an accessory vessel was present, it was also treated with the neurotropic agent by injection.

The entire procedure was completed in 20 min, similar to renal angioplasty. There was no significant pain experienced by the patients during the procedure compared to radiofrequency or ultrasound energy-based transluminal renal denervation procedures; 0.5 mg of morphine was given to mitigate mild pain observed with a few patients. To date, the five patients have been enrolled in the study with 100 % technical success. Two patients demonstrated greater than 30 mmHg drop in systolic pressure at the 30-day follow up. Patient follow-up occur at 1-, 3-, 6- and 12-month time points. We intend to continue enrollment of an additional 10–15 patients to gain more clinical experience.

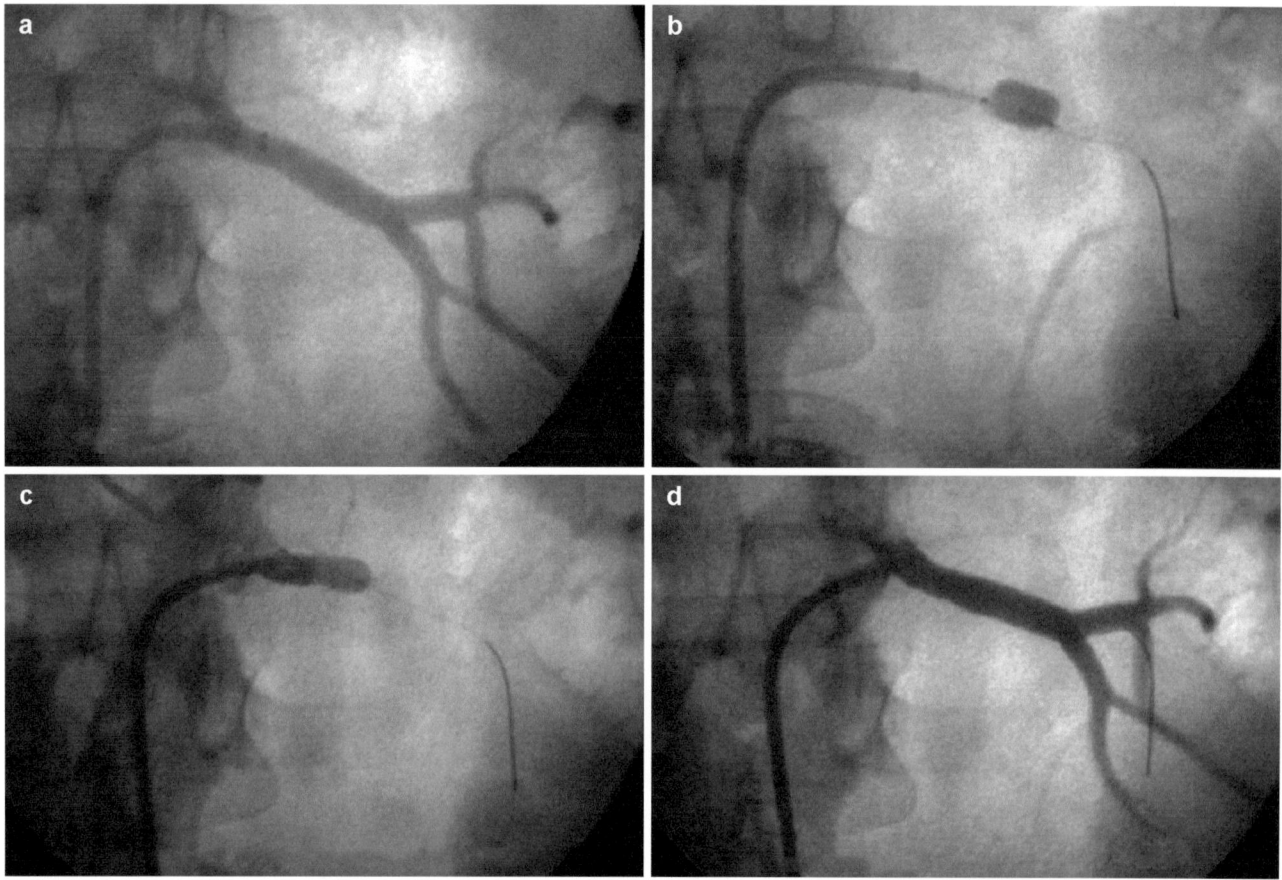

Fig. 16.6 Angiographic images showing the left renal arteries of patient-005, (**a**) prior to treatment, (**b**) inflation of the balloon and advancement of the microneedle into the vessel wall, (**c**) verification of needle advancement by balloon of the vessel, evidenced by no flow of contrast, and (**d**) final angiogram after treatment showing minimal damage to the vessel wall- no spasm, dissections or perforations

Concluding Remarks

Results from this study demonstrated that the administration of small volume, low dose neurotropic pharmacologic agent into the wall of renal arteries can induce highly localized, nerve-specific degenerative changes. The pharmacologic agents evaluated were determined to be safe for the renal arterial wall and surrounding renal tissues. Moreover, these agents were efficacious and induced nerve block, local neuronal apoptosis, and promoted the reduction of norepinephrine levels in kidney tissue. The focal neurodegenerative effects were sustained over a period of 90-days indicating the potential for this approach to be a durable treatment for refractory hypertension.

Early clinical results also demonstrate that targeted renal nerve deactivation using local delivery of neurotropic agents is safe and feasible with no acute injury to the vessel wall (for example, no dissections, spasm or perforations). It is a promising therapy that offers advantages over energy-based denervation methods in terms of its specificity (targets nerves), less pain (minimal use of an analgesic) and cost effectiveness (no energy system). Long-term clinical data are needed to evaluate safety and durability.

Acknowledgements The authors would like to thank Drs. Jorge Garcia, Félix Vega and Michelle Kelly (ISIS Services) for conducting preclinical studies and Drs. Narayan Raju (Pathology Research Laboratories) and Dr. Renu Virmani (CVPath Institute) for conducting histopathology and preparing immunohistochemical stains and pathology reports.

In addition, the authors thank the clinical investigators Drs. Konstantine Kipiani, Vakhtang Kipiani and Tea Mukhuradze (The Center for Vascular and Heart Diseases of Georgia, Tbilisi, Georgia); Dr. Horst Sievert (CardioVasculares Centrum, St. Katharinen-Krankenhaus, Frankfurt, Germany); Dr. Nicholas Kipshidze (Lenox Hill Hospital, New York, NY and General Director and Physician-in-Chief, Kipshidze University Hospital, Tbilisi, Georgia); and Dr. Michael Wholey for conducting the study and providing the clinical data for this manuscript. The Investigators plan to publish the results once follow-up data from all patients become available.

References

1. Bertog SC, et al. Renal denervation for hypertension. JACC Cardiovasc Interv. 2012;5:249–58.
2. Symplicity HTN-1 Investigators. Catheter-based renal sympathetic denervation for resistant hypertension. Hypertension. 2011;57:911–7.
3. Kandzari DE, et al. Catheter-based renal denervation for resistant hypertension: rationale and design of the SYMPLICITY HTN-3 trial. Clin Cardiol. 2012;35:528–35.
4. Ormiston JA, et al. Renal denervation for resistant hypertension using an irrigated radiofrequency balloon: 12-month results from the Renal Hypertension Ablation System (RHAS) trial. EuroIntervention. 2013;9:70–4.
5. Rocha-Singh KJ. Renal artery denervation: a brave new frontier-emerging therapies for treating patients with severe, treatment-resistant hypertension. Endovasc Today. 2012;6:45–53.
6. Brinton, et al. Externally focused ultrasound for sympathetic renal denervation. WAVE 1 First-In-Man Study, TCT 2012, Miami, 2012.
7. Ahmed H, et al. Renal sympathetic denervation using an irrigated radiofrequency ablation catheter for management of drug-resistant hypertension. JACC Cardiovasc Interv. 2012;5:758–65.
8. Waxman, Barbash. Renal artery brachytherapy for sympathetic renal denervation for the treatment of resistant hypertension: preclinical safety study. CRT 2013, Washington, DC, 2013.
9. Templin C, et al. Vascular lesions induced by renal nerve ablation as assessed by optical coherence tomography: pre- and post-procedural comparison with the Simplicity catheter system and the EnligHTN multi-electrode renal denervation catheter. Eur Heart J. 2013;34:2141–8.
10. Vonend O, et al. Secondary rise in blood pressure after renal denervation. Lancet. 2012;380:778.
11. Kaltenbach B, et al. Renal artery stenosis after renal sympathetic denervation. JACC. 2012;60:2694–5.
12. Melder et al. Renal denervation in stented porcine arteries. EuroPCR 2013, Paris, 2013.
13. Scheffers IJ, et al. Novel baroreflex activation therapy in resistant hypertension: results of a European multi-center feasibility study. JACC. 2010;15:1254–8.
14. Scott B. Percutaneous AV fistula for resistant hypertension. EuroPCR 2012, Paris, 2012.
15. Stefanadis C, et al. Chemical denervation of the renal artery by vincristine in swine. A new catheter based technique. Int J Cardiol. 2012;167:4215–5.
16. Owens CD. Adventitial drug-induced renal artery denervation in refractory hypertension: preclinical experience and first-in-human plans. TCT 2010, Washington, DC, 2010.
17. Fischell TA, et al. Ethanol-mediated perivascular renal sympathetic denervation: preclinical validation of safety and efficacy in a porcine model. EuroIntervention. 2013;9:140–7.
18. Herring N, Paterson DJ. Neuromodulators of peripheral cardiac sympatho-vagal balance. Exp Physiol. 2009;94(1):46–53.
19. Shanks J, Townend JN. Peripheral cardiac sympathetic hyperactivity in cardiovascular disease. Am J Physiol Regul Integr Comp Physiol. 2013;305(12):R1411–20.
20. Russell JA. Bench-to-bedside review: vasopressin in the management of septic shock. Crit Care. 2011;15(4):226.
21. Osborn JL, et al. Long-term increases in renal sympathetic nerve activity and hypertension. Clin Exp Pharmacol Physiol. 1997;24(1):72–6.
22. Maiter D. Pheochromocytoma: a paradigm for catecholamine-mediated hypertension. Acta Clin Belg. 2004;59(4):209–19.
23. Oparil S. The sympathetic nervous system in clinical and experimental hypertension. Kidney Int. 1986;30(3):437–52.
24. Schlaich MP, et al. International expert consensus statement: percutaneous transluminal renal denervation for the treatment of resistant hypertension. J Am Coll Cardiol. 2013;62(22):2031–45.
25. Mancia G, et al. 2013 ESH/ESC guidelines for the management of arterial hypertension. J Hypertens. 2013;31:1281–357.

Stefan C. Bertog, Laura Vaskelyte, Ilona Hofmann, Sameer Gafoor, and Horst Sievert

Device Description

The Vessix™ Renal Denervation System (Boston Scientific Corporation, Natick, MA, USA) consists of a denervation catheter and radiofrequency generator. The catheter is a 90 cm long balloon-tipped catheter. The balloon is 25 mm long. The balloon diameters depend on the vessel size (4 mm, 5 mm, 6 mm and 7 mm). Mounted on the surface of the balloon are (4–8, depending on the balloon size) bipolar radiofrequency electrodes distributed in a helical fashion emitting radiofrequency energy to a depth of a few millimeters into the renal artery. The catheter can be delivered over the wire into the renal artery via an 8F guide sheath (more common) or 9F guide catheter.

The performance of the procedure is similar to renal artery balloon angioplasty. First, femoral arterial access (e.g. with a 4, 5 or 6F sheath) is obtained and an abdominal aortogram performed (e.g. with a 4, 5 or 6F pigtail or omniflush catheter). The renal arteries are visualized and accessory renal arteries, if present, identified. Heparin is administered. Subsequently, the access sheath is exchanged over a 0.035 in. J-tipped guidewire for an 8F delivery sheath (e.g. Cook sheath, Cook Medical, Bloomington, IN, USA) positioned with the tip at the take-off of the renal arteries. If the anatomy is favorable (straight or superior take-off), the renal arteries are wired directly with a 0.014 in. coronary support (e.g. Hi-Torque Iron Man, Abbott Vascular, Abbott Park, Il, USA) or 0.018 in. peripheral wire (e.g. V-14™ControlWire®, Boston Scientific Corporation, Natick, MA, USA). If the take-off is inferior and wiring proves difficult, a 6F guide catheter (e.g. internal mammary, Judkins right or renal double curve) can be advanced via the sheath into the aorta over a J-tipped 0.035 in. guidewire. The guide catheter is positioned close to the renal artery ostia and the guidewire is removed, typically allowing the guide catheter to engage the renal artery ostium. The coronary or peripheral wire is advanced into a distal segmental renal artery branch and the 8F guidesheath follows over the guide catheter into the proximal renal artery. The guide catheter is removed while maintaining the guide sheath position in the renal artery and the Vessix balloon delivered into the renal artery. Radiofrequency energy is applied to all electrodes simultaneously at ~1 W for a duration of 30 s (via a temperature controlled algorithm keeping the temperature at 68 °C). In case of an early bifurcating renal artery, the respective branches can be denervated separately, or, alternatively, the balloon can be left partially in the renal artery with radiofrequency energy delivery to only those electrodes with wall apposition to the renal artery (the system will sense lack of contact of the electrodes that are protruding in the aorta causing deactivation of these electrodes).

Given the fairly straight tip of guide sheath, it can be difficult to deliver a wire or the Vessix balloon in to the renal artery, particularly if it has an inferior take-off. The Vessix balloon as it exits the guide sheath tip tends to further straighten the sheath with the balloon pointing towards the roof of the renal artery. Once again, in this situation, either a guide catheter can be advanced into the renal artery first followed by the guide sheath in a telescoping manner or an extra support wire can be advanced to improve guide sheath stability and balloon delivery.

The balloon sizes are chosen to match the vessel size and a 4 mm balloon can be used for vessels with diameters of 3–3.5 mm. The largest acceptable vessel diameter is 7 mm as larger diameters would not allow sufficient electrode contact.

Once the (non-compliant) balloon is at an optimal position, it is inflated with a standard inflation device to three ATM. Contrast is injected during inflation to assure cessation of

S.C. Bertog, MD, FACC, FSCAI • L. Vaskelyte, MD
I. Hofmann, MD • S. Gafoor, MD
H. Sievert, FESC, FACC, FSCAI (✉)
CardioVascular Center Frankfurt, Sankt Katharinen, Seckbacher Landstrasse 65, Frankfurt 60389, Germany
e-mail: sbertog@aol.com; info@cvcfrankfurt.de

R.R. Heuser et al. (eds.), *Renal Denervation: A New Approach to Treatment of Resistant Hypertension*,
DOI 10.1007/978-1-4471-5223-1_17, © Springer-Verlag London 2015

flow indicating adequate wall apposition. Then radiofrequency energy is applied by activating a single button on the generator. One or two (if the renal artery length allows) ablations are typically performed.

The advantages are the short ablation time, ease of delivery via an over the wire system similar to renal artery balloon angioplasty and the use of bipolar electrodes without the need for grounding. A potential disadvantage is the incompatibility of the Vessix balloon with conventional 6F guide catheters and the not infrequent need for above described maneuvers to allow proper guide sheath positioning for balloon delivery. However, the manufacturer is in the process of developing a dedicated guide sheath. If there are significant discrepancies in right and left renal artery sizes more than one Vessix balloon may have to be used.

The device has CE mark (approved in 4/2012) and is undergoing a number of clinical trials. Most recently (11/2013), data combining patients (n = 146) from the first-in-man (FIM) study (n = 18) and the post market surveillance (PMS) trial (n = 128) were presented at Trans-Catheter Therapeutics (TCT). Patients with resistant hypertension (≥3 antihypertensive medications) and an office systolic blood pressure of ≥160 mmHg (FIM study) or ≥160/90 mmHg (PMS trial) and renal arteries ≥3.5 mm in diameter and ≥15 mm (PMS trial) or ≥20 mm (FIM study) were enrolled including patients with accessory renal arteries provided they were of adequate size. The primary

endpoints were office and ambulatory systolic blood pressure reduction at 6 months follow-up. At the time of presentation, 139 patients had completed 6-month follow-up. Clinical characteristics were similar to other renal denervation trials (mean age: 59 years, 27 % diabetics, 38 % with a history of coronary artery disease baseline blood pressure 182/100 mmHg, average number of antihypertensive medications: 5.2). At 6-month follow-up, a significant blood pressure reduction of 26/13 mmHg was demonstrated along with a significant ambulatory blood pressure reduction of 9/6 mmHg. Those patients (n = 41) who underwent 12-month follow-up achieved a significant 30/14 mmHg office and 11/6 mmHg ambulatory blood pressure reduction. The response rate (defined as an at least 10 mmHg systolic office blood pressure reduction) was 76 % at 6 months and 85 % at 12 months. A target systolic office blood pressure (<140 mmHg) was reached in 19 and 34 % at 6 and 12 months, respectively. There was also a significant blood pressure reduction in those (24) patients who had accessory renal arteries, albeit slightly less pronounced at 21/12 mmHg at 6 months. Importantly, significant blood pressure reductions were seen regardless of age, gender and presence or absence of diabetes.

A number of trials studying renal denervation with the Vessix system are underway including patients with hypertension, renal insufficiency, atrial fibrillation and heart failure.

Radiofrequency and Irrigated Ablation: Principles and Potential for Renal Artery Denervation (RDN) in the Treatment of Resistant Arterial Hypertension

18

Kenichi Sakakura, Elena Ladich, Kristine Fuimaono, Renu Virmani, and Michael Joner

Key Points

1. Although renal denervation (RDN) is now considered as a valid interventional option for the treatment of patients with resistant hypertension, there is a need for improvement of this technology.
2. To this end, irrigated -tip ablation catheters are being developed that address these requirements – particularly with regard to avoiding complications that may compromise optimal lesion formation in the target renal arteries.
3. Specifically, irrigated-tip RF ablation enables those undertaking RDN procedures to effectively manage temperature, RF energy and power levels.
4. In turn, this shifts effective treatment zones of ablative energy into deeper tissue regions, where peri-arterial sympathetic nerves are targeted without damaging the renal arterial wall.
5. The development of cooled-tip ablation for RDN is still at a relatively early stage. However, this is an area of endovascular therapy that is expected to expand rapidly in the near future.

Introduction

Renal artery denervation (RDN) represents a relatively new technique for treating patients whose arterial hypertension persists despite three or more antihypertensive medications [1]. The main principle underlying RDN dates back 50 years or more and gave rise to surgical sympathectomy procedures [2]. Radiofrequency (RF) catheter ablation is a therapeutic procedure that delivers a controlled source of energy in order to create a lesion at the site of the target tissue. Lesion formation is restricted to a limited volume of tissue close to the ablation electrode. Since this technique was first introduced, it has become one of the most useful and widely accepted therapies in the field of cardiac electrophysiology, later followed by application in renal denervation procedures. Modifications in RF delivery and improvements in electrode design have resulted in a significant expansion of its indication such as chronic kidney disease (CKD), arrhythmias, obstructive sleep apnoea and glucose control [3, 4].

Novel therapeutic advances in this field have been developed exponentially in the last few years. Essentially, the aim is to develop new endovascular catheters that are simpler, faster and safer than those currently available. Much interest is now being devoted to irrigated renal artery ablation using cooled-tip percutaneous RF catheters in order to achieve optimal outcomes in patients with resistant arterial hypertension.

Renal Artery RF Ablation: Background and Practical Issues

The basis of RDN technology is characterised by deliberate tissue injury caused by heat generated by RF energy. Injury is aimed to be limited to the peri-arterial renal sympathetic nerve fibres that are more sensitive to heat than the surrounding tissue [5]. RF energy is delivered and monitored by a generator that allows the energy level to be adjusted

K. Sakakura, MD • E. Ladich, MD
R. Virmani, MD • M. Joner, MD (✉)
CVPath Institute, Inc., 19 Firstfield Road,
Gaithersburg, MD 20878, USA
e-mail: mjoner@cvpath.org

K. Fuimaono, BS
Cordis Corporation/Biosense Webster, Inc.,
3333 Diamond Canyon Road,
Diamond Bar, CA 91765, USA

R.R. Heuser et al. (eds.), *Renal Denervation: A New Approach to Treatment of Resistant Hypertension*,
DOI 10.1007/978-1-4471-5223-1_18, © Springer-Verlag London 2015

according to the individual requirements of the patient. The resulting lesion formation is achieved either through:

(i) Resistive heating, in which the natural resistance of the tissue generates heat, thereby forming the core of the lesion

(ii) Conductive heating, in which the heat generated by resistive heating is distributed to adjacent tissue and to the ablation electrode

The effects of RF energy on vascular tissue depend on multiple factors such as temperature, duration of energy delivery, power, electrode size, quality of electrode-tissue contact and histological characteristics of the tissue, including blood supply and proximity to major blood vessels that determine the degree of heat dissipation. Temperature is critical to the success or failure of the ablation technique. As RF energy is applied to tissue, it generates heat. When the tissue temperature reaches approximately 50° centigrade, protein denaturation destroys signal conducting nerve cells, causing tissue to become necrotic [6].

The degree of power delivered to the target site determines the tissue temperature. In turn, tissue temperature determines lesion size. As a general rule, therefore, higher power delivers higher tissue temperature, creating larger lesions. The power delivered to the tissue is significantly less than the output power of the generator, mainly because of power loss into the blood. Longer duration of RF ablation allows the temperature in the tissue to rise to a steady state and, therefore, penetrate more deeply into the tissue.

In general, a target tissue temperature of 50–70° centigrade is used for conventional RF ablation [7]. At temperatures above 100° centigrade, boiling will occur in the tissue surrounding the electrode. This results in denaturation of plasma proteins, while coagulation may be activated resulting in charring or coagulum formation, which increases the risk of thromboembolism [8]. An important sign indicating charring or coagulum formation is a sudden rise of impedance. The optimal duration of radiofrequency application in order to obtain effective ablation in RDN procedures remains a topic of debate, a minimum duration of 30–60 s may be needed with most available devices to obtain effective ablation.

The extent of successfully ablated tissue is proportional to the applied power of the radiofrequency source. Electrode size influences the volume of the ablation lesion and probably the clinical efficacy of RF ablation as well. As tissue is heated, there is a temperature-dependent drop in electrical impedance. A significant positive correlation between pre-ablation impedance and heating efficacy was demonstrated, and a similar association has been observed between maximum drop in impedance during energy delivery and heating efficacy [9]. Temperature monitoring also provides useful information about the quality of electrode/tissue contact. It has been reported that temperature rise is greater and faster

with properly engaged electrodes [10]. At the tissue level, convective heat dissipation removes heat from the tissue limiting the penetration depth of radiofrequency current [11].

Tissue and Electrode Temperature

The potential to increase energy output in order to achieve a larger lesion is limited by the risk of over-heating the electrode-tissue interface, ablation electrode and tissue itself. Overheating can lead to a number of adverse events that would compromise the success of the ablation technique.

Of note, the electrode is a source of power, but not of heat. The temperature of the ablation electrode only increases due to conductive heat transfer from the tissue. Therefore, the temperature of the adjacent tissue is always higher than that of the electrode during the ablation process. The temperature of the electrode is measured by temperature sensors in the electrode of the ablation catheter. Lesion formation correlates with a number of parameters that are monitored by the RF generator, including impedance, time, ablation electrode temperature and output power. The latter can be selected by the physician, as can the duration of RF delivery. Additional parameters affecting lesion formation include passive electrode cooling by blood flow, electrode-tissue orientation, electrode-tissue contact pressure and the physical properties of the tissue itself. In temperature control mode, electrode temperature is monitored by the RF generator to regulate output power in order to reach and maintain target temperature. High target temperatures are associated with a higher risk of adverse events. In power control mode, the output power delivered by the RF generator is chosen by the operator. The generator then delivers the pre-set level of power independently of the temperature of the ablation electrode. As a safety feature, if the ablation electrode temperature reaches a pre-determined cut-off value, energy delivery is terminated. In this mode, power can be delivered either constantly for the duration of the ablation procedure, or titrated manually (not a standard option).

Blood Flow and Passive Cooling

During ablation, blood flowing through the renal arteries cools the section of the ablation electrode not in contact with the tissue. Since the temperature of the blood is lower than that of the heated electrode, heat is removed from the electrode. The higher the blood flow, the more heat is removed – a phenomenon known as passive electrode cooling by blood flow. Passive cooling is also influenced by the degree of surface area exposed to the blood flow, which in turn is related to the size and orientation of the electrode, and the fraction of electrode surface area in contact with the tissue being ablated [6]. The effects of passive cooling must be taken into account when planning an ablation strategy because the blood flow will influence the choice of electrode size.

With respect to lesion size, the effects of passive cooling by blood flow are most pronounced in temperature control mode, because the ablation electrode temperature influences output power. When blood flow is low, the electrode is only slightly cooled – therefore, target temperature is reached with low output power. Only limited power enters the tissue, thereby creating a small lesion. When blood flow is high, more heat is removed from the electrode, and more power is required to reach and maintain target temperature. This higher output power will result in a larger lesion [12]. This phenomenon may have substantial impact on RDN efficacy when patients with low cardiac output are being treated, as target temperature will likely be reached sooner as compared to patients with normal cardiac output.

Renal Artery RF Ablation: Clinical Evidence and Complications

The feasibility of RF ablation of the renal arteries using a conventional, non-irrigated catheter is now well established. Krum et al. have reported 3 year follow up data from the Symplicity HTN-1 trial, which was designed to elucidate the long-term safety and effectiveness of RDN in a single arm registry [13]. Symplicity HTN-1 demonstrated blood pressure reduction in 93 % of patients at 36 months follow-up [13]. Worthley, et al. reported the results of the EnligHTN I trial, which included 46 patients in a single-arm registry [14]. Blood pressure reduction from baseline to 1, 3, and 6 months was 28/10, 27/10, 26/10 mmHg, respectively [14].

Esler et al. reported the results of the Symplicity HTN-2 trial, which was a multicentre, prospective, randomised clinical trial to test the efficacy of RDN [15] against standard treatment. In this trial, 106 patients were allocated to renal denervation and compared to an equally sized control group receiving standard drug treatment. Office-based blood pressure measurements in the renal denervation group was reduced by 32/12 mmHg (SD 23/11, baseline of 178/96 mmHg, p<0.0001), whereas no difference compared to baseline was observed in the control group [15].

Symplicty HTN-3 is the most recent randomized trial conducted in the USA. This trial was designed as a prospective, randomized, single-blind trial evaluating the safety and effectiveness of RDN for the treatment of uncontrolled hypertension in comparison to a sham-control group [16]. Contrary to expectations, the mean change in systolic blood pressure at 6 months was −14.13±23.93 mmHg in the denervation group as compared with −11.74±25.94 mmHg in the sham-procedure group (P<0.001 for both comparisons of the change from baseline), for a difference of −2.39 mmHg

(P=0.26 for superiority with a margin of 5 mmHg) [17]. While different factors may have contributed to this treatment failure, special focus of future clinical efforts should be on achieving complete circumferential ablation of the renal artery. Future clinical studies to elucidate the true efficacy of RF denervation are still needed.

Since most RF renal denervation procedures are performed via the renal artery, vascular safety is of critical concern. In the acute phase after renal denervation, Templin et al. reported that vasospasm was observed in 42 % of renal arteries, and endothelial-intimal edema was noted in 96 % of renal arteries following RF denervation [18]. Furthermore, intraluminal thrombus formation was observed in 67 % of renal arteries after RND (Fig. 18.1). These results suggest the need for appropriate antiplatelet therapy during RDN. In addition, Kaltenbach et al. reported renal artery stenosis secondary to RDN after 5 months [5], which highlights the need for long-term monitoring after RDN procedures. In the Symplicity HTN-1 trial, 2 renal artery stenosis were treated by stents (one was a progression from pre-existing mild stenosis, and the other one was a newly developed stenosis) from 150 enrolled patients during 3 year follow-up [13]. In light of these reports and the fact that clinical experience with this technology is limited to a very small number of patients treated world-wide in randomized studies, rigorous surveillance of patients undergoing these procedures is warranted.

Irrigated RF Ablation: Active Cooling

More recently, irrigated ablation has been investigated as a new technique for active cooling during the ablation procedure. Active cooling lowers the temperature of the ablation electrode and adjacent tissue to reduce the incidence of coagulum formation. It helps to achieve a more controllable ablation and allows for higher power delivery, resulting in larger lesions [4]. With active cooling, the basis for irrigated RF ablation, room temperature irrigation fluid is infused through an irrigation catheter designed specifically to cool the ablation electrode. Whereas passive cooling is pulsatile, and dependent upon cardiac output, active cooling can override the inconsistent and unknown characteristics of passive cooling.

With the irrigation catheter used in RDN procedures, irrigation fluid flows through the catheter and exits through small holes (irrigation ducts) around the electrode. The fluid is in direct contact with the electrode, blood and the surrounding tissue surface, and irrigation facilitates cooling of the electrode-tissue interface. When there is adequate irrigation flow rate, the temperature of this interface is lower, thus reducing the risk of thrombus or char formation [4]. Irrigated RF ablation creates renal artery lesions

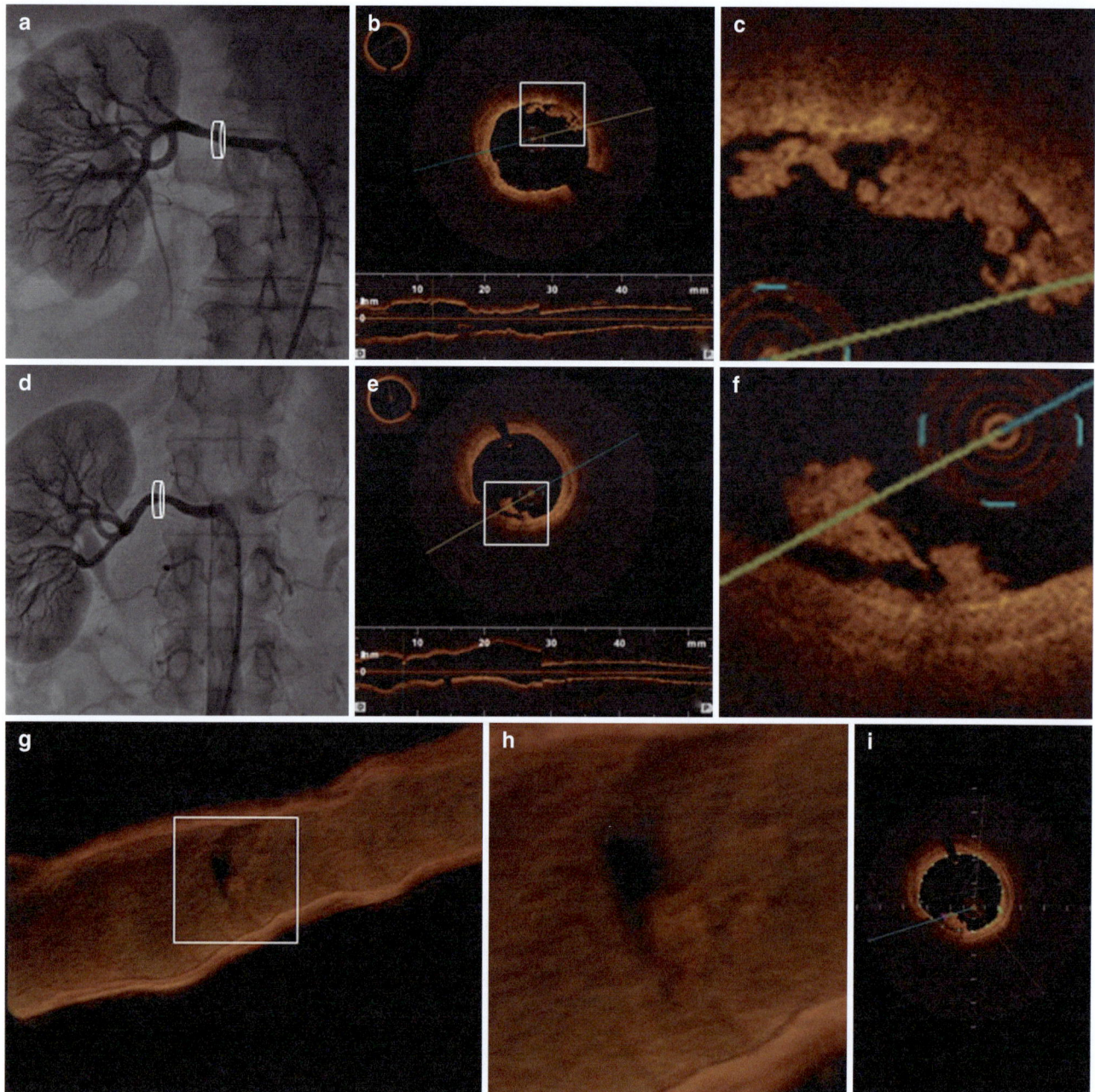

Fig. 18.1 Thrombus formation after renal nerve ablation. Significant intraluminal thrombus formation after renal nerve denervation are unapparent by angiography (**a**, **d**), however displayed in different OCT cross-sections (**b**, **c**, **e**, **f** and **i**) and in three-dimensional reconstructed renal artery (**g**, **h**) (Reproduced with permission from Templin et al. [18])

based on the same principles as conventional RF ablation. During lesion formation, the hottest tissue temperature is generated by resistive heating just below the surface of the tissue. Conduction transfers heat from this zone to the adjacent tissue and ablation electrode, allowing the lesion to form and grow. Increasing the power causes the tissue temperature to rise, resulting in a larger lesion [4]. Saline irrigation during power delivery cools both the electrodes

and the surface of the tissue, dissipating some of the excess heat [4].

During RF ablation, even with irrigation, not all the power is delivered to the tissue. A significant percentage is always lost into the blood and saline. The distribution of power along one of two pathways – blood and saline surrounding the electrode, or the tissue in contact with the electrode – depends on their respective impedances and the electrode-to-tissue contact. Optimal contact reduces power loss into the blood and increases lesion size [4].

Active cooling of the ablation electrode and the adjacent tissue influences lesion shape and vessel wall viability. With conventional RF ablation, the largest lesion diameter is close to the surface of the tissue. Resistive heating in the tissue is only cooled by the blood – therefore, stagnant blood can prevent optimal cooling. The resultant lesion damages a very wide section of the vessel media layer [4]. With irrigated catheter tip ablation, the surface adjacent to the electrode is cooled not only by blood, but also by irrigation solution (which has better cooling properties than blood). Thus, the surface diameter of the lesion is smaller. Increased energy delivery to tissue can be achieved by active cooling. Experimental studies have shown that active cooling results in higher tissue temperature resulting in larger and deeper lesions compared to conventional RF ablation [12, 19, 20].

Irrigated vs. Non-irrigated Radiofrequency Ablation: Preclinical Experience

There are substantial histopathological differences between irrigated and non-irrigated RF ablation. These differences refer to parameters of efficacy such as injury of peri-arterial nerves and parameters of safety such as arterial and peri-arterial tissue damage. Semi-quantitative ordinal grading schemes are useful, when changes in the nerve, renal artery, and peri-arterial soft tissue are evaluated following denervation [21].

Nerve damage can be semi-quantitated using an ordinal grading system of 0–4: 0 = none, 1 = minimal, 2 = mild, 3 = moderate, and 4 = severe [21]. It is important to mention that tissue damage may affect the peri-neuronal and/or endoneuronal portions of the renal nerves. In the assessment of peri-neuronal injury, inflammation and fibrosis are recognized as important signs of peri-neuronal injury. While acute-phase nerve injury may not necessarily be accompanied by peri-neuronal inflammation or fibrosis, chronic-phase nerve injury usually exhibits peri-neuronal fibrosis. Vacuolisation and digestion chambers are unique findings after endoneuronal injury. Vacuolisation is defined by the presence of vacuolated areas, which contain loose connective tissue with rare areas of homogenous eosinophilic staining of cell cytoplasm along with compressed and deformed nuclei (pyknotic nuclei) [22]. Digestion chambers are characterized by variable amounts of aggregated myelin (eosinophilic hyaline globules) and vacuolated spaces with occasional cells interspersed [22]. Also, depending upon the RF energy used there may be necrosis of the nerves bundles as well as calcification. Since minimal or mild injury can be seen even in untreated animals, moderate and severe injury is considered as definite

injury caused by thermal damage or toxins. Additional important parameters of renal peri-arterial nerve ablation procedures refer to the assessment of circumferential dimension and depth penetration of radiofrequency energy. These parameters are relevant for the examination of nerve injury and peri-arterial tissue damage.

Immunohistochemical stains may help to distinguish the morphological or functional presence of neuronal markers relevant to efferent sympathetic or afferent sensory activity. It is important to mention that most markers applied to date are not specific for sympathetic nerves, neither are they specific as markers of unidirectional neuronal signal transduction (afferent vs. efferent). Stains against tyrosine hydroxylase (TH), which is the enzyme for converting tyrosine to DOPA (dihydroxyphenylalanin), are used for the confirmation of norepinephrine synthesis [23]. Sensory nerve (afferent) as well as sympathetic nerve (efferent) fibers play a crucial role for the overall renal sympathetic nerve activity [24]. Immunostaining against calcitonin gene-related peptide (CGRP), which is a neurotransmitter in sensory nerves, can be used as a marker of afferent fibers [25]. The intensity and distribution of staining can be semi-quantified using a scoring system of 0–3; 0 = no reaction, 1 = very weak and/or patchy reaction, 2 = weak reaction, 3 = strong reaction [21].

To assess treatment reactions of the vascular and perivascular tissue including adjacent organs (kidney, lymph nodes, ureters, and renal veins), ordinal data can be collected for multiple parameters including endothelial loss, arterial and venous medial injury (depth and circumference), inflammation, degenerative changes and necrosis. Endothelial cells remain an important luminal barrier against activation of coagulation pathways and adhesion of thrombocytes. Endothelial loss can be observed in the treated vessel but also in adjacent non-treated vessels within the latitude of radiofrequency energy. Inflammation can be a sign of reversible or irreversible tissue damage and needs to be judged in association with the presence of degenerative changes or necrosis. These parameters can be semi-quantified using a scoring system of 0–4: 0 = none; 1 = minimal, 2 = mild; 3 = moderate; and 4 = marked [21]. In addition, distances from affected nerves to the intimal surface of the closest arterial segment through which RF energy was delivered can be measured with digital morphometry from histological slides stained with haematoxylin and Eosin.

In our laboratory, we compared the histopathology following irrigated, cooled-tip ablation and non-irrigated ablation in the swine model. In this regard, the overall nerve damage was comparable between irrigated and non-irrigated ablation. Furthermore, immunoreactivity to tyrosine hydoxylase, an efferent neuronal marker was also similar between

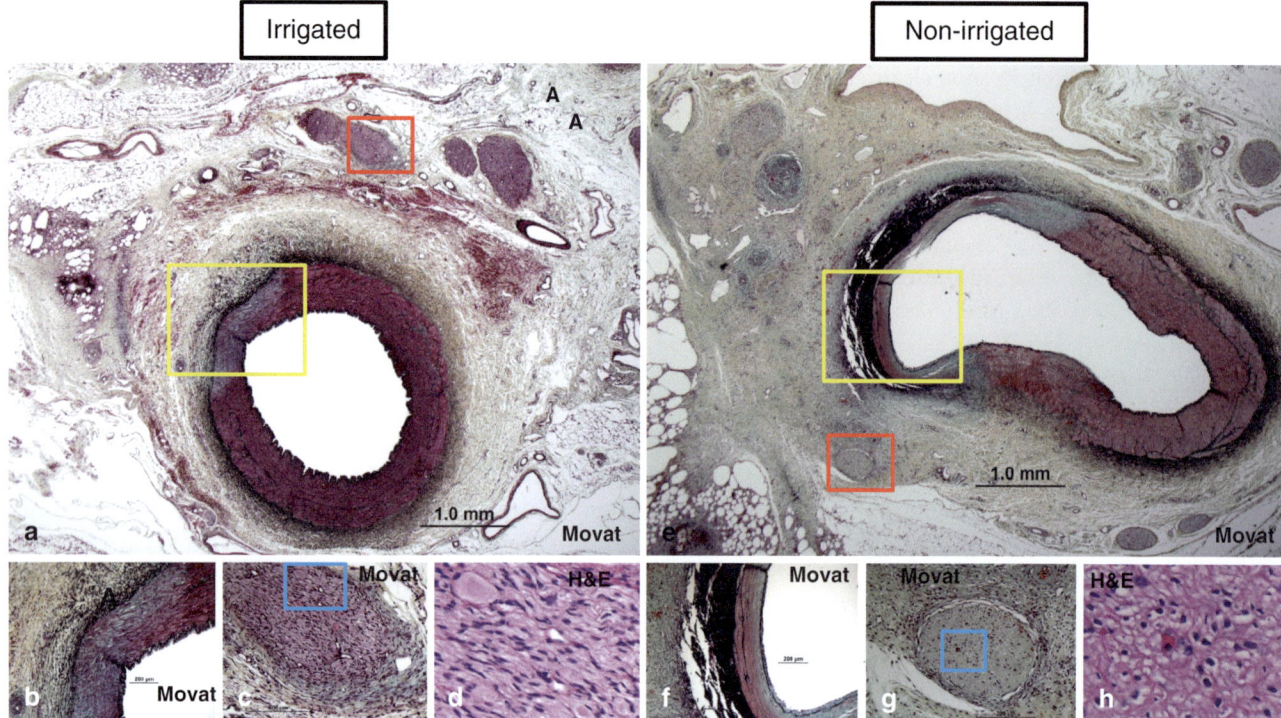

Fig. 18.2 (**a**) Low magnification image of renal artery and surrounding tissue treated by irrigated radiofrequency ablation. (**b**) High magnification image of renal arterial wall (*yellow boxed* area in panel **a**). Proteoglycan replacement (*green* tissue) in the media is observed, however, media thickness is preserved. (**c**) High magnification image of injured nerve (*red boxed* area in panel **a**; Movat stain). Perineurium fibrosis is observed. (**d**) High magnification image of injured nerve (*blue boxed* area in panel **c**; H&E stain). Endoneurium damage (digestion chambers) are observed. (**e**) Low magnification image of renal

artery and surrounding tissue treated by non-irrigated radiofrequency ablation. (**f**) High magnification image of renal arterial wall (*yellow boxed* area in panel **e**). Severe media damage with thinning and severe adventitial damage (denatured collagen) was observed. (**g**) High magnification image of injured nerve (*red boxed* area in panel **e**; Movat stain). (**h**) High magnification image of injured nerve (*blue boxed* area in Panel **g**; H&E stain). Swelling of endoneuronal tissue and pyknotic nuclei are observed

irrigated and non-irrigated ablation groups. On the other hand, renal arterial media damage was significantly less in the irrigated ablation group as compared to non-irrigated ablation group (Fig. 18.2).

However, an important remaining concern with irrigated RDN relates to the question whether the effective temperature registered at the catheter tip truly reflects intramural tissue condition or rather an inconclusive product of heat dissemination secondary to radiofrequency application and active cooling through irrigation. To answer this question, it is extremely important to simultaneously monitor acute and chronic effects within the arterial and peri-arterial tissue. In this regard, our experience with irrigated vs non-irrigated catheter ablation of renal peri-arterial nerves suggests that the latter may achieve similar nerve injury without jeopardizing safety by excess tissue damage. Preservation of peri-arterial tissue is another important factor contributing to long-term efficacy and safety in peri-renal nerve ablation procedures and our data are in line with a favourable effect towards peri-arterial tissue protection in irrigated ablation.

Irrigated RF Ablation: Clinical Experience

To date, there are several clinical studies using irrigated RF catheters for renal denervation. Ahmed et al. enrolled ten patients with resistant arterial hypertension to be treated with saline-irrigated RF denervation [26]. They used a 3.5-mm-tip internally irrigated RF catheter (Celsius Thermocool, Biosense Webster, Diamond Bar, CA, USA). From a total of 91 ablation lesions in these patients, an average of 5 ± 1 (range 2–6) and 4 ± 2 (range 1–7) ablations were performed in the left and right renal artery in each patient, respectively. The mean duration of ablation was 242 ± 98 s per patient (range 117–390 s). At 6 months, blood pressure decrease determined by ambulatory blood pressure measurement was -21 ± 15 mmHg in systolic blood pressure (range −10 to −40 mmHg; $P = 0.003$) and -11 ± 9 mmHg (range 0 to −26 mmHg; $P = 0.005$) in diastolic blood pressure [26]. In five patients, blood sampling for renal hormones was performed, and a significant decrease was observed in the levels of metanephrines, normetanephrines, and aldosterone [26].

Kiuchi et al. investigated blood pressure reduction and renal function in patients with chronic kidney disease and resistant hypertension using a standard irrigated cardiac ablation catheter [27]. A total of 24 patients with a mean baseline blood pressure of 151 ± 18 mmHg/92 ± 11 mmHg (ambulatory blood pressure) were treated by a 7-Fr irrigated ablation catheter (AlCath Flux eXtra Gold Full Circle 270°; VascoMed GmbH, Binzen, Germany) [27]. At 6 months follow-up, mean ABPM decreased to $132 + 15$ mmHg/$85 + 11$ mmHg, and median urine albumin:creatinine ratio decreased from base line (48.5 mg/g) to 6 months (15.7 mg/g) [27].

Recently, Remo et al. reported a case series using RDN as adjunctive therapy for refractory ventricular tachycardia (VT) in patients with underlying cardiomyopathy [28]. Four patients with cardiomyopathy with recurrent VT despite antiarrhythmic therapy and prior cardiac ablation underwent RDN ± repeat VT ablation using either a non-irrigated (6 W at 50 °C for 60 s) or irrigated ablation catheter (10–12 W for 30–60 s) [28]. The number of VT episodes was decreased from 11.0 ± 4.2 to 0.3 ± 0.1 per month after ablation with the combined approach (VT ablation + RDN using either irrigated or non-irrigated) [28].

Summary

It is clear that RDN does not result in a universal decrease of blood pressure– possibly because the procedure does not achieve complete denervation of the target renal arteries. It is also possible that renal sympathetic activity has a subordinate role in certain hypertensive patients with normal renal sympathetic tone [29]. Sympathetic nervous system activity appears to be of most importance during the early stages of hypertension, therefore, early modification of such activity may be a realistic goal.

Obesity and insulin resistance are frequent complications of hypertension. Given the high incidence of cardiovascular events in patients with insulin resistance and impaired glucose metabolism, and the favourable impact of reduced sympathetic drive, lower cardiovascular event rates after RDN may well be achievable. Studies evaluating the effect sympathetic RDN on diabetes control and cardiovascular events are ongoing [30]. Further studies of the long-term impact of RDN on renal haemodynamics – in particular, comparing RDN to conventional medical therapy – are warranted before a truly informed opinion regarding the protective, neutral or harmful effect of RDN in resistant hypertension and related disorders can be made.

Improvements in percutaneous catheter design with enhanced stability, modification of RF delivery and electrode design have clearly helped to improve clinical results in the broad spectrum of electrophysiological applications for RDN [4]. This has been exemplified in the introduction of cooled-tip percutaneous catheters, since conventional RF ablation catheters share the limitation of over-heating which may increase the risk of endothelial injury and thrombus formation [4].

External irrigation affords the additional advantage of locally cooling the blood/tissue interface, which has been demonstrated to reduce thrombus formation. At a technical level, temperature and impedance monitoring has been shown to be critical in predicting optimal catheter-tissue contact. With the introduction of cooled-tip catheters, professional appreciation and understanding of temperature monitoring will be further enhanced [4]. In the long-term, the combined efforts of engineers, researchers and clinicians will be crucial in order to facilitate increased knowledge of success and failure with regard to RDN procedures.

References

1. Calhoun DA, Jones D, Textor S, et al. Resistant hypertension: diagnosis, evaluation, and treatment. A scientific statement from the American Heart Association Professional Education Committee of the Council for High Blood Pressure Research. Hypertension. 2008;51:1403–19.
2. Chris SM. Sympathectomy for hypertension. Br Med J. 1951;1: 665–70.
3. Linz D, Hohl M, Nickel A, et al. Effect of renal denervation on neurohumoral activation triggering atrial fibrillation in obstructive sleep apnea. Hypertension. 2013;62:767–74.
4. Ammar S, Ladich E, Steigerwald K, Deisenhofer I, Joner M. Pathophysiology of renal denervation procedures: from renal nerve anatomy to procedural parameters. EuroIntervention. 2013;9:R89–95.
5. Kaltenbach B, Id D, Franke JC, et al. Renal artery stenosis after renal sympathetic denervation. J Am Coll Cardiol. 2012;60:2694–5.
6. Lustgarten DL, Spector PS. Ablation using irrigated radiofrequency: a hands-on guide. Heart Rhythm. 2008;5:899–902.
7. Haines DE. The biophysics of radiofrequency catheter ablation in the heart: the importance of temperature monitoring. Pacing Clin Electrophysiol. 1993;16:586–91.
8. Erez A, Shitzer A. Controlled destruction and temperature distributions in biological tissues subjected to monoactive electrocoagulation. J Biomech Eng. 1980;102:42–9.
9. Ko WC, Huang SK, Lin JL, Shau WY, Lai LP, Chen PH. New method for predicting efficiency of heating by measuring bioimpedance during radiofrequency catheter ablation in humans. J Cardiovasc Electrophysiol. 2001;12:819–23.
10. Avitall B, Mughal K, Hare J, Helms R, Krum D. The effects of electrode-tissue contact on radiofrequency lesion generation. Pacing Clin Electrophysiol. 1997;20:2899–910.
11. Otomo K, Yamanashi WS, Tondo C, et al. Why a large tip electrode makes a deeper radiofrequency lesion: effects of increase in electrode cooling and electrode-tissue interface area. J Cardiovasc Electrophysiol. 1998;9:47–54.
12. Nakagawa H, Yamanashi WS, Pitha JV, et al. Comparison of in vivo tissue temperature profile and lesion geometry for radiofrequency ablation with a saline-irrigated electrode versus temperature control in a canine thigh muscle preparation. Circulation. 1995;91: 2264–73.
13. Krum H, Schlaich MP, Bohm M, et al. Percutaneous renal denervation in patients with treatment-resistant hypertension: final 3-year report of the Symplicity HTN-1 study. Lancet. 2014;383:622–9.

14. Worthley SG, Tsioufis CP, Worthley MI, et al. Safety and efficacy of a multi-electrode renal sympathetic denervation system in resistant hypertension: the EnligHTN I trial. Eur Heart J. 2013;34: 2132–40.

15. Esler MD, Krum H, Sobotka PA, Schlaich MP, Schmieder RE, Bohm M. Renal sympathetic denervation in patients with treatment-resistant hypertension (the Symplicity HTN-2 trial): a randomised controlled trial. Lancet. 2010;376:1903–9.

16. Kandzari DE, Bhatt DL, Sobotka PA, et al. Catheter-based renal denervation for resistant hypertension: rationale and design of the SYMPLICITY HTN-3 trial. Clin Cardiol. 2012;35:528–35.

17. Bhatt DL, Kandzari DE, O'Neill WW, et al. A controlled trial of renal denervation for resistant hypertension. N Engl J Med. 2014. doi:10.1056/NEJMoa1402670.

18. Templin C, Jaguszewski M, Ghadri JR, et al. Vascular lesions induced by renal nerve ablation as assessed by optical coherence tomography: pre- and post-procedural comparison with the simplicity(R) catheter system and the EnligHTN multi-electrode renal denervation catheter. Eur Heart J. 2013;34:2141–8.

19. Nakagawa H, Wittkampf FH, Yamanashi WS, et al. Inverse relationship between electrode size and lesion size during radiofrequency ablation with active electrode cooling. Circulation. 1998;98: 458–65.

20. d'Avila A, Houghtaling C, Gutierrez P, et al. Catheter ablation of ventricular epicardial tissue: a comparison of standard and cooled-tip radiofrequency energy. Circulation. 2004;109:2363–9.

21. Sakakura K, Ladich E, Edelman ER, et al. Methodological standardization for the preclinical evaluation of renal sympathetic denervation. JACC Cardiovasc Interv. 2014. doi:10.1016/j.jcin.2014.04.024.

22. Whitney KM, Schwartz Sterman AJ, O'Connor J, Foley GL, Garman RH. Light microscopic sciatic nerve changes in control beagle dogs from toxicity studies. Toxicol Pathol. 2011;39: 835–40.

23. Burgi K, Cavalleri MT, Alves AS, Britto LR, Antunes VR, Michelini LC. Tyrosine hydroxylase immunoreactivity as indicator of sympathetic activity: simultaneous evaluation in different tissues of hypertensive rats. Am J Physiol Regul Integr Comp Physiol. 2011;300:R264–71.

24. DiBona GF, Esler M. Translational medicine: the antihypertensive effect of renal denervation. Am J Physiol Regul Integr Comp Physiol. 2010;298:R245–53.

25. Tellez A, Rousselle S, Palmieri T, et al. Renal artery nerve distribution and density in the porcine model: biologic implications for the development of radiofrequency ablation therapies. Transl Res. 2013;162:381–9.

26. Ahmed H, Neuzil P, Skoda J, et al. Renal sympathetic denervation using an irrigated radiofrequency ablation catheter for the management of drug-resistant hypertension. JACC Cardiovasc Interv. 2012;5:758–65.

27. Kiuchi MG, Maia GL, de Queiroz Carreira MA, et al. Effects of renal denervation with a standard irrigated cardiac ablation catheter on blood pressure and renal function in patients with chronic kidney disease and resistant hypertension. Eur Heart J. 2013;34:2114–21.

28. Remo BF, Preminger M, Bradfield J, et al. Safety and efficacy of renal denervation as a novel treatment for ventricular tachycardia storm in patients with cardiomyopathy. Heart Rhythm. 2013. doi:10.1016/j.hrthm.2013.12.038.

29. Bertog SC, Sobotka PA, Sievert H. Renal denervation for hypertension. JACC Cardiovasc Interv. 2012;5:249–58.

30. Mahfoud F, Ewen S, Ukena C, et al. Expanding the indication spectrum: renal denervation in diabetes. EuroIntervention. 2013;9: R117–21.

Renal Denervation: Potential Future Implications Beyond Resistant Hypertension

Markus P. Schlaich

Introduction

Sympathetic nervous system (SNS) activation is a common feature of arterial hypertension and has been demonstrated to contribute to the development and progression of the hypertensive state. Persuasive evidence suggests a strong association between SNS over-activity and variety of disease states including chronic renal failure, insulin resistance, congestive heart failure, sleep apnea, ventricular arrhythmias and others. While sympatholytic agents are available to target SNS over-activity pharmacologically, they are not widely used in clinical practice leaving the SNS unopposed in many patients. The recent introduction of catheter-based renal denervation as an alternative approach to target the SNS therapeutically has been trialed primarily in patients with resistant hypertension, Preliminary data obtained from small and mostly uncontrolled studies in related disease states often characterised by over-activity of the SNS are promising but require confirmation in appropriately designed clinical trials.

A Brief History of the Sympathetic Nervous System

While the first identifiable description of the anatomy of the sympathetic nervous system by Thomas Willis dates back to 1664, it was not until 1727 that the neural control of blood vessel caliber became apparent as a physiological concept through the work of du Petit, who demonstrated conjunctival vessel dilatation after section of cervical sympathetic nerves [1]. More than a century later, Stelling in 1840 suggested that the vasomotor fibers were sympathetic nerves originating in the central nervous system and supplying the peripheral blood vessels. In 1852, Claude Bernard and others observed dilatation of blood vessels by sectioning sympathetic nerves and a rise in blood pressure upon electrical stimulation of the cut nerves, thereby identifying these as "pressor nerves" [2]. However, it was not until 1932 that Adrian described actual sympathetic discharges from direct recording of electrical impulses in both pre- and post-ganglionic sympathetic fibers of cats and rabbits [3]. Von Euler in 1946 then identified nor-adrenaline as the major neurotransmitter of sympathetic nerves [4]. In the early decades of the twentieth century, Cannon [5] popularized the concept of the 'fight and flight' response to stress through his research on sympathetic nerves. Experimental and humans studies from the past three decades not only confirmed the critical role of the SNS in cardiovascular control but also provided conclusive evidence for a role of an overactive SNS in the pathophysiology of a variety of clinically relevant conditions such as essential hypertension [6–9], insulin resistance [10], congestive heart failure [11], renal disease [12], and others.

The Specific Role of Renal Nerves

Renal efferent and afferent nerves lie within the adventitia of the renal arteries and form a network that constitutes a significant control system for the physiological regulation of blood pressure and renal function, as summarized by Bertog et al. [13].

Efferent Renal Sympathetic Nerve

The efferent renal sympathetic nerves originate from the intermediolateral column of the spinal cord from T_8 to L_1. Nerves carrying fibers that project to the kidney are derived from the celiac plexus and its subdivisions [6]. The kidney, including the renal vasculature [14], the tubules [15, 16], the juxtaglomerular cells [17], and the renal pelvic wall

M.P. Schlaich, MD, FAHA
Neurovascular Hypertension and Kidney Disease Laboratory,
Baker IDI Heart and Diabetes Institute,
St Kilda Road Central, 6492, Melbourne, VIC 8008, Australia
e-mail: markus.schlaich@bakeridi.edu.au

R.R. Heuser et al. (eds.), *Renal Denervation: A New Approach to Treatment of Resistant Hypertension*,
DOI 10.1007/978-1-4471-5223-1_19, © Springer-Verlag London 2015

[18] all have a rich supply of efferent sympathetic nerves. The release of noradrenaline from renal sympathetic nerve terminals has three major consequences: (i) it stimulates β_1-adrenoceptors on juxtaglomerular granular cells to release renin [19] thereby increasing activity of the renin-angiotensin–aldosterone system [19, 20]; (ii) it decreases urinary sodium and water excretion via enhanced tubular reabsorption [21], and (iii) it reduces renal blood flow and glomerular filtration rate via constriction of the renal vasculature [22].

Afferent Renal Nerves

The kidneys also have abundant afferent sensory innervation, with sensory nerve fibers projecting from the kidney to the central nervous system via the dorsal root ganglia. The cell bodies of the afferent renal nerves are located in ipsilateral dorsal root ganglia predominantly from T_{12} to L_3 [23]. In contrast to the widespread distribution of the efferent sympathetic nerve fibers in the kidney, the major locations of the afferent renal sensory nerves are in the renal pelvic area [18, 24]. The pelvic pressure is a major determinant of afferent renal nerve activity and increments in urine flow rate increase the firing rate of renal afferent fibers [25]. This in turn results in a decrease in efferent renal sympathetic nerve activity and an increase in urinary sodium excretion, a reno-renal reflex response [26]. An increase in efferent renal nerve activity modulates afferent renal activity by the release of noradrenaline, which activates α_1-adrenoceptors (ARs) and α_2-ARs on renal sensory nerves [18].

From the above considerations it is conceivable that activation of renal nerves contributes substantially to both acute and long term blood pressure changes, but may also have important implications beyond blood pressure control.

Sympathetic Nerve Activity and Hypertension

While the pathogenesis of essential hypertension is multifactorial, sympathetic nervous system activation has been established as a major contributor to the development of hypertension. Based on direct recordings of muscle sympathetic nerve activity and measurement of the release of noradrenaline from organs critically involved in circulatory control such as the kidney and the heart, it is now well established that arterial hypertension, is commonly neurogenic, the blood pressure rise being initiated and sustained by increased sympathetic activity [7, 27]. The increase in the number of sympathetic bursts to the skeletal muscle circulation has been related directly to the degree of blood pressure elevation [28].

Studies employing radiotracer dilution methodology to measure overflow of noradrenaline (NE) from the kidneys to plasma have provided unequivocal evidence for increased renal noradrenaline spillover rates in patients with essential hypertension [7, 29]. Furthermore, elevated NE spillover from the heart is also often present and is commensurate with the typical hemodynamic profile seen in hypertensive patients [30, 31]. Importantly, sympathetic activation is commonly present in subjects with borderline hypertension and even in normotensive individuals with a strong genetic predisposition to develop hypertension, indicative of a causal role of sympathetic activation in blood pressure elevation [32].

The consequences of increased sympathetic outflow to the kidneys, perhaps most important in this context and described above in more detail include volume retention via tubular sodium re-absorption [21], reduced renal blood flow through neutrally mediated vasoconstriction [22, 33], and release of renin from the juxtaglomerular apparatus [20], all of which can contribute to blood pressure elevation, both acutely and in the long term. Accordingly, targeting the sympathetic nervous system appears to be a logical therapeutic approach for the treatment of hypertension.

Surgical Sympathectomy for the Treatment of Hypertension

The concept of targeting (renal) sympathetic nerves for the treatment of hypertension is an old one. It has long been recognized that RDN results in diuresis and natriuresis in animal studies [34, 35]. Bello-Reuss et al. [36] found that diuresis and natriuresis after acute RDN was caused by a depression of sodium and water reabsorption in the proximal tubule with partial compensation in more distal nephron segments. Indeed, bilateral RDN has been shown in many experimental models to reduced blood pressure or prevent the development of hypertension and has been carried out in many models of experimental hypertension, as previously summarized [6].

In the human setting, prior to the availability of effective pharmacologic drug therapy, surgical RDN was applied since the early 1920s and 1930s with thoraco-lumbar splanchnicectomy being the most commonly used form of surgical sympathectomy. It has been reported that the average survival time of patients in the malignant phase of hypertension at the time was only 8 months [37]. Although the results of sympathectomy in hypertension were not subjected to rigorous scientific analysis, a relatively high rate of long-term improvement of hypertension was reported [37–40]. Sympathectomy at the time was performed in either one or two stages and required a prolonged hospital stay (2–4 weeks) with a long recovery period (1–2 months). In a large population study including 1,266 hypertensive patients who underwent splanchnicectomy and 467 hypertensive control subjects treated by low salt diet only, the 5-year mortality rates were 19 and 54 %, respectively. Fourty-five percent of those who survived the surgery had significantly lower blood pressure afterwards, and the antihypertensive effect lasted 10 years or more [41]. Another large observational study of more than 2,000 patients 1,506 of whom underwent splanchnicectomy demonstrated a satisfactory blood pressure response in about half of the patients who underwent splanchnicectomy [42]. Interestingly, sympathectomy rendered blood pressure more sensitive to antihypertensive drugs, allowing a reduction in the number and doses of administered drugs. While surgical sympathectomy was effective in lowering blood pressure and improve outcomes in many cases it carried severe postoperative complications: prolonged hospitalisation, orthostatic hypotension, syncope, incontinence (both urinary and faecal) and difficulties in walking. As a consequence and due to the advent of effective pharmacological antihypertensive therapies, surgical sympathectomy for the treatment of hypertension was soon abandoned.

Endovascular Radiofrequency Ablation of the Renal Nerves

With the advances in technology and the availability of minimally invasive procedures, the concept of selective sympathectomy, or more specifically, renal sympathetic denervation, was recently revisited and resulted in the development of a catheter-based device using radiofrequency energy for ablation of renal nerves via the lumen of the renal artery, as described in detail in other chapters in this book. Given the relevance of renal sympathetic nerve activity for many other conditions commonly characterized by increased sympathetic drive, several preliminary and mostly uncontrolled studies have been performed and are briefly reviewed below.

End–Stage Renal Failure

Increased activity of the sympathetic nervous system has clearly been demonstrated to contribute substantially to elevated blood pressure levels commonly seen in patients with ESRD on dialysis [12, 43–45]. Very recently, preliminary data on the feasibility of renal denervation and its effects on blood pressure and sympathetic nerve activity in ESRD patients have been reported [46].

In this initial safety and proof-of-concept study RDN was performed in 12 patients with ESRD and uncontrolled blood pressure (BP). Standardized BP measurements were obtained in all patients on dialysis free days at baseline and

follow up and measures of renal noradrenaline spillover and muscle sympathetic nerve activity were available from five patients at baseline and from two patients at 12 month follow up and beyond. The average office BP was 170.8 ± 16.9/89.2 ± 12.1 mmHg despite the use of 3.8 ± 1.4 antihypertensive drugs in these patients. All five patients in whom muscle sympathetic nerve activity and noradrenaline spillover was assessed at baseline displayed substantially elevated levels, confirming high sympathetic tone in patients with ESRD. Of note, 3 out of 12 patients could not undergo RDN due to atrophic renal arteries, which made it impossible to position the RF treatment catheter appropriately. Compared to baseline, office systolic BP was significantly reduced at 3, 6, and 12 months after RDN (from 166 ± 16.0 to 148 ± 11, 150 ± 14, and 138 ± 17 mmHg, respectively), whereas no change was evident in the three non-treated patients. While preliminary in nature, these data indicate that RDN is feasible in patients with ESRD and appears to be associated with a sustained reduction in systolic office BP. In this patient cohort, technical issues may arise owing to atrophic renal arteries which may pose a problem for application of this technology in some patients with ESRD. Further studies are required to confirm these initial findings and assess the best technical approach to RDN treatment of this patient cohort.

Congestive Heart Failure

Whilst hypertension is an important etiological factor in the subsequent development of systolic chronic heart failure (CHF), patients with established systolic CHF generally have normal, and usually low, systemic blood pressure values. They do, however, have a markedly and chronically activated sympathetic nervous system which is strongly linked to progression of underlying disease processes as well as poor clinical outcomes in this setting [47]. Furthermore, it has been demonstrated that renal sympathetic nerve activity predicts outcomes in patients with heart failure, lending further support to the potentially beneficial concept of specifically targeting renal nerves in this scenario [48]. This is supported further by animal studies which have demonstrated improved cardiac function and reduced pathological fibrosis following renal denervation [49], as well as improved renal blood flow in the heart failure setting with potentially significant implications for the cardio-renal syndrome [50].

The effects of RDN in patients with heart failure are currently assessed in various studies and the results of a small pilot study including seven patients with chronic mild to moderate systolic heart failure have been published recently. In these seven patients with a mean ejection fraction of 43 ± 15 % no procedural or safety concerns were encountered [51] particularly no major drop in BP despite low baseline levels and no change in renal function. A mild improvement in the 6-min walking test could be detected, while ejection fraction and other cardiac structural and functional parameters were not changed significantly at 6 months after the procedure.

Currently, there are two ongoing clinical trials, Symplicity-HF (RDN in Patients with Chronic Heart Failure and Renal Impairment Clinical Trial) and REACH (Renal Artery Denervation in Chronic Heart Failure), investigating the safety and efficacy of RDN in patients with systolic CHF. The results of these clinical trials will provide important physiological information on the impact of RDN on cardiac function, as well as information to determine the safety, feasibility, efficacy, and durability of such an approach and whether there is therapeutic value of RDN in patients with CHF.

Insulin Resistance

Hypertension is more common in patients with diabetes than in the general population and is associated with impaired glucose metabolism and insulin resistance. Activation of the SNS may contribute to either condition. There are three major lines of evidence to indicate that sympathetic nervous system activation plays a critical role in the genesis and/or progression of insulin resistance and the risk associated with the condition.

Sympathetic activation causes peripheral vasoconstriction through release of the neurotransmitter noradrenaline from sympathetic nerve terminals and subsequent activation of vascular smooth muscle adrenoceptors. In the human forearm, increased noradrenaline release results in a substantial reduction in forearm blood flow and is associated with a markedly reduced forearm uptake of glucose, highlighting the adverse effect of sympathetic activation on the ability of the cell to transport glucose across its membrane, a hallmark of insulin resistance [52]. This is probably the result of a reduced number of open capillaries due to vasoconstriction and an increase in the distance that insulin must travel to reach the cell membrane from the intravascular compartment. This situation may be enhanced further if insulin resistance is already established, a state in which the ability of insulin to increase muscle perfusion has been demonstrated to be reduced by approximately 30 % [53]. These observations indicate that sympathetic nervous system activation modulates insulin sensitivity through alterations in regional haemodynamics and effects on glucose transport across the cell via non-hemodynamic effects, such as increased adipose tissue lipolysis, which releases free fatty acids into the circulation, thereby engaging a mechanism that directly inhibits glucose transport across the cell membrane.

Based on these considerations it is perhaps not surprising that reducing sympathetic activation may beneficially influence glucose homeostasis and insulin resistance. Indeed, a recent report demonstrated potential beneficial effects on glucose metabolism and insulin sensitivity with RDN [54]. In this study, 37 resistant hypertensive patients underwent bilateral catheter-based RDN, while 13 untreated patients served as controls. Office blood pressure was reduced by −28/−10 mmHg (p<0.001) and −32/−12 mmHg (P<0.001) at 1 and 3 months in the RDN group. Most relevant in this context, levels of fasting glucose (P=0.039), insulin (P=0.006), C-peptide (P=0.002) and HOMA index (P=0.001) were all reduced significantly, as were mean 2-h glucose levels during oral glucose tolerance test (P=0.012). In contrast, there were no significant changes in blood pressure or metabolic markers in the control group.

Clearly, additional studies are required to confirm these initial findings and the currently ongoing DREAMS (Denervation of the Renal Artery in Metabolic Syndrome) study will assess changes in insulin resistance at 1-year follow-up after RDN in patients with metabolic syndrome and elevated fasting glucose.

Obstructive Sleep Apnea

It has been suggested that up to 80 % of patients with resistant hypertension suffer from obstructive sleep apnea (OSA), defined as an apnea/hypopnea index (AHI) >5 events per hour [55–57]. Current guidelines therefore recommend screening for and treatment of sleep apnea in patients with resistant hypertension [58]. While several pathophysiologial mechanisms have been suggested to contribute to this detrimental relationship, there is general agreement that a major mechanism is an increase in sympathetic activity during the apneas [59].

Perhaps not unexpectedly, preliminary data indicates potential favorable effects on sleep apnea severity in patients with resistant hypertension and concomitant sleep apnea, as recently reported by Witkowski and colleagues [60]. In this proof-of-concept study, a total of ten patients with refractory hypertension and sleep apnea (seven men and three women; median age: 49.5 years) underwent renal denervation and completed 3-month and 6-month follow-up evaluations, including polysomnography. Antihypertensive regimens were not changed during the 6 months of follow-up. Three and 6 months after denervation, decreases in office systolic and diastolic BPs were observed (median: −34/−13 mmHg at 6 months; both P<0.01). A decrease in AHI at 6 months after renal denervation was observed in eight out of ten patients (median: 16.3 versus 4.5 events per hour; P=0.059).

These preliminary data suggest that catheter-based renal sympathetic denervation may lower OSA severity and confirmed previously described beneficial effects on glucose metabolism, indicating that patients with co-morbid resistant hypertension, glucose intolerance, and obstructive sleep apnea, may specifically benefit from this procedure. While no direct mechanistic insights could be obtained from this study, it is conceivable that renal denervation reduces salt avidity by efferent sympathetic renal nerve disruption and might reduce total body fluid, which is thought to contribute to obstructive episodes through peripharyngeal fluid accumulation that may predispose to upper airway obstruction [61]. Furthermore, venous capacitance remains under the control of the sympathetic nervous system and it is likely that renal denervation affects venous capacitance and blood pooling [62], thereby providing a further potential mechanism through which renal denervation could reduce OSA severity in resistant hypertension.

Atrial Fibrillation

Both animal and human studies suggest that the autonomic nervous system plays an important role in initiation and maintenance of atrial fibrillation (AF). Chen et al. documented that simultaneous sympatho-vagal activation was the most common trigger of paroxysmal atrial fibrillation (PAF) in dogs [63], which is consistent with several other reports [64, 65]. In human studies, Huang et al. [66] suggested that idiopathic PAF is primarily dependent on vagal withdrawal, while organic PAF is triggered by sympathetic excitation. Some studies observed increased sympathetic tone or a loss of vagal tone before the onset of AF [67, 68]. More recently, Pokushalov et al. [69] reported that RDN reduced AF recurrence when combined with pulmonary vein isolation (PVI). In this study, 27 hypertensive patients with a history of symptomatic paroxysmal or persistent AF were enrolled, 14 of whom underwent PVI only, and 13 were treated with PVI and RDN. At 12 months follow-up, patients in the PVI + RDN group not only experienced a significant reduction in systolic (181 ± 7 to 156 ± 5 mmHg; $p < 0.001$) and diastolic blood pressure (97 ± 6 to 87 ± 4 mmHg; $p < 0.001$) but also had a substantially lower rate of recurrence of AF. Nine of the 13 patients (69 %) treated with PVI plus renal denervation were AF-free versus 4 (29 %) of the 14 patients in the PVI-only group (p = 0.033). Although optimized blood pressure control might play a considerable role in the reduction of AF recurrence, this study raises the possibility that reducing sympathetic drive with RDN may reduce the rate of AF recurrence in resistant hypertensive patients.

Conclusions

Renal denervation has emerged as a novel treatment option for patients with resistant hypertension whose blood pressure cannot be controlled by optimal combinations of lifestyle modification and pharmacotherapy. Based on the

mechanisms underpinning several other relevant conditions commonly associated with hypertension, benefits beyond improved BP control could potentially be expected in the context of end stage renal disease, heart failure, impaired glucose metabolism, obstructive sleep apnea, and others. However, at this stage there is not sufficient evidence to support its use in any of these potential indications. Appropriately designed prospective randomized controlled trials will be required to explore this further.

References

1. Esler M. The sympathetic nervous system through the ages: from Thomas Willis to resistant hypertension. Exp Physiol. 2011;96:611–22.
2. Ackerknecht EH. The history of the discovery of the vegatative (autonomic) nervous system. Med Hist. 1974;18:1–8.
3. Adrian ED, Bronk DW, Phillips G. Discharges in mammalian sympathetic nerves. J Physiol. 1932;74:115–33.
4. Von Euler US. A substance with sympathin E properties in spleen extracts. Nature. 1946;157:369.
5. Cannon WB. Chemical mediators of autonomic nerve impulses. Science. 1933;78:43–8.
6. DiBona GF, Kopp UC. Neural control of renal function. Physiol Rev. 1997;77:75–197.
7. Schlaich MP, Lambert E, Kaye DM, Krozowski Z, Campbell DJ, Lambert G, Hastings J, Aggarwal A, Esler MD. Sympathetic augmentation in hypertension: role of nerve firing, norepinephrine reuptake, and angiotensin neuromodulation. Hypertension. 2004; 43:169–75.
8. Grewal RS, Kaul CL. Importance of the sympathetic nervous system in the development of renal hypertension in the rat. Br J Pharmacol. 1971;42:497–504.
9. Smith PA, Graham LN, Mackintosh AF, Stoker JB, Mary DA. Relationship between central sympathetic activity and stages of human hypertension. Am J Hypertens. 2004;17:217–22.
10. Masuo K, Rakugi H, Ogihara T, Esler MD, Lambert GW. Cardiovascular and renal complications of type 2 diabetes in obesity: role of sympathetic nerve activity and insulin resistance. Curr Diabetes Rev. 2010;6:58–67.
11. Cohn JN, Levine TB, Francis GS, Goldsmith S. Neurohumoral control mechanisms in congestive heart failure. Am Heart J. 1981;102:509–14.
12. Grassi G, Quarti-Trevano F, Seravalle G, Arenare F, Volpe M, Furiani S, Dell'Oro R, Mancia G. Early sympathetic activation in the initial clinical stages of chronic renal failure. Hypertension. 2011;57:846–51.
13. Bertog SC, Sobotka PA, Sievert H. Renal denervation for hypertension. JACC Cardiovasc Interv. 2012;5:249–58.
14. Barajas L, Liu L, Powers K. Anatomy of the renal innervation: intrarenal aspects and ganglia of origin. Can J Physiol Pharmacol. 1992;70:735–49.
15. Barajas L, Powers KV. Innervation of the thick ascending limb of Henle. Am J Physiol. 1988;255:F340–8.
16. Barajas L, Powers K, Wang P. Innervation of the late distal nephron: an autoradiographic and ultrastructural study. J Ultrastruct Res. 1985;92:146–57.
17. Barajas L, Muller J. The innervation of the juxtaglomerular apparatus and surrounding tubules: a quantitative analysis by serial section electron microscopy. J Ultrastruct Res. 1973;43:107–32.
18. Kopp UC, Cicha MZ, Smith LA, Mulder J, Hokfelt T. Renal sympathetic nerve activity modulates afferent renal nerve activity by

PGE2-dependent activation of alpha1- and alpha2-adrenoceptors on renal sensory nerve fibers. Am J Physiol Regul Integr Comp Physiol. 2007;293:R1561–72.

19. DiBona GF. Nervous kidney. Interaction between renal sympathetic nerves and the renin-angiotensin system in the control of renal function. Hypertension. 2000;36:1083–8.

20. Zanchetti AS. Neural regulation of renin release: experimental evidence and clinical implications in arterial hypertension. Circulation. 1977;56:691–8.

21. Bell-Reuss E, Trevino DL, Gottschalk CW. Effect of renal sympathetic nerve stimulation on proximal water and sodium reabsorption. J Clin Invest. 1976;57:1104–7.

22. Kirchheim H, Ehmke H, Persson P. Sympathetic modulation of renal hemodynamics, renin release and sodium excretion. Klin Wochenschr. 1989;67:858–64.

23. Weiss ML, Chowdhury SI. The renal afferent pathways in the rat: a pseudorabies virus study. Brain Res. 1998;812:227–41.

24. Liu L, Barajas L. The rat renal nerves during development. Anat Embryol (Berl). 1993;188:345–61.

25. Genovesi S, Pieruzzi F, Wijnmaalen P, Centonza L, Golin R, Zanchetti A, Stella A. Renal afferents signaling diuretic activity in the cat. Circ Res. 1993;73:906–13.

26. Morsing P, Persson AE. Pelvic pressure and tubuloglomerular feedback in hydronephrosis. Ren Physiol Biochem. 1990;13:181–9.

27. Esler M, Straznicky N, Eikelis N, Masuo K, Lambert G, Lambert E. Mechanisms of sympathetic activation in obesity-related hypertension. Hypertension. 2006;48:787–96.

28. Grassi G, Cattaneo BM, Seravalle G, Lanfranchi A, Mancia G. Baroreflex control of sympathetic nerve activity in essential and secondary hypertension. Hypertension. 1998;31:68–72.

29. Esler M, Jennings G, Biviano B, Lambert G, Hasking G. Mechanism of elevated plasma noradrenaline in the course of essential hypertension. J Cardiovasc Pharmacol. 1986;8 Suppl 5:S39–43.

30. Esler M, Jennings G, Lambert G. Noradrenaline release and the pathophysiology of primary human hypertension. Am J Hypertens. 1989;2:140S–6.

31. Schlaich MP, Kaye DM, Lambert E, Sommerville M, Socratous F, Esler MD. Relation between cardiac sympathetic activity and hypertensive left ventricular hypertrophy. Circulation. 2003;108:560–5.

32. Anderson EA, Sinkey CA, Lawton WJ, Mark AL. Elevated sympathetic nerve activity in borderline hypertensive humans. Evidence from direct intraneural recordings. Hypertension. 1989;14:177–83.

33. Kon V. Neural control of renal circulation. Miner Electrolyte Metab. 1989;15:33–43.

34. Surtshin A, Mueller CB, White HL. Effect of acute changes in glomerular filtration rate on water and electrolyte excretion; mechanism of denervation diuresis. Am J Physiol. 1952;169:159–73.

35. Kamm DE, Levinsky NG. The mechanism of denervation natriuresis. J Clin Invest. 1965;44:93–102.

36. Bello-Reuss E, Colindres RE, Pastoriza-Munoz E, Mueller RA, Gottschalk CW. Effects of acute unilateral renal denervation in the rat. J Clin Invest. 1975;56:208–17.

37. Parkes WE. Thoracolumbar sympathectomy in hypertension. Br Heart J. 1958;20:249–52.

38. Newcombe CP, Shucksmith HS, Suffern WS. Sympathectomy for hypertension; follow-up of 212 patients. Br Med J. 1959;1:142–4.

39. Peet MM. Results of bilateral supradiaphragmatic splanchnicectomy for arterial hypertension. N Engl J Med. 1947;236:270–7.

40. Abbott AC. The surgical treatment of hypertension; 17 years in retrospect. Can Med Assoc J. 1952;66:211–4.

41. Smithwick RH, Thompson JE. Splanchnicectomy for essential hypertension; results in 1,266 cases. J Am Med Assoc. 1953;152:1501–4.

42. Smithwick RH. Hypertensive vascular disease; results of and indications for splanchnicectomy. J Chronic Dis. 1955;1:477–96.

43. Lilley JJ, Golden J, Stone RA. Adrenergic regulation of blood pressure in chronic renal failure. J Clin Invest. 1976;57:1190–200.

44. Degli Esposti E, Sturani A, Santoro A, Zuccala A, Chiarini C, Zucchelli P. Effect of bromocriptine treatment on prolactin, noradrenaline and blood pressure in hypertensive haemodialysis patients. Clin Sci (Lond). 1985;69:51–6.

45. Schlaich MP, Socratous F, Hennebry S, Eikelis N, Lambert EA, Straznicky N, Esler MD, Lambert GW. Sympathetic activation in chronic renal failure. J Am Soc Nephrol. 2009;20:933–9.

46. Schlaich MP, Bart B, Hering D, Walton A, Marusic P, Mahfoud F, Bohm M, Lambert EA, Krum H, Sobotka PA, Schmieder RE, Ika-Sari C, Eikelis N, Straznicky N, Lambert GW, Esler MD. Feasibility of catheter-based renal nerve ablation and effects on sympathetic nerve activity and blood pressure in patients with end-stage renal disease. Int J Cardiol. 2013;168(3):2214–20.

47. Floras JS. Clinical aspects of sympathetic activation and parasympathetic withdrawal in heart failure. J Am Coll Cardiol. 1993;22:72A–84.

48. Petersson M, Friberg P, Eisenhofer G, Lambert G, Rundqvist B. Long-term outcome in relation to renal sympathetic activity in patients with chronic heart failure. Eur Heart J. 2005;26:906–13.

49. Sobotka PA, Krum H, Bohm M, Francis DP, Schlaich MP. The role of renal denervation in the treatment of heart failure. Curr Cardiol Rep. 2012;14:285–92.

50. Villarreal D, Freeman RH, Johnson RA, Simmons JC. Effects of renal denervation on postprandial sodium excretion in experimental heart failure. Am J Physiol. 1994;266:R1599–604.

51. Davies JE, Manisty CH, Petraco R, Barron AJ, Unsworth B, Mayet J, Hamady M, Hughes AD, Sever PS, Sobotka PA, Francis DP. First-in-man safety evaluation of renal denervation for chronic systolic heart failure: primary outcome from REACH-pilot study. Int J Cardiol. 2013;162:189–92.

52. Jamerson KA, Julius S, Gudbrandsson T, Andersson O, Brant DO. Reflex sympathetic activation induces acute insulin resistance in the human forearm. Hypertension. 1993;21:618–23.

53. Laakso M, Edelman SV, Brechtel G, Baron AD. Decreased effect of insulin to stimulate skeletal muscle blood flow in obese man. A novel mechanism for insulin resistance. J Clin Invest. 1990;85:1844–52.

54. Mahfoud F, Schlaich M, Kindermann I, Ukena C, Cremers B, Brandt MC, Hoppe UC, Vonend O, Rump LC, Sobotka PA, Krum H, Esler M, Bohm M. Effect of renal sympathetic denervation on glucose metabolism in patients with resistant hypertension: a pilot study. Circulation. 2011;123:1940–6.

55. Logan AG, Perlikowski SM, Mente A, Tisler A, Tkacova R, Niroumand M, Leung RS, Bradley TD. High prevalence of unrecognized sleep apnoea in drug-resistant hypertension. J Hypertens. 2001;19:2271–7.

56. Baguet JP, Barone-Rochette G, Pepin JL. Hypertension and obstructive sleep apnoea syndrome: current perspectives. J Hum Hypertens. 2009;23:431–43.

57. Ruttanaumpawan P, Nopmaneejumruslers C, Logan AG, Lazarescu A, Qian I, Bradley TD. Association between refractory hypertension and obstructive sleep apnea. J Hypertens. 2009;27:1439–45.

58. Mancia G, De Backer G, Dominiczak A, Cifkova R, Fagard R, Germano G, Grassi G, Heagerty AM, Kjeldsen SE, Laurent S, Narkiewicz K, Ruilope L, Rynkiewicz A, Schmieder RE, Boudier HA, Zanchetti A, Vahanian A, Camm J, De Caterina R, Dean V, Dickstein K, Filippatos G, Funck-Brentano C, Hellemans I, Kristensen SD, McGregor K, Sechtem U, Silber S, Tendera M, Widimsky P, Zamorano JL, Erdine S, Kiowski W, Agabiti-Rosei E, Ambrosioni E, Lindholm LH, Viigimaa M, Adamopoulos S, Bertomeu V, Clement D, Farsang C, Gaita D, Lip G, Mallion JM, Manolis AJ, Nilsson PM, O'Brien E, Ponikowski P, Redon J, Ruschitzka F, Tamargo J, van Zwieten P, Waeber B, Williams B.

2007 Guidelines for the management of arterial hypertension: the task force for the management of arterial hypertension of the european society of hypertension (ESH) and of the european society of ardiology (ESC). J Hypertens. 2007;25:1105–87.

59. Narkiewicz K, Somers VK. Sympathetic nerve activity in obstructive sleep apnoea. Acta Physiol Scand. 2003;177:385–90.

60. Witkowski A, Prejbisz A, Florczak E, Kadziela J, Sliwinski P, Bielen P, Michalowska I, Kabat M, Warchol E, Januszewicz M, Narkiewicz K, Somers VK, Sobotka PA, Januszewicz A. Effects of renal sympathetic denervation on blood pressure, sleep apnea course, and glycemic control in patients with resistant hypertension and sleep apnea. Hypertension. 2011;58:559–65.

61. Friedman O, Bradley TD, Chan CT, Parkes R, Logan AG. Relationship between overnight rostral fluid shift and obstructive sleep apnea in drug-resistant hypertension. Hypertension. 2010;56:1077–82.

62. Pang CC. Autonomic control of the venous system in health and disease: effects of drugs. Pharmacol Ther. 2001;90:179–230.

63. Chen PS, Tan AY. Autonomic nerve activity and atrial fibrillation. Heart Rhythm. 2007;4:S61–4.

64. Sharifov OF, Fedorov VV, Beloshapko GG, Glukhov AV, Yushmanova AV, Rosenshtraukh LV. Roles of adrenergic and cholinergic stimulation in spontaneous atrial fibrillation in dogs. J Am Coll Cardiol. 2004;43:483–90.

65. Shen MJ, Choi EK, Tan AY, Han S, Shinohara T, Maruyama M, Chen LS, Shen C, Hwang C, Lin SF, Chen PS. Patterns of baseline autonomic nerve activity and the development of pacing-induced sustained atrial fibrillation. Heart Rhythm. 2011;8:583–9.

66. Huang JL, Wen ZC, Lee WL, Chang MS, Chen SA. Changes of autonomic tone before the onset of paroxysmal atrial fibrillation. Int J Cardiol. 1998;66:275–83.

67. Dimmer C, Tavernier R, Gjorgov N, Van Nooten G, Clement DL, Jordaens L. Variations of autonomic tone preceding onset of atrial fibrillation after coronary artery bypass grafting. Am J Cardiol. 1998;82:22–5.

68. Wen ZC, Chen SA, Tai CT, Huang JL, Chang MS. Role of autonomic tone in facilitating spontaneous onset of typical atrial flutter. J Am Coll Cardiol. 1998;31:602–7.

69. Pokushalov E, Romanov A, Corbucci G, Artyomenko S, Baranova V, Turov A, Shirokova N, Karaskov A, Mittal S, Steinberg JS. A randomized comparison of pulmonary vein isolation with versus without concomitant renal artery denervation in patients with refractory symptomatic atrial fibrillation and resistant hypertension. J Am Coll Cardiol. 2012;60:1163–70.

Renal Denervation for Congestive Heart Failure

Claire E. Raphael and Justin E. Davies

Key Points
- Chronic heart failure is associated with global increase in sympathetic activity, a marker of adverse outcome.
- The sympathetic nervous system activates the renin-angiotensin-aldosterone system via the efferent renal nerves
- The afferent renal nerves create positive feedback, further increasing global sympathetic tone
- Pharmacological agents (ACE inhibitors, beta blockers, aldosterone inhibitors) act to decrease the global sympathetic tone and renin-angiotensin-aldosterone pathway but optimal doses are rarely achieved in clinical practice
- Pilot data suggests renal denervation is safe in heart failure and causes only a small decrease in blood pressure in this population
- Randomised controlled trials of renal denervation in heart failure are underway and due to report in 2014/2015

The Global Burden of Heart Failure

Heart failure is an increasing epidemic within the developed world. Twenty percent of people over 40 will develop heart failure over their lifetime and over 650,000 cases are diagnosed annually. The total cost of heart failure care in the

USA is in excess of $30 billion a year [1]. Despite improvements in treatment, survival rates remain poor with a 50 % mortality at 5 years after diagnosis and a high burden of morbidity [2]. Heart failure is the most common cause for hospital admission in the elderly and admissions are often prolonged [3]. Patients are often significantly limited by shortness of breath and quality of life is impaired [4]. While pharmacological treatments have improved outcomes, there is still a significant unmet need for treatments that improve survival and symptoms.

Heart Failure with Preserved Ejection Fraction

Heart failure with preserved ejection fraction (HF-PEF) constitutes up to half of heart failure with an increasing prevalence in the community [5]. Patients with HF-PEF have signs and symptoms consistent with heart failure but with an ejection fraction within normal limits or only mildly reduced. The diagnosis of HF-PEF is challenging, with co-morbidities contributing to shortness of breath, such as lung disease and obesity, more prevalent in HF-PEF [6]. Compared to the systolic heart failure population, patients with HF-PEF are more likely to be female, tend to be older and the underlying aetiology is more commonly hypertension with a lower rate of ischaemic heart disease. The precise definition of HF-PEF is variable between trials, usually including patients with an ejection fraction of 45 % and above in patients with signs and symptoms consistent with heart failure.

Heart Failure and the Sympathetic Nervous System

The presence of increased sympathetic activity has been well demonstrated in both systolic heart failure [7, 8] and heart failure with preserved [9] or mildly reduced ejection fraction [10, 11]. These patients have on-going maladaptive

C.E. Raphael, MA, BSc, MRCP (✉)
Department of Cardiology, Royal Brompton and Harefield NHS Foundation Trust, Sydney Street, London SE9 5AP, UK
e-mail: Claire.raphael@gmail.com

J.E. Davies, MBBS, BSc, MRCP, PhD
Department of Cardiology, Hammersmith Hospital,
Imperial College London, Du Cane Road,
3rd Floor ICTEM Building, London, UK
e-mail: justin.davies@imperial.ac.uk

R.R. Heuser et al. (eds.), *Renal Denervation: A New Approach to Treatment of Resistant Hypertension*,
DOI 10.1007/978-1-4471-5223-1_20, © Springer-Verlag London 2015

hyper-stimulation of the neurohormonal and sympathetic nervous systems [12–14] as a result of reduced cardiac output. The sympathetic nervous system is activated earlier than the renin-angiotensinogen-aldosterone system, with increased sympathetic stimulation particularly to the heart and kidneys [15]. This increased sympathetic tone is accompanied by decreased parasympathetic tone [16]. Initially, these systems act to compensate for the underlying myocardial impairment, allowing maintenance of cardiac homeostasis. This is beneficial in situations of acute myocardial impairment, for example with an acute infarction, however in chronic disease, the long term neurohormonal and sympathetic activation have deleterious effects.

Sympathetic over-activity causes an increase in heart rate, cardiac contractility and peripheral vasoconstriction. Activation of the sympathetic nervous system occurs via multiple mechanisms. The central and peripheral chemoreceptors detect changes in oxygen and carbon dioxide concentration and act to stimulate the SNS if hypoxia or hypercapnia are detected. Inhibition occurs via baroreceptors located in the carotid sinuses and aortic arch. A decrease in blood pressure detected by the baroreceptors causes a reflex increase in heart rate, allowing maintenance of cardiac output. Finally, sympathetic activity stimulates the release of renin and increased activity of the renin-angiotensin-aldosterone system. Angiotensin II produced as a result of this causes positive feedback with further stimulation of the sympathetic nervous system (Fig. 20.1) [15].

In heart failure, sympathetic stimulation leads to activation of the renin-angiotensin-aldosterone system with increased sodium re-absorption from the distal and proximal tubules within the nephrons. Renin release and resultant angiotensin II generation results in activation of the sodium/hydrogen exchange transporters and sodium bicarbonate co-transporters, leading to re-absorption of sodium in the proximal tubules [17]. Water re-absorption is further increased through vasoconstriction of the efferent renal arteriole, increasing the hydrostatic gradient across the renal tubules [18]. Aldosterone acts on the distal tubule and collecting duct, activating the sodium-potassium pumps and further increasing sodium retention within the body's circulation. This leads to an increase in circulating volume, with water re-absorbed with the sodium and potentially resulting in pulmonary and peripheral oedema.

Separately, sympathetic signalling to the heart itself is increased [19]. Release of norepinephrine from the right stellate ganglion results in an increased heart rate through actions on the sinus and atrioventricular nodes [12]. Increased sympathetic stimulation of the heart increases oxygen consumption by the myocardium and increases propensity to arrhythmia. The sympathetic nervous system also alters the chemoreceptor sensitivity to carbon dioxide, leading to an

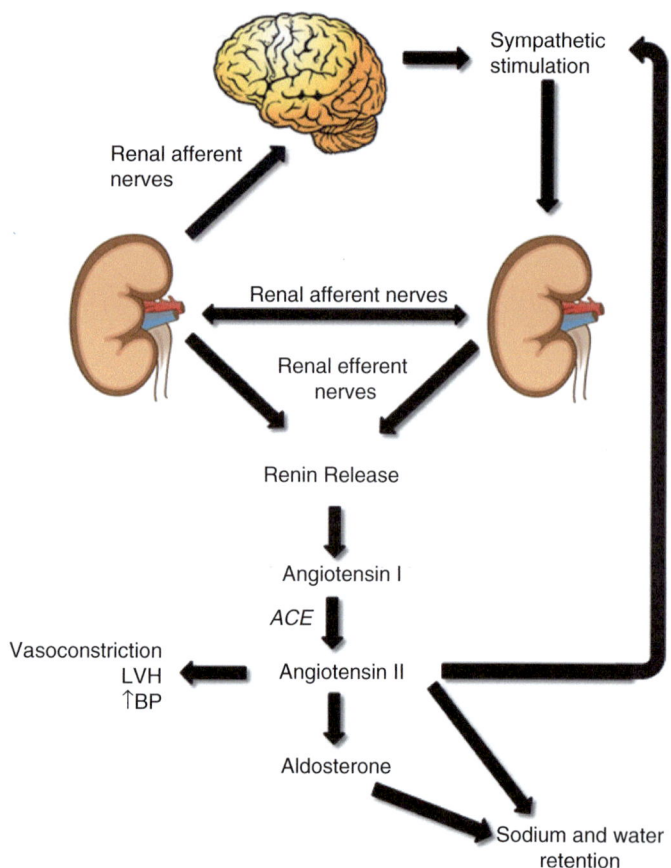

Fig. 20.1 Interaction of the sympathetic nervous system, kidney and activation of the renin-angiotensin-aldosterone pathway

increased perception of shortness of breath and sleep disturbances such as periodic breathing. The increased sympathetic tone results in peripheral vasoconstriction, with a resultant increase in afterload which, over time, results in further myocardial impairment.

It is therefore not surprising that the level of sympathetic over-activity is predictive of adverse prognosis in heart failure. Plasma norepinephrine, the principal neurotransmitter in the sympathetic nervous system, was first shown to predict outcome in 1984 [20]. High renal norepinephrine levels measured invasively were later shown to be predictive of adverse outcome in a population of chronic heart failure patients followed for 6 years with a combined endpoint of all-cause mortality and heart transplantation [21]. Norepinephrine can be measured either globally (plasma norepinephrine) or regionally e.g. renal norepinephrine spillover, via invasive catheterisation. Renal norepinephrine in this study was independently predictive of outcome when entered into a model with total body norepinephrine spillover, glomerular filtration rate and ejection fraction. Patients with high sympathetic over-activity are also more symptomatic with a poorer functional capacity [22, 23] and an increased predisposition to arrhythmia [24]. Non invasive markers of high sympathetic tone, including heart rate variability [25, 26] have also been shown to predict adverse outcome in heart failure.

Tablets that target the sympathetic nervous system and the renin-angiotensin-aldosterone system have a strong prognostic benefit in systolic heart failure. There is less evidence for benefit in patients with heart failure and preserved ejection fraction, although trial data which included patients with mildly impaired systolic function did show some prognostic benefit.

Pharmacological Trials in Systolic Heart Failure

Inhibitors of the Renin-Angiotensin-Aldosterone Pathway

Inhibitors of the angiotensin converting enzyme (ACE) reduce the production of angiotensin II and aldosterone levels with a corresponding increase in renin. In systolic heart failure, treatment with ACE inhibitors leads to an improvement in levels of circulating plasma norepinephrine [27] thought to occur as a result of improved haemodynamics and the reduced angiotensin II leading to decreased stimulation of the sympathetic nervous system. Reduction in angiotensin II, a potent vasoconstrictor, causes improvement in the afterload through relaxation of the peripheral vascular system and reduction in venous dilatation decreases pulmonary congestion and the preload. Prognostic benefit of ACE inhibitors in systolic heart failure was shown in the SOLVD [28] and CONSENSUS [29] trials.

Aldosterone antagonists such as spironolactone reduce production of aldosterone, reducing retention of water and sodium. This was shown to have a prognostic benefit in systolic heart failure in the RALES trial, with a 30 % reduction in death compared to the placebo group and a 35 % decrease in hospitalization following commencement of spironolactone [30].

Direct renin inhibitors such as aliskiren have also been shown to reduce B-type natriuetic peptide in patients with chronic heart failure [31], although in a large double blinded randomised controlled trial, addition of aliskiren to standard therapy in a cohort of 1,639 patients with a recent heart failure hospitalisation did not reduce CV death or HF rehospitalization at 6 months or 12 months after discharge [32].

Beta blockers were initially thought to be harmful in systolic heart failure as administration to patients who were acutely fluid overloaded often caused haemodynamic decompensation. However in chronic systolic heart failure, beta blockers decrease total sympathetic activity, leading to improvement in symptoms and reduction in mortality. The β_1 receptors on the myocardium are down-regulated in heart failure as a result of the excess sympathetic tone with loss of the force-frequency relationship and these changes are reversed by beta blocker therapy [33]. Cardiac Insufficiency Bisoprolol Study (CIBIS) was the first trial to demonstrate a prognostic benefit of beta blockage in chronic systolic heart failure [34]. This was confirmed in the CIBIS-II which demonstrated a significant reduction in all cause and sudden death in patients treated with bisoprolol compared with placebo [35]. Beta blockers have also been shown to reduce plasma renin activity in heart failure [36].

Centrally Acting Inhibitors of the Sympathetic Nervous System

Interest in global sympathetic activation led to the investigation of centrally acting inhibitors of the sympathetic nervous system. Small studies in the late 1990s in systolic heart failure demonstrated that administration of clonidine, a centrally acting agent causing a decrease in global sympathetic tone, led to a decrease in cardiac and global norepinephrine spillover [37]. This promising finding led to the multicentre randomised double blinded Moxonidine in Congestive Heart Failure (MOXCON) trial, which randomised patients with NYHA class II–IV heart failure and reduced ejection fraction to a sustained release preparation of monoxidine or placebo. Measurement of plasma norepinephrine demonstrated a significant decrease in total sympathetic nervous activity, with a 19 % decrease in the monoxidine group compared to a small increase (7 %) in the placebo group.

However, the trial was terminated prematurely due to an excess of deaths in the monoxidine group after 1,934 patients were entered. As well as an excess in all cause mortality, there were increased rates of hospitalisation for heart failure and acute myocardial infarction in the monoxidine group [38]. Questions were raised regarding the up-titration regimen of the trial and whether the doses used were too high, however in view of the excess of mortality in the trial, no further investigation of centrally acting sympathetic antagonists are currently planned.

Pharmacological Trials in Heart Failure with Preserved Ejection Fraction

The evidence base for pharmacological treatment in patients with heart failure and preserved ejection fraction is much smaller. Trials in HF-PEF are challenging as accurate identification of patients is less clear-cut than for systolic heart failure, due to clustering of disease processes leading to shortness of breath [39]. Most trials included patients with mild systolic left ventricular impairment (EF of 45 % or greater) on the basis that diastolic impairment is likely to be accompanied by systolic heart failure.

The PEP-CHF trial [40] enrolled patients aged 70 or greater with a clinical diagnosis of heart failure due to LV diastolic dysfunction, based on signs and symptoms of heart failure, left atrial enlargement, left ventricular hypertrophy and echocardiographic markers of impaired LV filling based on E/A ratio and isovolaemic relaxation time. Patients with atrial fibrillation were considered to have LV impaired filling. This trial showed a significant reduction in hospitalization for heart failure at 1 year with improvement in functional class and 6-min walk distance, although the trial was hampered by a high number of patients withdrawing from the trial to take open-label ACE-inhibitors, reducing its power.

I-PRESERVE [41] studied a population of 4,128 patients with a diagnosis of HF-PEF, defined as an ejection fraction of 45 % or greater with a hospitalisation in the previous 6 months and NYHA class II-IV. Patients had a mean blood pressure of $137\pm15/79\pm9$. Patients were randomised to 300 mg irbesartan or placebo. During a mean follow-up of 50 months, the primary outcome occurred in 742 patients in the irbesartan group and 763 in the placebo group with no difference in outcome between the two groups.

The CHARM-Preserved trial [42] randomised 3,023 patients with LVEF greater than 40 % and New York Heart Association functional class II-IV to candesartan (titrated up to a target of 32 mg) or placebo. There was no difference in rates of cardiovascular between the groups but fewer patients assigned to candesartan had heart failure admissions compared to the placebo group (230 vs 279, p=0.017).

The SENIORS (Study of Effects of Nebivolol Intervention on Outcomes and Rehospitalization in Seniors With Heart Failure) trial [43], assessed the effect of nebivolol in a cohort of 2,111 patients aged 70 and above. The study cohort was examined to assess cohorts of impaired ejection fraction (<35 %) and "preserved ejection fraction" with an EF of 35 % or above. The primary endpoint of all-cause mortality and cardiovascular hospitalization was reached in a similar proportion of patients in both groups. Both groups showed similar benefit from nebivolol treatment.

The DIG-PEF trial enrolled 988 patients with symptomatic heart failure with an ejection fraction greater than 45 %. Digoxin had no effect on all cause or cause specific mortality or all-cause or cardiovascular hospitalisation [44]. By contrast, in the reduced ejection fraction cohort of the same trial, while digoxin had no effect on mortality, it did lead to a significant decrease in rates of hospitalisation [45].

Pharmacological treatment of heart failure is challenging in both systolic heart failure and HF-PEF. In systolic heart failure, few patients attain maximal doses of beta blockers, ACE inhibitors or aldosterone antagonists with up-titration often limited by renal impairment, symptomatic hypotension and other side effects. In HF-PEF, the evidence base for treatment is much smaller and may therapies have not been shown to improve survival.

There is therefore an unmet need in both pathologies for novel treatments. Therapy that is able to target the maladaptive signal processes at an early stage, reducing chronic sympathetic stimulation would theoretically be of benefit.

The Role of the Kidney in Pathogenesis of Heart Failure

The kidney plays a key role in heart failure pathophysiology, both responding to increased sympathetic tone, via the efferent signalling pathways and also in stimulation of increased sympathetic tone, via the afferent signalling pathways. The reduced cardiac output of heart failure increases both renal efferent and afferent nerve discharge. The renal sympathetic supply innervates the renal arteries and veins, the juxtaglomerular apparatus and the renal tubules.

Discharge of norepinephrine from the renal efferent nerves activates the renin-angiotensin system, reducing renal blood flow and leading to increased sodium reabsorption from the proximal tubules and water retention. There is an increase in renal vascular resistance resulting from the relatively greater constriction of the afferent compared to the efferent renal arterioles to the glomeruli, resulting in a decreased glomerular filtration rate.

Meanwhile, increased afferent nerve discharge enhances central sympathetic drive increasing heart rate, arterial tone, and myocardial oxygen consumption. These afferent fibres transmit sensory information from the kidney to the central nervous system [46, 47], largely the brain stem and hypothalamus. The afferent renal sensory nerves are stimulated by hypoxia, renal ischaemia and oxidative stress. Increased afferent sympathetic signalling is likely to lead to a reflex increase in renal sympathetic tone, known as the reno-renal reflex [15].

Cardio-Renal Syndrome

Most patients hospitalised for acute decompensated heart failure have renal impairment [48]. Cardiorenal syndrome describes the complex interaction of the heart and the kidney (Fig. 20.2). The failing heart can cause a previously normally functioning kidney to behave as though it were intrinsically diseased and vice versa. For the failing heart, renal impairment and dysfunction may occur as a result of decreased renal perfusion, but there are a number of neurohormonal, immune and cytokine mediated mechanisms that link the two organs. Treatment of the underlying heart failure in the presence of significant renal impairment is further complicated by the adverse effect of ACE inhibitors on

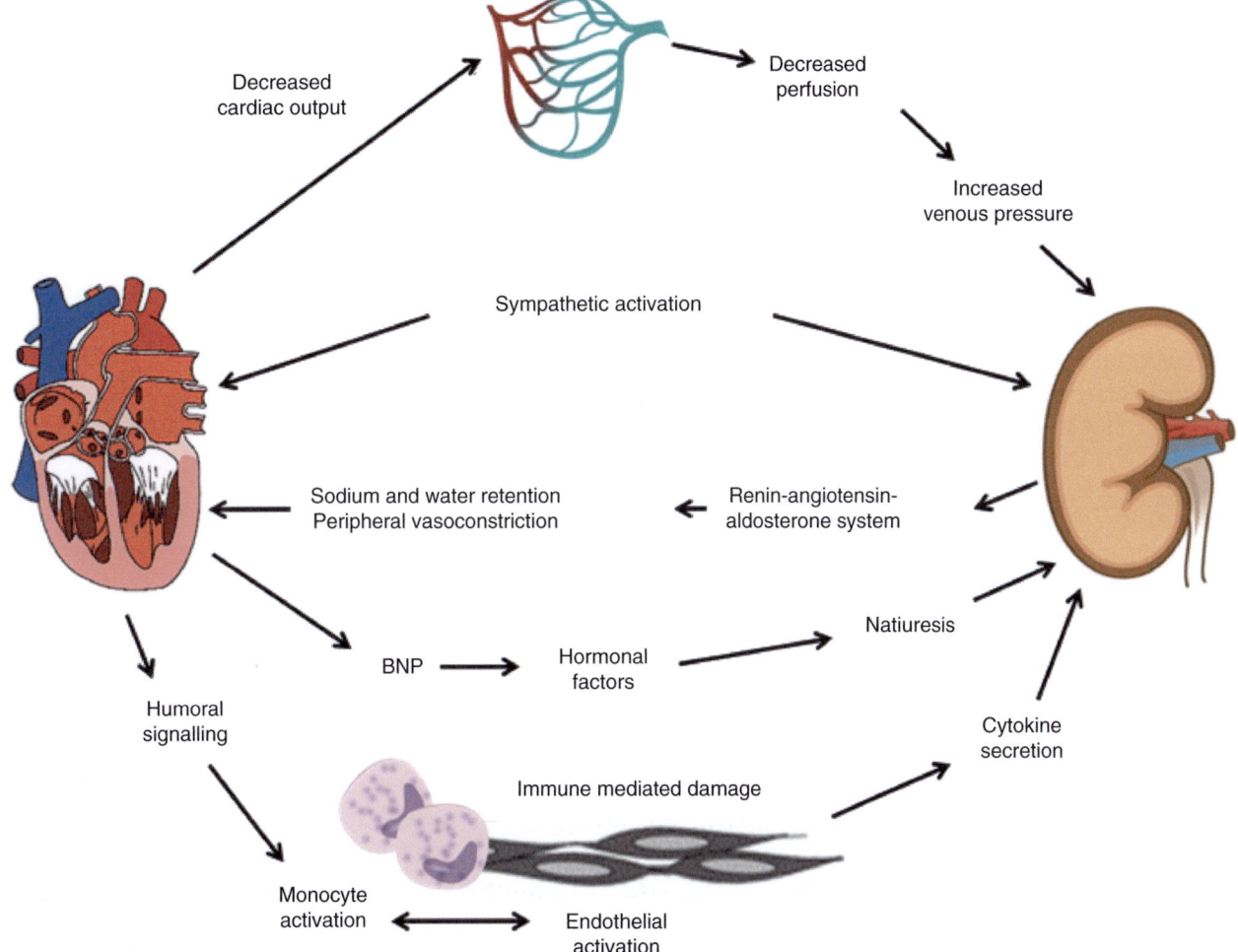

Fig. 20.2 Complex interaction of the heart and the kidney. The interplay between the two describes the cardiorenal syndrome (Adapted from Ronco et al. [49])

renal function, in particular requiring caution to avoid hyperkalaemia. While sympathetic activity has a deleterious effect on both organs, this is only a small part of the interaction [49].

Chemoreceptors: A Further Source of Increased Sympathetic Tone

Sympathetic over-activity in heart failure is also mediated by the baro- and chemo-receptors. The arterial baroreceptor reflexes, which inhibit the sympathetic nervous system, are suppressed, whereas the chemoreceptor reflexes, which increase sympathetic activity, are augmented [12, 50]. As well as modulating overall sympathetic activity, the chemoreceptors are likely to also impact on patient perception of symptoms. Increased chemoreceptor sensitivity to carbon dioxide leads to an increased perception of shortness of breath and sleep disturbances such as periodic breathing

[51, 52]. Enhanced chemosensitivity to hypercapnia is an adverse prognostic marker in chronic systolic heart failure and is known to be associated with greater neurohormonal activation [53]. There is therefore a potential role for renal denervation not only in modulation of sympathetic tone but also in resultant reduction in chemoreceptor sensitivity, leading to improvement in shortness of breath.

Evidence for Renal Denervation as a Potential Treatment for Heart Failure

Animal Models

Small animal models of denervation use surgical ligation of the renal nerves rather than radiofrequency energy. Selective division of the dorsal spinal nerve roots prevented hypertension in a rat model of renal failure, demonstrating that afferent nerve fibres were implicated in development of hypertension in chronic renal failure [54]. Conversely, direct renal injury using phenol resulted in an acute increase in renal sympathetic efferent and afferent nerve discharge and an increase in norepinephrine secretion, resulting in hypertension [55] and demonstrating the effect of renal efferent signalling in global increase in sympathetic tone with a corresponding increase in blood pressure.

Rats with heart failure produced by ligation of the left anterior descending artery showed a reduction in sodium retention following surgical renal denervation [56]. Rabbits with pacing-induced heart failure have also allowed assessment of the effects of renal denervation. Those with surgical renal denervation prior to pacing did not exhibit changes in renal vascular resistance or expression of angiotensin II receptors compared to the non-denervated population [57].

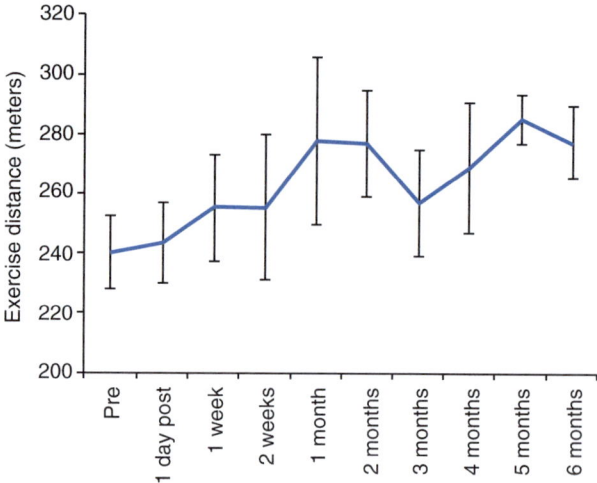

Fig. 20.3 Six minute walk distance increased over the 6 months following renal denervation in the REACH pilot study (Reprinted from Davies et al. [58] with permission from Elsevier)

Data from the Hypertension Trials of Renal Denervation

Radiofrequency ablation of the renal sympathetic nerves has been shown to lead to a decrease in both renal efferent and afferent outflow in hypertensive patients [46]. If the same holds true in heart failure, reduction in efferent outflow will lead to activation of the renin-angiotensin-aldosterone system, while decrease in the afferent signalling will decrease further positive feedback via the hypothalamus, leading to a decrease in total sympathetic activity. Data from the hypertensive population demonstrated a marked decrease in renal norepinephrine spillover following bilateral percutaneous denervation (47 % reduction at 1 month) and a corresponding 50 % decrease in plasma renin. These results suggest a successful reduction in both renal efferent and afferent activity post denervation [47].

Pilot Data in Chronic Heart Failure

REACH-pilot was an open label study which explored the safety of renal denervation in chronic systolic heart failure [58]. Seven patients in NYHA class III or IV on maximal tolerated medical therapy, including a beta-blocker, ACE inhibitor or angiotensin receptor blocker, and spironolactone underwent bilateral renal denervation. Patients were admitted for 5 days for inpatient monitoring to assess for any change in haemodynamics following the procedure.

All seven patients successfully completed the procedure and all felt symptomatically improved. There was a small but significant increase in the 6 min walk distance (by 27 ± 10 m, Fig. 20.3). No patients had symptomatic hypotension as a result of the procedure and blood pressure remained stable

over the 6 month follow up with only a small trend to blood pressure reduction (−7/−0.6 mmHg) immediately post procedure (Fig. 20.4) and a similar, non significant, decrease in heart rate ($\Delta HR -4 \pm 4.6$ beats per minute). No patients were re-admitted for heart failure symptoms or complications as a result of the procedure. Renal function remained stable over the 6 month period following the procedure.

Four patients had their loop diuretic stopped following renal denervation due to a reduction in peripheral odema. There was a need to decrease prognostically important heart failure medications (ACE inhibitors and beta blockers) in four (57 %) of the patients, although two other patients had their beta blocker and ACE inhibitor up-titrated over the 6 months following renal denervation.

The **OLOMOUC study**, presented at the European Society of Cardiology in 2012, compared patients with advanced heart failure (NYHA class III–IV) assigned to either renal denervation or standard medical therapy [59]. The primary endpoint was rehospitalisation at 12 months and change in left ventricular end diastolic dimensions. Of the 26 patients assigned to renal denervation, there was one complication, an arterio-venous fistula in the renal artery, requiring surgical revision. At 12 months, patients assigned to renal denervation showed significant improvement in their ejection fraction (25 ± 12 % rising to 31 ± 14 %, $p < 0.001$) and improvements in the end diastolic dimensions (LVEDD 68 ± 5 mm increased to 60 ± 7 mm, $p < 0.001$). There was no evidence of remodelling in the group undergoing standard therapy. The full data are awaiting publication.

The overriding conclusions coming from REACH-pilot and OLOMOUC trials was that renal denervation could be

Fig. 20.4 Blood pressure over 6 month follow up following renal denervation in chronic heart failure in the REACH-pilot study (Reprinted from Davies et al. [58] with permission from Elsevier)

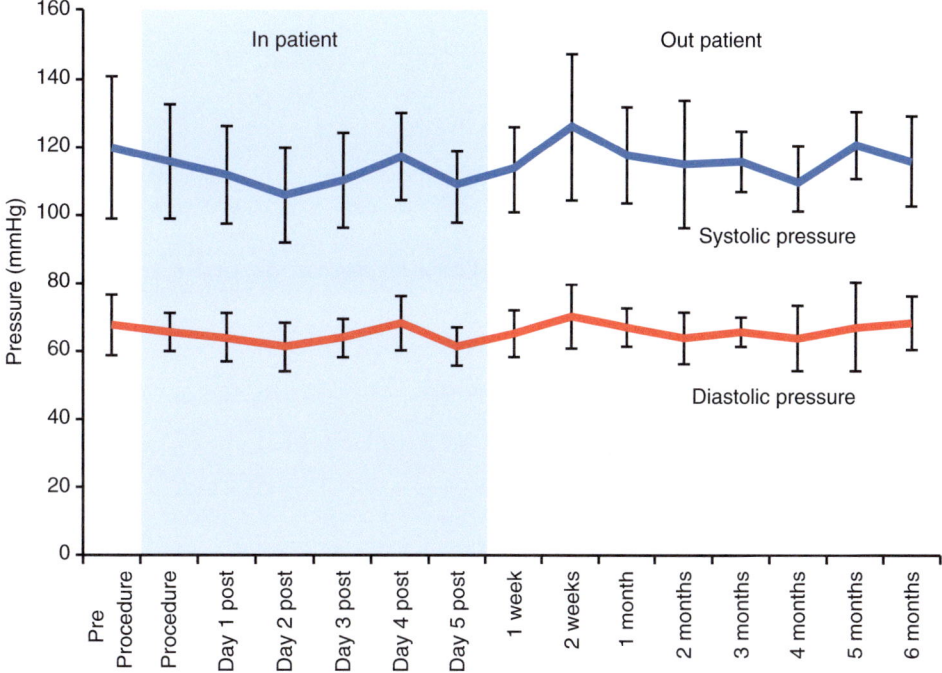

performed safely in patients with systolic heart failure and that theoretical concerns regarding hypotension post procedure were not borne out in practice. Renal function also remained stable in both populations, despite renal impairment at baseline.

While no trials of renal denervation recruiting exclusively heart failure with preserved ejection fraction have yet reported, Brand et al. studied patients with hypertension and left ventricular hypertrophy, demonstrating regression of LVH at 6 months following the procedure [60]. Enrolled patients were hypertensive with an office blood pressure of ≥160 mmHg (≥150 mmHg for type 2 diabetics) or more, despite treatment with at least three antihypertensive drugs including a diuretic. There was a significant reduction in left ventricular mass from 53.9 ± 15.6 g/m^2 at baseline to 44.7 ± 14.9 g/m^2 at 6 months (p<0.001). There was also an improvement in diastolic function with reduction in the mitral E wave deceleration time and improvement in the iso-volaemic relaxation time. Tissue Doppler imaging parameters also improved, with a statistically significant reduction in lateral E/E′ seen at 1 month and with further improvement at 6 months.

In this study, the percentage of patients with normal LV filling pressures, (an E/E′ ratio ≤8) increased from 39 % at baseline to 68 % at 6 months post renal denervation and the percentage of patients with an E/E′ ratio ≥12, indicating elevated filling pressures, declined from 29 % at baseline to 4 % after 6 months. The left atrial size also significantly reduced in the renal denervation group compared to an increase in the control group.

Ongoing Trials of Renal Denervation in Heart Failure

Further trials are in progress. The Symplicity-HF trial will recruit 40 patients with NYHA class II to III systolic heart failure with an ejection fraction less than 40 %, a glomerular filtration rate of 30–75 ml/min/1.73 m^2 and on optimal stable medical therapy [61]. The study is an open label Phase 4 clinical trial of the Symplicity catheter, due to report on the primary endpoint in 2017. The primary end point is safety data as measured by adverse events at 6 month follow up. Secondary measures of change in ventricular function and renal function at 6 months will also be assessed.

The Renal Artery Denervation in Chronic Heart Failure Study (REACH) trial, a double blinded prospective trial of renal denervation (RDN) in chronic systolic heart failure with a sham arm (3:2, treatment : sham), will assess the effect of RDN on symptomatology and exercise capacity [62] in a population of 100 patients with symptomatic systolic heart failure, NYHA class II or higher, with an ejection fraction less than 40 % and on maximal medical therapy. Denervation will also be performed using the Symplicity catheter. The primary endpoint is change in symptomatology at 6 months as assessed using the Kansas City Questionnaire. Secondary endpoints will be change in peak VO2 on cardiopulmonary exercise testing, improvement in 6 min walk test, change in chemoreflex sensitivity and change in NYHA functional classification at 12 months. The trial will report in early 2015.

Trials are also underway in diastolic heart failure. The Denervation of the renal sympathetic nerveS in hearT Failure

Table 20.1 Trials of renal denervation in heart failure

	Population	End point	Design	n	Results
Trials reported					
REACH-Pilot	Systolic heart failure	Safety	Open label	7	No adverse events Improvement in 6MWT
OLOMOUC	Systolic heart failure NYHA III/IV	Rehospitalisation LV dimensions	Renal denervation vs medical therapy	51	Improvement in EF and LV dimensions
Trials in progress					
REACH	Systolic heart failure NYHA class II or greater Ejection fraction <40 % Maximal medical therapy	Change in symptoms	Double blinded	100	Due to report 2015
Symplicity-HF	Systolic heart failure Ejection fraction <40 % GFR 30–75 ml/min/1.73 m^2	Safety	Open label	40	Due to report 2017
DIASTOLE	HF-PEF Hypertension on 2 agents Ejection fraction ≥50 %	Change in E/E$'$	Open label	60	Due to report 2015

With nOrmalLv Ejection Fraction (DIASTOLE) underway in Utrechtis will recruit patients with heart failure and preserved ejection fraction and co-existent hypertension into an open label single group assignment safety and efficacy study. Study patients will have signs or symptoms of heart failure with normal or mildly abnormal systolic function, defined as an ejection fraction of 50 % or greater and evidence of left ventricular diastolic dysfunction, hypertension (defined as BP of 140/90 or greater and treated with two or more antihypertensive agents and be clinically stable prior to recruitment. The primary outcome measure is change in E/E$'$ at 12 months with a secondary safety outcome. The trial will report in December 2014.

The Renal Denervation in Heart Failure With Preserved Ejection Fraction (RDT-PEF) is a randomised open label trial comparing renal denervation to medical therapy in heart failure with preserved ejection fraction. The primary endpoint is a composite of symptoms, change in exercise capacity measured by cardiopulmonary exercise testing, change in B-type natriuretic peptide and measures of left ventricular remodelling, with change in left ventricular mass index and left atrial volume measured by cardiovascular magnetic resonance and diastolic function by echocardiography [63].

Finally, long term safety of renal denervation is still unknown and a large comprehensive safety study is underway at University Hospital, Saarland [64]. This will assess the long term safety and effectiveness of renal denervation in patients with hypertension and other conditions characterised by elevated sympathetic drive, including chronic heart failure, with a target recruitment of 1,000 patients. Different catheter systems will be evaluated, using the Symplicity flex Medronic catheter, EnligHTN St Jude Medical, Paradise Recor and V2 Vessix systems. Secondary

outcomes assessed will include myocardial function and volumes, heart rate, arrhythmia incidence, effect on glucose metabolism, blood pressure and hospitalisation rates (Table 20.1).

Potential Difficulties of Renal Denervation in Heart Failure

While pilot data seems encouraging, there are several considerations within the heart failure population that may limit efficacy of treatment with renal denervation.

Firstly, the most common cause of systolic heart failure is ischaemic heart disease. Although targeting sympathetic over-activity in this population may lead to improvements in fluid retention and peripheral vasoconstriction, the damage to the myocardium itself is currently irreversible. Treatment with renal denervation may not have a significant additive role in patients already on good doses of ACE inhibitors, beta blockers and spironolactone and if the trend to reduction in blood pressure seen in the REACH trial is borne out in larger trial data, this may limit uptitration of these proven prognostically beneficial medications.

Secondly, treatment of patients with heart failure with centrally acting agents to reduce sympathetic activity showed similar promising early data to that of renal denervation, with improvement in symptomatology and haemodynamic parameters. However, when assessed in a large, prospective double blinded randomised controlled trial, monoxidine was actually associated with an excess of mortality and hospitalisation compared to the control group, resulting in early trial termination [38]. While renal denervation is more selective, targeting only sympathetic outflow from the kidneys and not global sympathetic tone, improvements in symptoms in small studies may not be mirrored in prognostic data.

In patients with severe heart failure, the excess sympathetic tone, initially a maladaptive response, may now be required to maintain blood pressure and cardiac output: in patients with advanced heart failure, decrease in this sympathetic tone may result in decompensation. As with studies in hypertension, once safety data is established, larger trials are required to assess the impact of renal denervation on symptomatology and prognostic markers before treatment may be considered in routine clinical management.

Finally, impaired renal function is common in patients with heart failure, particularly in patients who are hospitalised or have more severe disease. The ongoing trials have all excluded patients with severe renal impairment, with an eGFR of <30 ml/min/1.73 m^2 excluded in SYMPLICITY-HF and DIASTOLE, an eGFR of <35 ml/min/1.73 m^2 in REACH and an eGFR of 45 ml/min/1.73 m^2 in RDT-PEF. If renal denervation does prove beneficial in these studies, further trials will be required to establish safety in patients with cardiac and renal impairment, as otherwise many heart failure patients will be ineligible for therapy.

Potential Prognostic Markers for Assessment of Response to Renal Denervation

Non-invasive markers of sympathetic over activity have been shown to predict responders to RDN in a cohort of 50 hypertensive patients who underwent renal denervation [65]. Continuous arterial blood pressure and high resolution electrocardiography recordings were performed prior to and after renal denervation. Assessment of the degree of fluctuation in arterial blood pressure and heart rate allows assessment of baroreflex sensitivity, relating the magnitude of changes in heart rate to changes in blood pressure. Impaired cardiac baroreflexes are linked to sympathetic overactivity both in hypertension [66] and heart failure [67].

Patients with reduced cardiac baroreflex sensitivity were more likely to respond to renal denervation, defined as a reduction of mean systolic blood pressure on ambulatory monitoring of 10 mmHg or more at 6 months after denervation. A further study in 35 patients demonstrated a significant reduction in muscle sympathetic nerve activity following renal denervation [68]. Assessment of these variables prior to the procedure may allow more favourable selection of patients with a high central sympathetic tone.

Other potential non-invasive variables that may predict patients with the most to gain from denervation includes assessment of the chemoreceptor sensitivity, which have been shown to identify heart failure patients with high sympathetic tone and which have been shown to predict outcome in chronic systolic heart failure [50]. The current trials in progress will also assess renal norepinephrine spillover (Symplicity-HF), chemoreceptor reflexes (REACH) and more conventional markers of prognosis in heart failure, including the 6 min walk test, cardiopulmonary exercise testing [69, 70] and parameters of left ventricular remodelling.

Conclusions

Chronic heart failure remains a condition with a high mortality and symptom burden. These patients have maladaptive signalling pathways with excess sympathetic tone predictive of adverse outcome. Pharmacological treatment targeting the sympathetic nervous system and the renin-angiotensin-aldosterone pathway have been shown to have prognostic benefit in systolic heart failure. Heart failure with preserved ejection fraction has also been shown to have a high sympathetic tone, although these medications have limited proven benefit in this population.

Renal sympathetic denervation offers the potential to intervene much earlier in the pathway, reducing efferent and afferent renal sympathetic signalling. Pilot data has shown that renal denervation appears safe in heart failure with no evidence of symptomatic hypotension post procedure and with early data suggesting improvement in symptoms, ejection fraction and left ventricular dimensions. A number of randomised controlled trials are underway in both systolic heart failure and heart failure with preserved ejection fraction and these are due to report in 2014 and 2015. However, if symptomatic benefit is established, larger trials to establish a mortality benefit will be required before this treatment is offered as part of clinical practice.

References

1. Hunt SA, Abraham WT, Chin MH, Feldman AM, Francis GS, Ganiats TG, Jessup M, Konstam MA, Mancini DM, Michl K, Oates JA, Rahko PS, Silver MA, Stevenson LW, Yancy CW, Antman EM, Smith Jr SC, Adams CD, Anderson JL, Faxon DP, Fuster V, Halperin JL, Hiratzka LF, Jacobs AK, Nishimura R, Ornato JP, Page RL, Riegel B, American College of Cardiology; American Heart Association Task Force on Practice Guidelines; American College of Chest Physicians; International Society for Heart and Lung Transplantation; Heart Rhythm Society. ACC/AHA 2005 guideline update for the diagnosis and management of chronic heart failure in the adult: a report of the American College of Cardiology/American Heart Association Task Force on practice guidelines (writing committee to update the 2001 guidelines for the evaluation and management of heart failure): developed in collaboration with the American College of Chest Physicians and the International Society for Heart and Lung Transplantation: endorsed by the Heart Rhythm Society. Circulation. 2005;112:e154–235.

2. Allman KC, Shaw LJ, Hachamovitch R, et al. Myocardial viability testing and impact of revascularization on prognosis in patients with coronary artery disease and left ventricular dysfunction: a metaanalysis. J Am Coll Cardiol. 2002;39:1151–8.

3. Shah AB, Morrissey RP, Baraghoush A, Bharadwaj P, Phan A, Hamilton M, Kobashigawa J, Schwarz ER. Failing the failing heart: a review of palliative care in heart failure. Rev Cardiovasc Med. 2013;14:41–8.

4. Schowalter M, Gelbrich G, Störk S, Langguth JP, Morbach C, Ertl G, Faller H, Angermann CE. Generic and disease-specific health-related quality of life in patients with chronic systolic heart failure: impact of depression. Clin Res Cardiol. 2013;102:269–78.

5. Bhatia RS, Tu JV, Lee DS, et al. Outcome of heart failure with preserved ejection fraction in a population-based study. N Engl J Med. 2006;355:260–9.

6. Owan TE, Hodge DO, Herges RM, Jacobsen SJ, Roger VL, Redfield MM. Trends in prevalence and outcome of heart failure with preserved ejection fraction. N Engl J Med. 2006;355:251–9.

7. Kaye DM, Lambert GW, Lefkovits J, Morris M, Jennings G, Esler MD. Neurochemical evidence of cardiac sympathetic activation and increased central nervous system norepinephrine turnover in severe congestive heart failure. J Am Coll Cardiol. 1994;23:570–8.

8. Eisenhofer G, Friberg P, Rundqvist B, Quyyumi AA, Lambert G, Kaye DM, Kopin IJ, Goldstein DS, Esler MD. Cardiac sympathetic nerve function in congestive heart failure. Circulation. 1996;93:1667–76.

9. Doi T, Nakata T, Hashimoto A, Yuda S, Wakabayashi T, Kouzu H, Kaneko N, Hase M, Tsuchihashi K, Miura T. Synergistic prognostic values of cardiac sympathetic innervation with left ventricular hypertrophy and left atrial size in heart failure patients without reduced left ventricular ejection fraction: a cohort study. BMJ Open. 2012;2(6):e001015. doi:10.1136/bmjopen-2012-001015.

10. Grassi G, Seravalle G, Cattaneo BM, Lanfranchi A, Vailati S, Giannattasio C, Del Bo A, Sala C, Bolla GB, Pozzi M. Sympathetic activation and loss of reflex sympathetic control in mild congestive heart failure. Circulation. 1995;92:3206–11.

11. Rundqvist B, Elam M, Bergmann-Sverrisdottir Y, Eisenhofer G, Friberg P. Increased cardiac adrenergic drive precedes generalized sympathetic activation in human heart failure. Circulation. 1997;95:169–75.

12. Triposkiadis F, Karayannis G, Giamouzis G, Skoularigis J, Louridas G, Butler J. The sympathetic nervous system in heart failure physiology, pathophysiology, and clinical implications. J Am Coll Cardiol. 2009;54:1747–62.

13. Packer M. The neurohormonal hypothesis: a theory to explain the mechanism of disease progression in heart failure. J Am Coll Cardiol. 1992;20:248–54.

14. Schrier RW, Abraham WT. Hormones and hemodynamics in heart failure. N Engl J Med. 1999;341:577–85.

15. Sobotka PA, Krum H, Böhm M, Francis DP, Schlaich MP. The role of renal denervation in the treatment of heart failure. Curr Cardiol Rep. 2012;14:285–92.

16. Osterziel KJ, Hänlein D, Willenbrock R, Eichhorn C, Luft F, Dietz R. Baroreflex sensitivity and cardiovascular mortality in patients with mild to moderate heart failure. Br Heart J. 1995;73:517–22.

17. Jessup M, Costanzo MR. The cardiorenal syndrome: do we need a change of strategy or a change of tactics? J Am Coll Cardiol. 2009;53:597–9.

18. Schrier RW. Body fluid volume regulation in health and disease: a unifying hypothesis. Ann Intern Med. 1990;113:155–9.

19. Hasking GJ, Esler MD, Jennings GL, Burton D, Johns JA, Korner PI. Norepinephrine spillover to plasma in patients with congestive heart failure: evidence of increased overall and cardiorenal sympathetic nervous activity. Circulation. 1986;73:615–21.

20. Cohn JN, Levine TB, Olivari MT, Garberg V, Lura D, Francis GS, Simon AB, Rector T. Plasma norepinephrine as a guide to prognosis in patients with chronic congestive heart failure. N Engl J Med. 1984;311:819–23.

21. Petersson M, Friberg P, Eisenhofer G, Lambert G, Rundqvist B. Long-term outcome in relation to renal sympathetic activity in patients with chronic heart failure. Eur Heart J. 2005;26:906–13.

22. Notarius CF, Ando S, Rongen GA, Senn B, Floras JS. Resting muscle sympathetic nerve activity and peak oxygen uptake in heart failure and normal subjects. Eur Heart J. 1999;20:880–7.

23. Kraemer MD, Kubo SH, Rector TS, Brunsvold N, Bank AJ. Pulmonary and peripheral vascular factors are important determinants of peak oxygen uptake in patients with heart failure. J Am Coll Cardiol. 1993;21:641–8.

24. Tomaselli GF, Zipes DP. What causes sudden death in heart failure? Circ Res. 2004;95:754–63.

25. Mortara A, La Rovere MT, Signorini MG, Pantaleo P, Pinna G, Martinelli L, Ceconi C, Cerutti S, Tavazzi L. Can power spectral analysis of heart rate variability identify a high risk subgroup of congestive heart failure patients with excessive sympathetic activation? A pilot study before and after heart transplantation. Br Heart J. 1994;71:422–30.

26. Woo MA, Stevenson WG, Moser DK, Middlekauff HR. Complex heart rate variability and serum norepinephrine levels in patients with advanced heart failure. J Am CollCardio. 1994;23:565–9.

27. Benedict CR, Francis GS, Shelton B, Johnstone DE, Kubo SH, Kirlin P, Nicklas J, Liang CS, Konstam MA, Greenberg B. Effect of long-term enalapril therapy on neurohormones in patients with left ventricular dysfunction. SOLVD Investigators. Am J Cardiol. 1995;75:1151–7.

28. SOLVD The Investigators. Effect of enalapril on survival in patients with reduced left ventricular ejection fractions and congestive heart failure. N Engl J Med. 1991;325:293–302.

29. The CONSENSUS Trial Study Group. Effects of enalapril on mortality in severe congestive heart failure: results of the Cooperative North Scandinavian Enalapril Survival Study (CONSENSUS). N Engl J Med. 1987;316:1429–35.

30. Pitt B, Zannad F, Remme WJ, Cody R, Castaigne A, Perez A, Palensky J, Wittes J. The effect of spironolactone on morbidity and mortality in patients with severe heart failure. Randomized aldactone evaluation study investigators. N Engl J Med. 1999;341:709–17.

31. McMurray JJ, Pitt B, Latini R, Maggioni AP, Solomon SD, Keefe DL, Ford J, Verma A, Lewsey J, Aliskiren Observation of Heart Failure Treatment (ALOFT) Investigators. Effects of the oral direct renin inhibitor aliskiren in patients with symptomatic heart failure. Circ Heart Fail. 2008;1:17–24.

32. Gheorghiade M, Böhm M, Greene SJ, Fonarow GC, Lewis EF, Zannad F, Solomon SD, Baschiera F, Botha J, Hua TA, Gimpelewicz CR, Jaumont X, Lesogor A, Maggioni AP, ASTRONAUT Investigators and Coordinators. Effect of aliskiren on postdischarge mortality and heart failure readmissions among patients hospitalized for heart failure: the ASTRONAUT randomized trial. JAMA. 2013;309:1125–35.

33. Just H. Pathophysiological targets for beta-blocker therapy in congestive heart failure. Eur Heart J. 1996;17(Suppl B):2–7.

34. CIBIS Investigators and Committees. A randomized trial of beta-blockade in heart failure. The Cardiac Insufficiency Bisoprolol Study (CIBIS). Circulation. 1994;90:1765–73.

35. CIBIS-II Investigators and Committees. The Cardiac Insufficiency Bisoprolol Study II (CIBIS-II): a randomised trial. Lancet. 1999;353:9–13.

36. Fung JW, Yu CM, Yip G, Chan S, Yandle TG, Richards AM, Nicholls MG, Sanderson JE. Effect of beta blockade (carvedilol or metoprolol) on activation of the renin-angiotensin-aldosterone system and natriuretic peptides in chronic heart failure. Am J Cardiol. 2003;92:406–10.

37. Azevedo ER, Newton GE, Parker JD. Cardiac and systemic sympathetic activity in response to clonidine in human heart failure. J Am Coll Cardiol. 1999;33:186–91.

38. Cohn JN, Pfeffer MA, Rouleau J, Sharpe N, Swedberg K, Straub M, Wiltse C, Wright TJ, MOXCON Investigators. Adverse mortality

effect of central sympathetic inhibition with sustained-release moxonidine in patients with heart failure (MOXCON). Eur J Heart Fail. 2003;5:659–67.

39. Pérez-Calvo JI, Montero-Pérez-Barquero M, Formiga F. Diagnosis of heart failure with preserved ejection fraction: still a challenge. J Am Coll Cardiol. 2013;61:1748–9.

40. Cleland JG, Tendera M, Adamus J, Freemantle N, Polonski L, Taylor J, PEP-CHF Investigators. The perindopril in elderly people with chronic heart failure (PEP-CHF) study. Eur Heart J. 2006;27:2338–45.

41. Massie BM, Carson PE, McMurray JJ, Komajda M, McKelvie R, Zile MR, Anderson S, Donovan M, Iverson E, Staiger C, Ptaszynska A, I-PRESERVE Investigators. Irbesartan in patients with heart failure and preserved ejection fraction. N Engl J Med. 2008;359:2456–67.

42. Yusuf S, Pfeffer MA, Swedberg K, Granger CB, Held P, McMurray JJ, Michelson EL, Olofsson B, Ostergren J, CHARM Investigators and Committees. Effects of candesartan in patients with chronic heart failure and preserved left-ventricular ejection fraction: the CHARM-Preserved Trial. Lancet. 2003;362:777–81.

43. van Veldhuisen DJ, Cohen-Solal A, Böhm M, Anker SD, Babalis D, Roughton M, Coats AJ, Poole-Wilson PA, Flather MD, SENIORS Investigators. Beta-blockade with nebivolol in elderly heart failure patients with impaired and preserved left ventricular ejection fraction: data from seniors (study of effects of nebivolol intervention on outcomes and rehospitalization in seniors with heart failure). J Am Coll Cardiol. 2009;53:2150–8.

44. Ahmed A, Rich MW, Fleg JL, Zile MR, Young JB, Kitzman DW, Love TE, Aronow WS, Adams Jr KF, Gheorghiade M. Effects of digoxin on morbidity and mortality in diastolic heart failure: the ancillary digitalis investigation group trial. Circulation. 2006;114:397–403.

45. Digitalis Investigation Group. The effect of digoxin on mortality and morbidity in patients with heart failure. N Engl J Med. 1997;336:525–33.

46. Schlaich MP, Lambert E, Kaye DM, Krozowski Z, Campbell DJ, Lambert G, Hastings J, Aggarwal A, Esler MD. Sympathetic augmentation in hypertension: role of nerve firing norepinephrine reuptake, and angiotensin neuromodulation. Hypertens. 2004;43:169–75.

47. Schlaich MP, Sobotka PA, Krum H, Lambert E, Esler MD. Renal sympathetic-nerve ablation for uncontrolled hypertension. N Engl J Med. 2009;361:932–4.

48. Heywood JT, Fonarow GC, Costanzo MR, Mathur VS, Wigneswaran JR, Wynne J, ADHERE Scientific Advisory Committee and Investigators. High prevalence of renal dysfunction and its impact on outcome in 118,465 patients hospitalized with acute decompensated heart failure: a report from the ADHERE database. J Card Fail. 2007;13:422–30.

49. Ronco C, Haapio M, House AA, Anavekar N, Bellomo R. Cardiorenal syndrome. J Am Coll Cardiol. 2008;52:1527–39.

50. Ponikowski P, Chua TP, Anker SD, Francis DP, Doehner W, Banasiak W, Poole-Wilson PA, et al. Peripheralchemoreceptor hypersensitivity: an ominous sign in patients with chronic heart failure. Circulation. 2001;104:544–9.

51. Wensel R, Francis DP, Georgiadou P, Scott A, Genth-Zotz S, Anker SD, Coats AJ, Piepoli MF. Exercise hyperventilation in chronic heart failure is not caused by systemic lactic acidosis. Eur J Heart Fail. 2005;7:1105–11.

52. Wensel R, Georgiadou P, Francis DP, Bayne S, Scott AC, Genth-Zotz S, Anker SD, Coats AJ, Piepoli MF. Differential contribution of dead space ventilation and low arterial pCO2 to exercise hyperpnea in patients with chronic heart failure secondary to ischemic or idiopathic dilated cardiomyopathy. Am J Cardiol. 2004;93:318–23.

53. Giannoni A, Emdin M, Bramanti F, Iudice G, Francis DP, Barsotti A, Piepoli M, Passino C. Combined increased chemosensi-

tivity to hypoxia and hypercapnia as a prognosticator in heart failure. J Am Coll Cardiol. 2009;53:1975–80.

54. Campese VM. Neurogenic factors and hypertension in chronic renal failure. J Nephrol. 1997;10:184.

55. Ye S, Zhong H, Yanamadala V, Campese VM. Renal injury caused by intrarenal injection of phenol increases afferent and efferent renal sympathetic nerve activity. Am J Hypertens. 2002;15:717–24.

56. DiBona GF, Sawin LL. Role of renal nerves in sodium retention of cirrhosis and congestive heart failure. Am J Physiol. 1991;260:R298–305.

57. Clayton SC, Haack KK, Zucker IH. Renal denervation modulates angiotensin receptor expression in the renal cortex of rabbits with chronic heart failure. Am J Physiol Renal Physiol. 2011;300:F31–9.

58. Davies JE, Manisty CH, Petraco R, Barron AJ, Unsworth B, Mayet J, Hamady M, et al. First-in-man safety evaluation of renal denervation for chronic systolic heart failure: primary outcome from REACH-Pilot study. Int J Cardiol. 2013;162:189–92.

59. Taborsky M, Lazarova ML, Vaclavik J. The effect of renal denervation in patients with advanced heart failure. Eur Heart J. 2012;33:A517.

60. Brandt MC, Mahfoud F, Reda S, Schirmer SH, Erdmann E, Böhm M, Hoppe UC. Renal sympathetic denervation reduces left ventricular hypertrophy and improves cardiac function in patients with resistant hypertension. J Am Coll Cardiol. 2012;59:901–9.

61. Medtronic Vascular. Renal denervation in patients with chronic heart failure & renal impairment clinical trial (SymplicityHF). In: Clinical Trials.gov [Internet]. Bethesda: National Library of Medicine (US); 2000, [20140903]. Available from: URL of the record NLM Identifier: NCT01392196.

62. Imperial College London. Renal Artery Denervation in Chronic Heart Failure study (REACH). In: Clinical Trials.gov [Internet]. Bethesda: National Library of Medicine (US); 2000, [20140903]. Available from: URL of the record NLM Identifier: NCT 01639378.

63. Royal Brompton & Harefield NHS Foundation Trust. Renal denervation in heart failure with preserved ejection fraction (RDT-PEE). In: Clinical Trials.gov [Internet]. Bethesda: National Library of Medicine (US); 2000, [20140903]. Available from: URL of the record NLM Identifier: NCT 01840059.

64. University Hospital, Saarland. Influence of Catheter-based renal denervation in disease with increased sympathetic activity. In: Clinical Trials.gov [Internet]. Bethesda: National Library of Medicine (US); 2000, [20140903]. Available from: URL of the record NLM Identifier: NCT 01888315.

65. Zuern CS, Eick C, Rizas KD, Bauer S, Langer H, Gawaz M, Bauer A. Impaired cardiac baroreflex sensitivity predicts response to renal sympathetic denervation in patients with resistant hypertension. J Am Coll Cardiol. 2013;62:2124–30. pii: S0735-1097(13)03077-5.

66. Bristow JD, Honour AJ, Pickering GW, Sleight P, Smyth HS. Diminished baroreflex sensitivity in high blood pressure. Circulation. 1969;39:48–54.

67. Kassis E. Baroreflex control of the circulation in patients with congestive heart failure. Dan Med Bull. 1989;36:195–211.

68. Hering D, Lambert EA, Marusic P, et al. Substantial reduction in single sympathetic nerve firing after renal denervation in patients with resistant hypertension. Hypertens. 2013;61:457–64.

69. Francis DP, Shamim W, Davies LC, Piepoli MF, Ponikowski P, Anker SD, Coats AJ. Cardiopulmonary exercise testing for prognosis in chronic heart failure: continuous and independent prognostic value from VE/VCO(2)slope and peak VO(2). Eur Heart J. 2000;21:154–61.

70. Ponikowski P, Francis DP, Piepoli MF, Davies LC, Chua TP, Davos CH, Florea V, Banasiak W, Poole-Wilson PA, Coats AJ, Anker SD. Enhanced ventilatory response to exercise in patients with chronic heart failure and preserved exercise tolerance: marker of abnormal cardiorespiratory reflex control and predictor of poor prognosis. Circulation. 2001;103:967–72.

Great Myths of Blood Pressure Effect Size in Renal Denervation

James P. Howard, Matthew J. Shun-Shin, and Darrel P. Francis

"Office Pressures Are More Clinically Relevant than Ambulatory"

False.

At the simplest level, far more strokes occur outside the doctor's office than inside it, which makes it embarrassing to claim that the size of the office reduction is more important than the size of the 24-h reduction. At a more sophisticated level, what matters to patients is the incremental effect on blood pressure of denervation (in comparison with not undergoing the procedure).

Designing a study to be unblinded and rely on office blood pressure measurements acquired and manually documented by clinicians has been shown in drug trials to produce exaggerated estimates of effect size [1].

'Anachronistic' is a word many may think unlikely to occur in an article about a technology that may be the biggest step forward in hypertension in several decades. But, with honest respect for our many friends involved, there seems no more succinct way to describe the design of renal denervation trials to date (December 2013). Despite originating in an era of where double-blinded randomised controls or automatic ambulatory measurements are recognised as essential for antihypertensive drug research to be considered credible, the designs of renal denervation trials so far have focused on uncontrolled or unblinded structures with office blood pressure as the primary endpoint.

Most readers will be able to respect the traditions of the Amish, even though they do not share their desire to eschew the fruits of science. In the same way, we in turn hope that future science historians accept non-judgementally that our community currently prefers effect sizes measured and documented manually rather than automatically, even if in years to come the reason for this preference may be a mystery.

"Office BP Is What Guidelines Use as Treatment Targets"

True but irrelevant.

The effect of blood pressure on risk is continuous with no clear and sharp demarcation between risky and risk-free. Targets are provided not to indicate the disappearance of blood-pressure-related risk but as an organisational convenience to help staff rapidly decide on starting (or uptitrating) therapy rather than having to consider global risk and patient disutility on each visit of each patient.

Readers of scientific papers play close attention to the methods so that they may judge the scientific rigor that has been applied to the task. Unfortunately, guidelines do not report the methods used in coming to a decision. Indeed, enquiry reveals that this is not a coincidence, but rather a conspiracy of silence. Guideline members seem to be forbidden to discuss the decision making process. The confidentiality agreement for AHA/ACC guideline writers appear not only to silence authors whilst the guideline is being developed, but to compel them to take the secrets to their graves:

> [I]ndication of areas of writing committee agreement or disagreement on any topic is prohibited. [2]
>
> Breach of confidentiality may result in removal from the guideline writing committee and possibly other consequences. [2]

Guidelinists know that automatically-stored and averaged ambulatory pressures are a better risk marker than clinician-documented office pressures [3, 4], but in most regions of the world they nevertheless set guidelines on office pressures rather than ambulatory. This is likely not because of some as-yet-undiscovered scientific superiority of office pressures, but rather a reflection of pragmatism. Population risk from hypertension is reduced broadly in proportion to the amount of antihypertensive medication taken by the

J.P. Howard, MA, MB BChir, MRCP
M.J. Shun-Shin, MA, BM BCh, MRCP
D.P. Francis, MA, MB BChir, FRCP (✉)
International Centre for Circulatory Health,
National Heart and Lung Institute, Imperial College London,
59-61 North Wharf Road, London W2 1LA, UK
e-mail: jphoward@doctors.org.uk; m@shun-shin.com;
Darrel@DrFrancis.Org

R.R. Heuser et al. (eds.), *Renal Denervation: A New Approach to Treatment of Resistant Hypertension*,
DOI 10.1007/978-1-4471-5223-1_21, © Springer-Verlag London 2015

population. Very large meta-analyses show the curve of risk against pressure is smooth (i.e. there is no distinct plateau where blood-pressure risk disappears) [5]. Therefore if a population that is generally hypertensive receives more therapy it does not matter greatly exactly which individual patients are the recipients; the population risk reduction is similar. The effect achievable by targeting automatic (ambulatory) blood pressures is therefore similar to that achieved by targeting clinician-documented (office) blood pressure, assuming the blood pressure target is set appropriately lower for ambulatory pressures, since they are on average lower. The exact individuals who receive therapy will differ between the two strategies (and indeed between two instances of the same strategy) but the net benefit on events will be similar. However, the practical wisdom of guidelines presenting cost-effective strategies suitable for application across millions of patients should not deflect us from using bias-resistant measurements for our research into effect size.

"We Should Be Identifying the Responders in Advance, So We Can Make a Special Effort to Target Them"

True but impractical

Most clinicians do not realise that the noisiness of office measurements makes it almost impossible to reliably quantify the effect size of any newly-added drug on a single patient basis by simply measuring in the office on one visit before initiation and one visit after initiation. The result of this unawareness is the continuing efforts to identify predictors of large office blood pressure response.

The test-retest variability of blood pressure can easily be more than the variability in the effect size between individuals. Clinicians wishing to quantify effect size within individuals would need to make patients attend for multiple visits, perhaps dozens [6], both before and after intervention, so that the inherent noise can be quenched away by averaging.

If noisy values are used, then it is inevitable that patients with higher values at baseline will tend to fall more: this process is known as regression to the mean.

Imagine a tray of dice representing a group of patients with similar blood pressures, but subject to variability. A "6" represents a patient having a "big day" in his blood pressure, while a "1" represents a day of lower pressure. If we select only the "6"s, and shake the tray again, the dice which previously showed "6"s will tend to drop in value, averaging 3.5. This fall is not because they have undergone treatment for hypertension, but merely the effect of having been selected as outlier values of a noisy variable.

Meanwhile, any dice which previously showed "1"s will tend to show higher values, again averaging 3.5. We do not see these initial "1"s in renal denervation trials because the trials only take patients with high values.

Studies would show that the higher the baseline values of dice, the greater the fall. This does not necessarily mean any therapy given to the patients in between was especially effective in patients with high baseline values. It may mean merely that the patients with the highest baseline values were those for whom the baseline values were most severely overestimating their true long-term mean values.

"Some Patients Respond, But Just Happen to Manifest in a Manner Other than Blood Pressure Reduction"

Not relevant to its role in blood pressure control

On this basis no therapy for any condition can ever be declared ineffective; since it may merely be effective for some other condition.

If renal denervation is being used to treat high blood pressure, the measurement of interest to referrers, payers and patients is a bias-resistant estimate of the average effect size on blood pressure. Of course renal denervation may have many effects beyond blood pressure lowering. For example, it has been reported to reduce arrhythmias and regress left ventricular hypertrophy. However, while these aims are worthy, we should not assume that if they occur they are mediated by blood pressure reduction, if the bias-resistant measures of blood pressure reduction do not show an effect of adequate size.

Meanwhile, testing of efficacy against non blood pressure targets is just as much in need of measurement conditions that are resistant to bias, for example by blinding.

Finally, we should be wary of attributing all instances of a variable changing in a favourable direction in a patient as evidence of benefit. Most variables are not identical when measured at two timepoints, and therefore half of patients show a change in a favourable direction. If there are three physiologically independent variables being measured, the probability in any individual patient that *at least one* of them changes in a favourable direction is $1 - (1/2)^3 = 87.5\%$. Thus if we count a favourable change in any one or more of three variables as evidence of response, any ineffective therapy would appear to deliver a favourable change in almost nine out of ten patients.

"It Doesn't Matter Whether the Blood Pressure Drop Is Due to the Denervation or Placebo: It Is the Total Effect that Matters"

False.

While charlatans and quacks happily claim credit for the healing force of nature or for natural biological variability, as physicians educated in the scientific era we should sense a responsibility to attribute cause and effect as correctly as we can. If there is a substantial effect that it is not caused by denervation then we should not claim it is.

Patient trust in their cardiologists could be damaged if it were discovered that we had been exaggerating the effect size of a therapy by several fold for several years. Unpleasant though such loss of trust might be, it would be justified. The blame would lie with us as the cardiovascular community for repeatedly dismissing the consistent signs of a more modest benefit in the measurements most resistant to bias.

"My Mercury Sphygmomanometer Doesn't Lie"

True.

It is not the sphygmomanometer that lies but the person operating it, although we emphasise that this is entirely out of good intentions. When faced with an unexpectedly undesirable value of a noisy variable, normal clinical practice is to discard that value and remeasure in the hope of obtaining a more "representative" value.

We have asked the question below of over 1,000 lecture attendees in Europe, Japan and USA. We invite the reader to give their own answer, and compare with the responses of colleagues shown at the end of this chapter.

> Imagine an elderly gentleman walks into your clinic with a BP of 160/88.
>
> You commence 5 mg amlodipine and bring him back for review after 1 week.
>
> After a week his BP is 162/88. He swears he has been taking his tablets, and you believe him.
>
> QUESTION: What do you do?

A) Document "reverse response"
B) Document "intolerance"
C) Review in 2 weeks
D) Measure BP again

This scenario is not uncommon, given the high variability of office blood pressures. A standard deviation of blood pressure between visits of 12 mmHg [6] means that on 28 % of occasions it is 7 mmHg above its long-term average. The standard deviation of difference between visits is $\sqrt{2}$ times larger than that, which means that on 28 % of occasions, the increment between two successive visits be 10 mmHg ($7\sqrt{2}$) or more. If a drug drops the true long-term blood pressure of a patient by 10 mmHg, this means that in 28 % cases of initiation, on returning to the clinic after starting the drug, the patient's blood pressure will actually be equal or *higher* than the baseline measurement (Fig. 21.1). This does not mean the drug is ineffective in that patient, rather this is a necessary consequence of biological variability.

When given the above question, 86 % of audience respondents replied with D. This re-measurement could well have

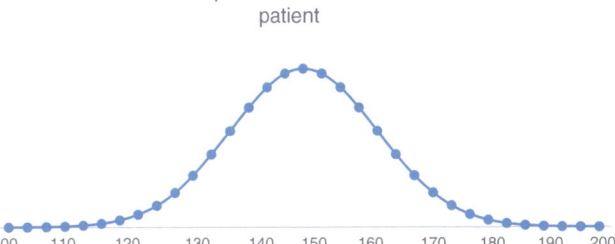

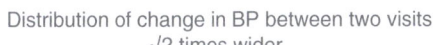

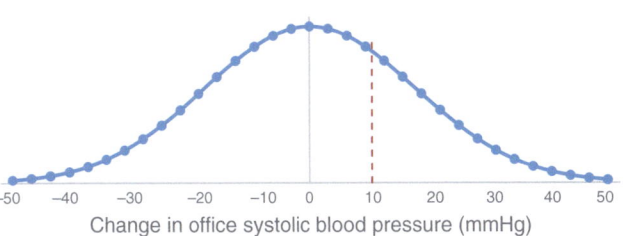

Fig. 21.1 *Top*: The normal distribution of blood pressures from repeated blood pressure measurements in a hypothetical patient presenting to the clinic with a 'true' mean blood pressure of 150 mmHg, and a standard deviation of 12 mmHg. *Bottom*: A graph showing a normal distribution of the changes in clinic-to-clinic blood pressures in the same patient. These changes do not reflect improvement in their hypertension; rather the nature of repeated measurements in a noisy variable. The measurements to the right of the *red line* represent the 28 % of repeat readings which may be wrongly interpreted as a rise in blood pressure of over 10 mmHg

resulted in a lower blood pressure which would no doubt be documented. This appears perfectly reasonable; indeed, isn't the second value just as valid as the first?

However, what would these 86 % of attendees have done had the patient not been started on a drug a week earlier? Almost all audience members agreed that the 162/88 could simply be accepted and documented.

What is concerning is the consequences of such behaviour in the context of unblinded and/or uncontrolled trials, where a physician's expectations of a treatment can influence their measurement strategy.

"Everyone Knows that Office BP Falls More than Ambulatory BP in Drug Trials"

True, but a hilariously self-destructing statement

Office blood does indeed fall more than ambulatory blood pressures in drug trials [7], but only when the office staff are unblinded to the study arm. When controlled and blinded, office and ambulatory pressure fall in direct parallel [1]. The amusing aspect of this myth is that it contains the seeds of its own destruction, by highlighting how powerful bias can be in unblinded blood pressure trials.

It is for this reason that since the turn of the century there has been pressure to abandon bias-susceptible office blood pressure measurement and rely instead on ambulatory monitoring [8], or alternatively to carry out strict blinding.

A good antidote to this myth is to restate it, but rename office blood pressure to "blood pressure documented by a person who knows which arm the patient is in", and ambulatory blood pressure to "blood pressure automatically documented by a machine which does not know which arm the patient is in". With such wording the myth is difficult to sustain.

"Office Effects Are Larger than Ambulatory Effects Because the Sympathetics Contribute More to Blood Pressure in the Daytime than in the Night"

Non-sequitur.

While intellectually persuasive in isolation, the reasoning was shown to be fallacious by the elegant work of Felix Mahfoud's group. Perhaps sympathetics do contribute more to blood pressure in the daytime than in the night, but careful automatic monitoring shows that unblinded renal denervation gives similar reductions in daytime pressure (10.2 mmHg) and night-time pressure (11.1 mmHg) [9].

Proponents of the sympathetic explanation for the human-versus-automatic discrepancy, having lost the battle for the defence of the city of daytime, may well retreat to make a last stand in the inner citadel of the office. However, the history of sieges tells us what happens next.

"RD Is One of the Most Exciting Developments in Medicine in the Last 10 Years"

True, but not only for its contribution to BP control.

Future medical historians may look back on this time as unique. Never before have large proportions of specialists have been so comfortable writing, reading and discussing manually-documented values that overestimated a biological variable to such a large extent in the face of contradiction by automatically-documented data.

A threefold overstatement, in other spheres of medicine, would be serum sodium levels consistently being reported as ~420 mmol/l, body temperatures as ~300°F, or heights as ~5 m.

Threefold overestimation of effect sizes, e.g. 30 rather than ~10 mmHg appears to be unique.

"ABPM Is Unnatural and Weird Because There is a Mechanical Pump Inside, Which Makes a Whizzing Noise"

True but irrelevant.

Any medical assessment, and certainly any measurement of blood pressure, is unnatural. Awareness that it is happening can affect physiology.

Machines lack the natural tendency of physicians to portray an optimistic view of the effect of an intervention they have carried out.

Moreover, machines generally do not have preference for particular digits such as 5 and 0. Humans do, and may be unable to resist rounding up pressures pre-intervention and rounding down pressures after intervention.

It is very rare for automatic equipment to exhibit digit preference. In research where this occurs [10], the effect size has been found to be greatly enhanced to the level seen in manual office measurements. One explanation for this might be mislabelling of office measurements as ambulatory by accident borne of excitement [1].

"I Don't Care What the Number Is, I Want to Treat Patients [11]"

Up to you.

There may be a group of physicians who do not care whether an effect is 30, 10, 1 or 0.1 mmHg. Should we not all strive to avoid being members of this group?

If the effect size was 1 mmHg (or 0.1 mmHg) nobody would read this book, or even write it.

In medicine almost everything affects everything else. We personally think the only question worth asking is: how much?

"10 mmHg Is Not Enough, It Needs to Be More"

False.

Biological values have no obligation to be any different from what they actually are, in the same way that π does not need to be larger than its current value.

Since politicians in the past have attempted to pass laws to change the ratio of the circumference of a circle to its diameter [12], we should not be surprised that they have medical counterparts attempting to change biological realities. We should ignore both categories of modern-day Canute.

A genuine 10 mmHg drop in BP equates to a 41 % reduction in stroke and a 22 % reduction in coronary heart disease events [13] which would be very useful to have.

"The Only Way to Quantify the Benefit of Renal Denervation on Stroke and Heart Attack Rates Is by Doing Trials with Those as Endpoints"

False.

It is well established in antihypertensive drug trials therapy that successfully and safely lowering blood pressure delivers predictable in cardiovascular events. So strong is the data for this that antihypertensive drugs are accepted on the basis of demonstration of safe reduction in blood pressure in randomised blinded trials. There is no requirement to conduct an endpoint trial.

The weakness of denervation at time of writing (December 2013) is that there are no randomised blinded data. There are only unblinded studies which show dramatically different effect size estimates depending on whether blood pressures are documented by unblinded staff or by automatically documented by machines. This means that the choice of values to use to calculate the expected event reduction is in very substantial dispute even within any single trial.

Denervation requires reliable values for a reasonable expectation of the average blood pressure reduction. Because some clinicians have distrust for automatic monitors used in ambulatory blood pressures, and office pressures are open to bias in unblinded trials, what is need is blinded randomized controlled trial data.

Unnecessary confusion about the relative merit of methods of documenting blood pressure may have motivated investigators to conduct the hard endpoint trials which are now recruiting [14].

"The Blood Pressure Effect of Denervation Expands with Time"

Yes, but strangely only when documented by humans.

Blood pressures documented by clinicians aware of the fact that the patient has undergone denervation have indeed been reported to be progressively lower at later time points (see Fig. 21.2, presented at ACC 2012 & TCTAP 2013).

However, readers should note that long-term data is only available for a particularly small subset of patients, namely those pioneer patients judged to have such severe hypertension to warrant the earliest procedures performed.

This effect is only impressive when different patient cohorts are demonstrated in different bars, as above. In contrast, when a consistent cohort is followed up over time, it is difficult to argue persuasively that there is increasing effect with time [15].

Perhaps astonishingly, when machines are used to document blood pressure, the pattern is a stable BP effect between 1, 3 and 6 months [16], as shown in Fig. 21.3.

"Novel Therapies Often Start with Large Effects that Get Smaller in Later Studies"

Tragically true.

It is sad that this phenomenon is true and even sadder that enthusiasts might highlight this.

The pattern of a slew of early reports of large effects, followed later by a recognition that the effect size is very much smaller than previously indicated, should invite not fatalism but curiosity.

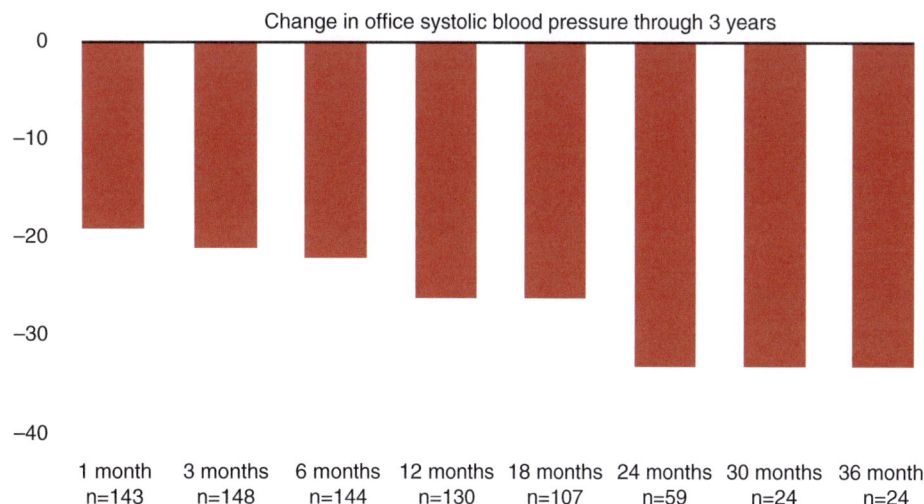

Fig. 21.2 "Expanding benefit?" SYMPLICITY HTN1: change in office systolic blood pressure through 3 years (Created using data presented by Sobotka et al., presented at ACC 2012 & TCTAP 2013)

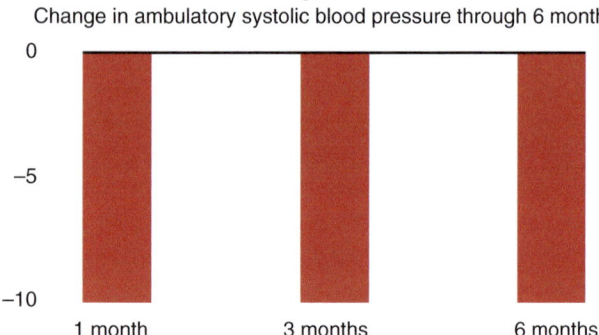

EnligHTN 1
Change in ambulatory systolic blood pressure through 6 months

Fig. 21.3 "Or not?" EnligHTN1: change in ambulatory systolic blood pressure through 6 months (Created using data published by Worthley et al. [16]

Why should early reports consistently overstate effect sizes? One explanation is that patients enrolled earliest in trials are those with the most severe disease and are unrepresentative of the patients more regularly encountered in medical practice.

Another explanation is that early reports are typically more susceptible to bias because the authors are broaching a new frontier and achieving a paradigm shift.

A third explanation is that most effects of most interventions are modest at best, and it is only reports that inadvertently overestimate the effect sizes which tend to be successful in the race to publication. This has been addressed by Ioannidis [17].

A final explanation is that the biological effect size really is somehow fading with the passing years. The bias-resistant automatically documented (ambulatory) measurements in renal denervation trials do not support this. In antibiotic chemotherapy, there is a process of evolution in the genomes of the microbes being combated, providing a plausible mechanism for the same intervention to have less effect in future years. However for renal denervation, and the other cardiac interventions for which this decline has been observed, there is neither a plausible biological basis nor any happiness in elucidating its cause.

References

1. Howard JP, Nowbar AN, Francis DP. Size of blood pressure reduction from renal denervation: insights from meta-analysis of antihypertensive drug trials of 4,121 patients with focus on trial design: the CONVERGE report. Heart. 2013;99:1579–87.

2. American Heart Association. Methodology manual and policies from the ACCF/AHA Task Force on practice guidelines. 2010;65.

3. Hansen TW, Jeppesen J, Rasmussen S, Ibsen H, Torp-Pedersen C. Ambulatory blood pressure monitoring and risk of cardiovascular disease: a population based study. Am J Hypertens. 2006;19:243–50.

4. Verdecchia P, Reboldi G, Porcellati C, et al. Risk of cardiovascular disease in relation to achieved office and ambulatory blood pressure control in treated hypertensive subjects. J Am Coll Cardiol. 2002;39:878–85.

5. Lewington S, Clarke R, Qizilbash N, Peto R, Collins R, Prospective Studies C. Age-specific relevance of usual blood pressure to vascular mortality: a meta-analysis of individual data for one million adults in 61 prospective studies. Lancet. 2002;360:1903–13.

6. Warren RE, Marshall T, Padfield PL, Chrubasik S. Variability of office, 24-hour ambulatory, and self-monitored blood pressure measurements. Br J Gen Pract. 2010;60:675–80.

7. Mancia G, Parati G. Office compared with ambulatory blood pressure in assessing response to antihypertensive treatment: a meta-analysis. J Hypertens. 2004;22:435–45.

8. O'Brien E, Coats A, Owens P, et al. Use and interpretation of ambulatory blood pressure monitoring: recommendations of the British hypertension society. BMJ. 2000;320:1128–34.

9. Mahfoud F, Ukena C, Schmieder RE, et al. Ambulatory blood pressure changes after renal sympathetic denervation in patients with resistant hypertension. Circulation. 2013;128:132–40.

10. Simonetti G, Spinelli A, Gandini R, et al. Endovascular radiofrequency renal denervation in treating refractory arterial hypertension: a preliminary experience. Radiol Med. 2012;117:426–44.

11. Deflating the hype: are we setting renal denervation up for disappointment? 2013. At http://www.massdevice.com/features/deflating-hype-are-we-setting-renal-denervation-disappointment.

12. Indiana Pi Bill. At http://en.wikipedia.org/wiki/Indiana_Pi_Bill.

13. Law MR, Morris JK, Wald NJ. Use of blood pressure lowering drugs in the prevention of cardiovascular disease: meta-analysis of 147 randomised trials in the context of expectations from prospective epidemiological studies. BMJ. 2009;338:b1665.

14. St. Jude Medical EnligHTNment Study Highlighted at EuroPCR during trials that may change clinical practice session. 2013. At http://www.sjm.com/corporate/media-room/media-kits/new-products/~/media/SJM/corporate/Media%20Kits/EnligHTN/for_0 5212013/052113EnligHTNmentNewsReleaseFINAL.ashx.

15. Esler MD, Krum H, Schlaich M, et al. Renal sympathetic denervation for treatment of drug-resistant hypertension: one-year results from the Symplicity HTN-2 randomized, controlled trial. Circulation. 2012;126:2976–82.

16. Worthley SG, Tsioufis CP, Worthley MI, et al. Safety and efficacy of a multi-electrode renal sympathetic denervation system in resistant hypertension: the EnligHTN I trial. Eur Heart J. 2013; 34:2132–40.

17. Ioannidis JP. Why most published research findings are false. PLoS Med. 2005;2:e124.

The Potential Role of Catheter-Based Renal Sympathetic Denervation in Chronic and End-Stage Kidney Disease

Markus P. Schlaich and Yusuke Sata

Introduction: Overview of Catheter-Based Renal Denervation and Its Potential Benefits

The introduction of catheter-based radiofrequency renal sympathetic denervation to clinical medicine has been considered to be a promising new avenue to the future device-based therapy of hypertension. Renal sympathetic efferent and afferent nerves located in the adventitia of the renal artery are the target of this procedure. On the basis of their crucial role in development and maintenance of systemic hypertension, renal sympathetic nerves have long been considered to be an attractive target for neuromodulation therapy [1].

The rationale for sympathetic modulation therapy has been assessed in various conditions associated with hypertension. Classic surgical sectioning of sympathetic nerves by thoracic and lumbar sympathectomy and splanchnicectomy have been successful in reducing blood pressure and improved the long-term outcome of patients with hypertension [2, 3]. Studies in animals have also demonstrated reduced sympathetic nervous activity [4], improvement in natriuresis [5], as well as improvement in left ventricular function [6] after renal sympathetic denervation.

In light of the promising results of renal denervation in human and animal studies, the Symplicity HTN trial program was initiated to assess the potential utility of this approach. The initial proof-of-concept study, Symplicity HTN-1 in 2009 [7], demonstrated the efficacy and safety of renal denervation in 45 patients with resistant hypertension. The study eligibility criteria were defined as uncontrolled office systolic blood pressure (>160 mmHg) despite being treated with at least three antihypertensive drugs (including

one diuretic) at optimal doses. This study proved not only the safety and efficacy of RDN but a substantial reduction in the office blood pressure. Among the participants, only a few minor procedure-related complications were reported; one renal artery dissection on placement of catheter before radiofrequency energy delivery and three femoral artery pseudoaneurysms at the access site [8]. Over the 12 months, the reduction in office systolic and diastolic blood pressure was −14/−10, −21/−10, −22/−11, −24/−11, and −27/−17 mmHg at 1, 3, 6, 9, and 12 months, respectively, from an average of 177/101 mmHg at baseline [7]. The sustained long-term effect of renal denervation on blood pressure reduction (−32/−14 mmHg) was recently reported in 36-month follow-up results [9] (Fig. 22.1). The release of norepinephrine from the renal sympathetic nerves was measured in ten patients with the isotope dilution renal norepinephrine spillover method [7]. In 15–30 days after the procedure, the renal norepinephrine spillover was decreased by 47 %, suggesting a substantial albeit incomplete reduction of renal efferent sympathetic nerve traffic [7].

Symplicity HTN-2 was designed as a randomized control study and results were reported in 2010 and 2012 [10, 11]. Enrolled resistant hypertensive patients with a baseline office systolic blood pressure >160 mmHg (>150 mmHg for patients with type 2 diabetes) were randomized to either undergo RDN ($n=52$) or to continue their established conventional pharmacological treatment ($n=54$). In line with the results of Symplicity HTN-1, renal denervation reduced office blood pressure −32±23/12±11 mmHg at 6 months [10], with sustained effect reported at 12-month follow-up (−28±25/10±11 mmHg) [11]. In contrast, no significant change was observed in the control group (1±21/0±10 in office blood pressure and 2±13/7±11 mmHg in home blood pressure) [10]. Mean estimated glomerular filtration ratio (eGFR) was unchanged in both groups at 6 months (0.2±11 ml/min/1.73 m [2] in the RDN group and 0.9±12 ml/min/1.73 m [2] in the control group) [10] (Fig. 22.2).

These trials had their origins in the three observations: (1) the renal sympathetic outflow is activated in patients with

M.P. Schlaich, MD, FAHA (✉) • Y. Sata, MD
Neurovascular Hypertension and Kidney Disease Laboratory,
Baker IDI Heart and Diabetes Institute,
St Kilda Road Central, 6492,
Melbourne, VIC 8008, Australia
e-mail: markus.schlaich@bakeridi.edu.au;
yusuke.sata@bakeridi.edu.au

R.R. Heuser et al. (eds.), *Renal Denervation: A New Approach to Treatment of Resistant Hypertension*,
DOI 10.1007/978-1-4471-5223-1_22, © Springer-Verlag London 2015

Fig. 22.1 Effects of RDN on BP (**a**) and changes in eGFR (**b**) over time in Symplicity HTN-1 with follow-up to 2 years (Reproduced from Symplicity HTN-1 Investigators [8], with permission)

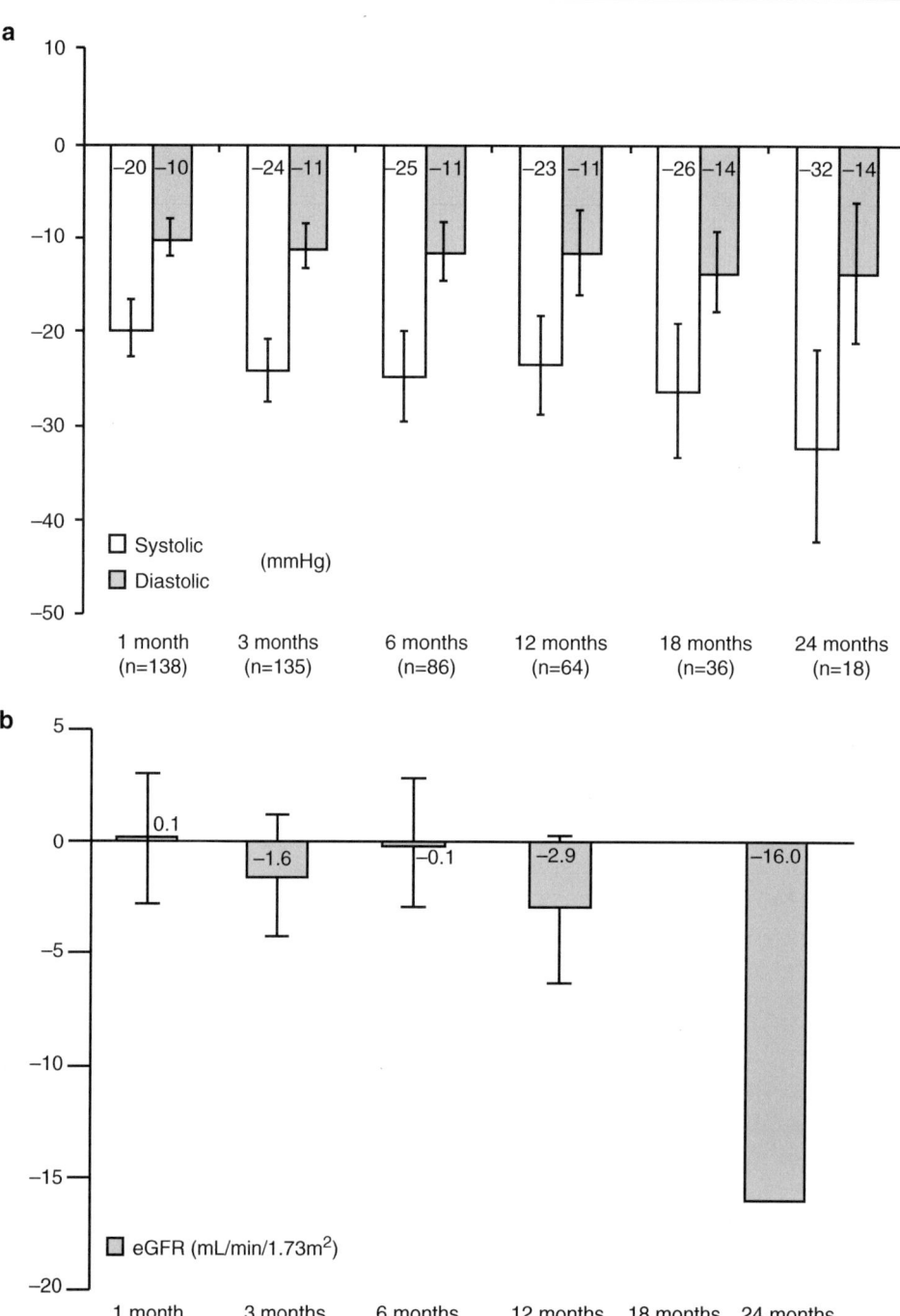

resistant hypertension; (2) overactivated renal sympathetic nerve results in higher blood pressure through the mechanisms of sodium and water retention, reducing renal blood flow, and activation of renin-angiotensin system; and (3) suppression of renal sympathetic nerve activity reduces blood pressure with sustained effects.

Symplicity HTN-3

The latest and the largest clinical trial of catheter-based renal denervation, Symplicity HTN-3, has been reported very recently [12]. This study was a rigorously designed randomized, blinded, sham-controlled trial. Patients in

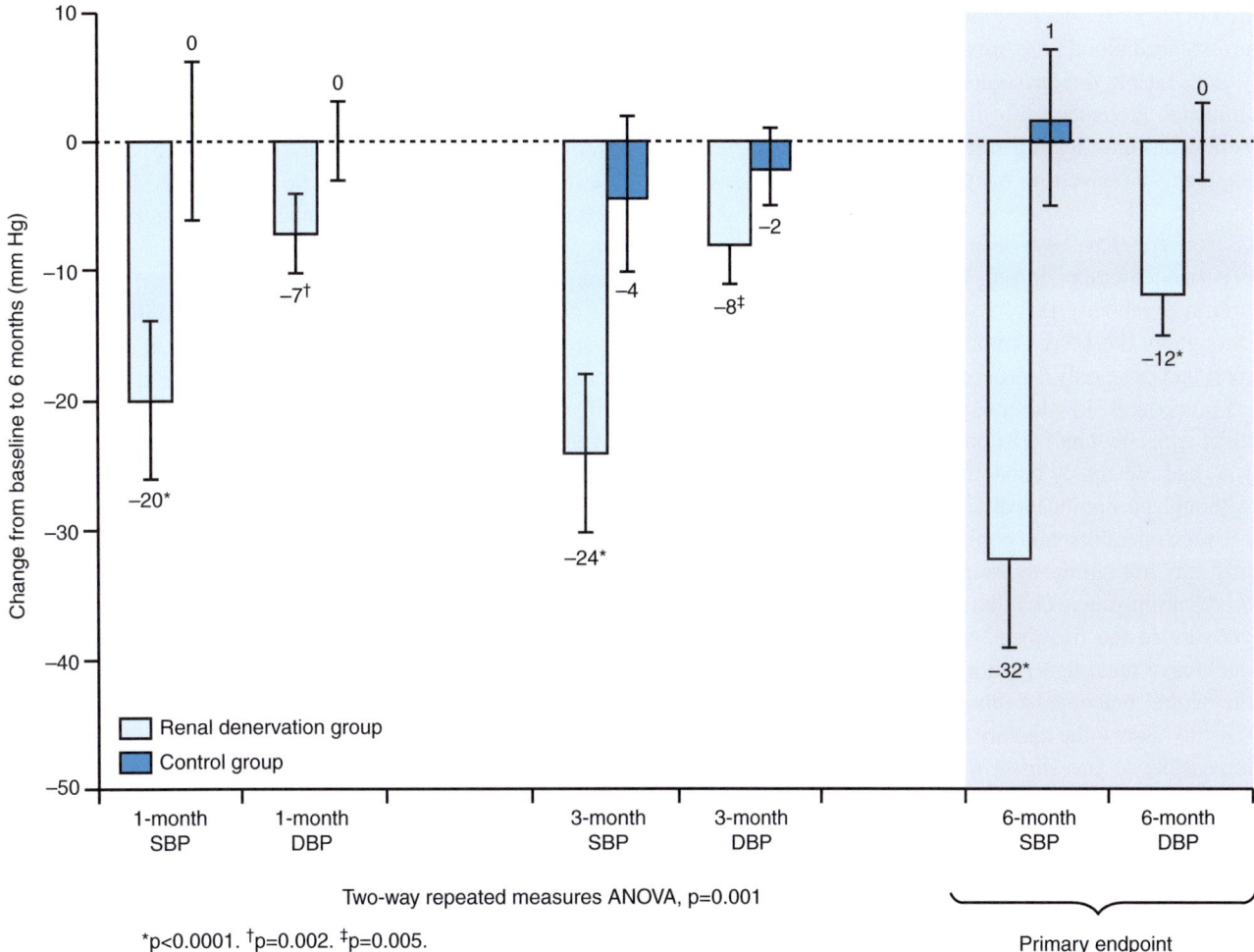

Fig. 22.2 BP reduction in Symplicity HTN-2 in the treatment and control group up at 3 and 6 months of follow-up (Reprinted from Esler et al. [10], Copyright (2010), with permission)

control group underwent renal angiogram, masked to mimic renal denervation. Patients' enrollment criteria were essentially the same as previous Symplicity trials. Patients had to be treated with at least three antihypertensive medications at maximally tolerated dose, and one of which should be a diuretic. The regimen had to be unchanged for 2 weeks before the enrollment. Subsequently, patients needed to fulfill the blood pressure criterion which was systolic blood pressure ≥160 mmHg on a day of office visit. Automated 24-h ambulatory blood pressure monitoring was performed to confirm an average 24-h systolic blood pressure ≥135 mmHg to rule out white-coat hypertension. The renal denervation was performed by means of Medtronic Symplicity renal denervation catheter. The safety and efficacy endpoints were examined at 6-month follow-up. During the 6-month follow-up period, the regimen of antihypertensive medication was not allowed to change unless there was clinical necessity.

Among 535 uncontrolled hypertensive patients, 364 patients were blindly allocated to treatment group and underwent renal denervation across the USA. At 6 months after the procedure, despite a significant drop in office systolic blood pressure from the baseline in the treatment group, this was not statistically significant when compared to that of the sham procedure group (-14.1 ± 23.9 vs. -11.7 ± 25.9 mmHg, $p = 0.26$).

In contrast to Symplicity HTN-1 and HTN-2, the reduction of office blood pressure in the treatment group was less pronounced ($-14.1 \pm 23.9/-6.6 \pm 11.9$ in HTN-3 vs. $-22/-11$ mmHg in HTN-1 [7], and $-32 \pm 23/-12 \pm 11$ mmHg in HTN-2) [10]. Furthermore, there was a large effect in the sham control group; the drop in office systolic blood pressure was prominent compared to that of HTN-2 (-11.7 ± 25.3 vs. 1 ± 21 mmHg in HTN-2) [10]. Although the pretreatment blood pressure was similar, greater range of standard deviation in the treatment group of HTN-3 indicates wider variation in response. Interestingly, African-Americans had a less pronounced blood pressure effect in response to renal denervation, raising the question whether racial background may influence the response to the procedure. Of note, African-Americans have less effective blood pressure reduction with angiotensin-converting enzyme (ACE) inhibitors and beta-blockers [13].

Concerns have also been raised in regard to the operator experience in this US trial. The procedure of renal denervation in Symplicity HTN-3 was performed by 111 operators throughout the USA. Among them, 31 % (about 34 operators) had done only 1 procedure, and 85 operators had done <5 procedures. In addition, among 364 patients in the treatment arm, about half (181 patients) were treated by operators who had previously done <5 (mostly 1–2) procedures [12]. Although no significant difference was observed in outcomes between operators who performed <5 procedures and others, this may not eliminate the possible influence of the operators' learning curve on relatively marginal reduction of blood pressure in the treatment group. From this point of view, ineffective renal denervation might be partly attributable to the neutral outcome of this study. However, the absence of tests to assess the quality of renal denervation makes it impossible to investigate this matter, unlike experimental renal denervation in animal studies.

The results raised some important issues that need to be resolved in future renal denervation studies. The procedure of catheter-based renal denervation is essentially different from traditional experimental denervation in animals, in which total renal denervation is accomplished by visually stripping and by painting phenol or xylocaine around the renal artery [5, 14, 15]. In contrast to animal experiments, a reliable test to confirm that renal denervation is successfully achieved is limited to the renal norepinephrine spillover and muscle sympathetic nerve activity (MSNA) in clinical studies [7, 16, 17], and the question remains what is accomplished by the catheter-based renal denervation.

While the evidence of the utility of renal denervation from experimental animal studies is very strong, it has to be considered together with outcomes of clinical research studies to inform future and better designed trials. In this regard, partial ineffectiveness of current clinical approaches to achieve successful renal denervation is a real possibility.

Irrespective of the results of Symplicity HTN 1–3, the therapeutic concept of renal denervation is likely to be most efficacious in conditions characterized by increased sympathetic drive, such as CKD, heart failure, and other cardiac-relating disorders. Below, we will discuss the potential roles of renal denervation in CKD from both a clinical and a basic science point of view.

Renal Denervation and Chronic Kidney Disease

CKD is one of the most important comorbidities of hypertension as CKD substantially contributes to the systemic fluid burden as well as sympathetic overactivity [18–21]. The mechanisms of renal sympathetic overactivity to elevate blood pressure include (i) urinary sodium retention and volume expansion, (ii) reduction in renal blood flow due to vasoconstriction, and (iii) activation of the renin-angiotensin system [1]. CKD therefore appears as a logical indication for renal denervation approaches [22]. Hering et al. reported the effects of catheter-based renal denervation on resistant hypertensive patients with moderate to severe CKD [23]. A significant drop in the office blood pressure (−34/−14, −25/−11, −32/−15, and −33/−19 mmHg at 1, 3, 6, and 12 months after RDN, respectively) was observed without deterioration in renal function and renal blood flow. These findings confirmed the safety and efficacy of catheter-based renal denervation in resistant hypertensive patients with CKD. Kiuchi et al. reported the beneficial effects of catheter-based renal denervation in 24 patients with CKD and refractory hypertension [24]. Using an irrigated cardiac ablation catheter, a significant improvement in eGFR (64.4 ± 23.9 to 85.4 ± 34.9 ml/min/1.73 m [2], at baseline and at 6 months after denervation, respectively), has been observed in addition to the reduction in the office blood pressure ($186 \pm 19/108 \pm 13$ to $135 \pm 13/88 \pm 7$ mmHg, at baseline and at 6 months after denervation). Improvement in albuminuria was also reported after catheter-based renal denervation in resistant hypertensive patients [25].

In animal experiments, Campese et al. reported that renal afferent denervation (dorsal rhizotomy) improved the NE turnover rate in posterior and lateral hypothalamic nuclei of chronic renal failure rats [26] and prevented the progression of renal failure [27]. These results indicate that renal afferent nerves play an important role in the development of hypertension and the progression of renal disease in renal failure model. Therefore, it appears that successful catheter-based renal denervation has a potential not only to improve hypertension but also slow progression of CKD.

CKD and Hypertension as Major Cardiovascular Risk Factors

Since the introduction of the concept of cardiorenal syndrome, CKD has been recognized as a risk factor of CVD, rather than just a precursor of end-stage renal disease (ESRD). Go et al. reported the graded association observed between a reduced estimated GFR and the risk of death, cardiovascular events, and hospitalization in a large, community-based population [28].

As a clinical manifestation of CKD, proteinuria and albuminuria are not only reliable markers of progression of CKD but also stimulate progression of CKD [29]. In the RENAAL and LIFE studies, the improvement of albuminuria was also associated with the reduction in the incidence of CVD [30, 31]. Accordingly, improvement in proteinuria and albuminuria are potentially important in the therapy of CKD, not only from the viewpoint of CVD prevention, but also regression of CKD [32, 33].

Increased CVD risk in CKD is predominantly attributable to the development of atherosclerosis [34]. The frequent comorbidities of CKD listed in Table 22.1 (classic risks), such as hypertension, diabetes, and dyslipidemia, are also well known as risk factors for atherosclerosis. Because of those comorbidities, CKD had not been identified as an independent risk factor of CVD. Recently, however, albuminuria and hyperhomocysteinemia have been characterized as CKD-specific risk factors (nonclassic risks) and showed that they are independently associated with the development of atherosclerosis [35–37].

Atherosclerosis also links CKD with hypertension. Through the development of atherosclerosis, CKD accelerates vascular remodeling which coincides with endothelial dysfunction. The vascular abnormalities increase systolic BP and pulse pressure, resulting in high cardiovascular mortality (Fig. 22.3). On the other hand, hypertension accelerates the progression of CKD. The risk of ESRD increases by 20–30 % with every 10 mmHg increase in systolic blood pressure [38]. In fact, a number of clinical studies suggest the strong relation between hypertension and CKD [18, 19].

As shown in Table 22.1, CKD and CVD have a lot of risk factors in common. Slowing progression of CKD therefore presents a means to reduce CVD morbidity and mortality. Indeed, the sub-analysis of HOPE study revealed that while angiotensin-converting enzyme (ACE) inhibitors reduced the events of CVD in patients with CKD to a similar extent to that in non-CKD patients [39, 40], the effect was more pronounced in more severe stages of CKD.

Improvement of albuminuria is potentially important to prevent the progression of CKD, as well as CVD, in the early stage. A recent study by Ott et al. showed that catheter-based renal denervation reduced micro- and macroalbuminuria in patients with treatment-resistant hypertension [25], demonstrating the

Table 22.1 Classic and nonclassic risk factors for

Classic risks	Nonclassic risk
Age	Albuminuria
Gender: male	Hyperhomocysteinemia
Hypertension	Lipoprotein, apoprotein
Low HDL	Low production of nitric oxide
Diabetes mellitus	Electrolyte abnormality
Lack of exercise	Oxidative stress
Menopausal	Inflammation
Familial history of CVD	Somnipathy
Left ventricular hypertrophy	Hemostatic/fibrinolytic abnormality

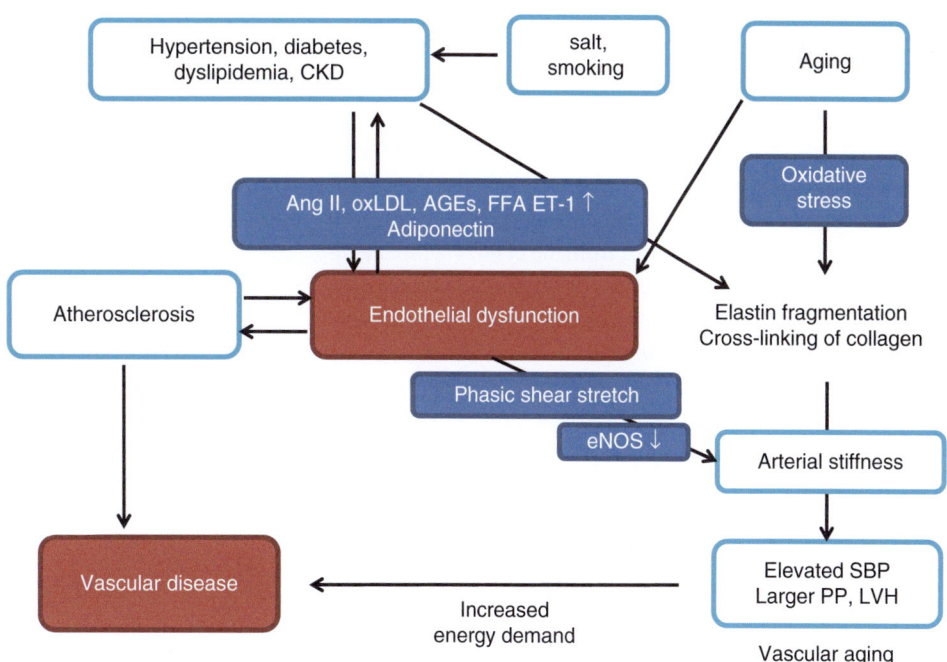

Fig. 22.3 Schematic relationship between CKD and CVD mechanisms

crucial role of sympathetic hyperactivity in both hypertension and CKD.

Sympathetic Nervous System and CKD

Elevated sympathetic nervous activity is well known to play a key role in cardiovascular complications in humans [41]. Although sympathetic hyperactivity has been consistently demonstrated in ESRD, it is already present from the early stage of renal disease [20, 42]. Urinary albumin excretion was positively correlated with the elevated plasma norepinephrine level in a cross-sectional study of 495 subjects from the general population [43]. The elevated plasma norepinephrine level may be associated with future renal injury in normotensive subjects [20], and higher plasma norepinephrine is an established prognostic predictor in patients with chronic heart failure [44]. As a treatment of hypertension associated with CKD, both metoprolol and enalapril decreased microalbuminuria in patients with type I diabetes mellitus [45]. Regarding the underlying mechanisms, Rao et al. proposed adrenergic mediation of early glomerular permeability from the study of adrenergic polymorphism and genetic predisposition [46]. These findings suggest that sympathetic nervous activation precedes early glomerular permeability alterations [21]. Modulation of overactivity of renal nerves might therefore prevent progression of CKD. The question remains, however, which nerve pathway (afferent or efferent or both) plays the key role in sympathetic hyperactivity in CKD.

The Specific Role of Renal Sympathetic Nerves in Hypertension and CKD

The renal sympathetic nerves consist of efferent sympathetic fibers and afferent sensory fibers [47]. The renal efferent nerves supply all renal relevant structures including the renal vasculature, the tubules, and the juxtaglomerular apparatus with direct physiological control from the central sympathetic nervous system [47]. Accordingly, sympathetic activation of renal efferent nerves results in (i) urinary sodium and water retention via enhanced tubular sodium reabsorption, (ii) reduction in renal blood flow and GFR through neurally mediated vasoconstriction, and (iii) release of renin by stimulation of β1-adrenoceptors on the juxtaglomerular apparatus with concomitant engagement of the renin-angiotensin-aldosterone system [48–50].

The renal afferent sensory nerves are predominantly located in the renal pelvic wall [1, 51]. In contrast to renal efferent nerves, afferent nerves project to the ipsilateral dorsal root ganglia at T6–L2 level with the majority of the nerve cell bodies being at the T9–L1 level. Being processed in the paraventricular nuclei in the brain, stimuli of renal afferent nerves end up deteriorating baroreceptor sensitivity, vagal

function, and endothelial function [52, 53]. Increase in renal afferent activity is also known to decrease renal efferent activity through the powerful negative feedback control of renal sympathetic activity via the activation of renorenal reflexes [51, 54, 55]. In contrast, increase in renal efferent activity increases renal afferent activity [56]. In experiments of rats, Kopp et al. showed that renal afferent denervation (efferent nerve remains intact) increased mean arterial pressure in rats [57], suggesting tonically active renal afferent nerves contributing to the maintenance of low efferent renal nerve activity. On the other hand, Campese et al. reported renal afferent denervation prevents the progression of hypertension in rats with chronic renal failure [26], indicating neurally mediated mechanisms of hypertension through renal afferent impulses from the kidneys of uremic rats.

In the context of neural control of renal function, as well as renal contribution to systemic sympathetic tone, neuromodulation therapy is theoretically beneficial in the treatment of hypertension with CKD. The overall goal of renal denervation is to maintain low renal efferent sympathetic nervous activity to achieve sustained reduction in blood pressure. In addition, renal afferent denervation contributes to maintain low systemic sympathetic activity in renal failure model. As summarized in Fig. 22.4, interaction of the kidney and brain involves multiple factors. Indeed, the etiology of hypertension tends to be multifactorial especially when accompanied by CKD. However, sympathetic overactivity is the fundamental hallmark of the disease. Given the above-mentioned rationale of renal denervation, hypertensive patients with CKD would be expected to experience benefits from catheter-based renal denervation.

Renal Denervation and Heart Failure and Electrophysiological Disorders

Among the various conditions of sympathetic activation, heart failure plays a crucial role in cardiovascular outcomes and is very common in CKD [44, 58]. Remarkably, sympathetic hyperactivation is known to occur in the early stage of asymptomatic heart failure with both preserved and reduced ejection fraction [59]. Given the role of renal denervation in sympathetic hyperactive condition, renal denervation may possibly improve the outcomes of patients with heart failure. Surgical renal denervation was shown to improve the LV function of heart failure Wistar rats induced by myocardial infarction [6]. Surgical renal denervation also restored natriuresis in response to atrial natriuretic peptide (ANP) in experimental ischemic heart failure dogs [60].

Several studies have suggested an improvement of left ventricular (LV) function after catheter-based renal denervation in resistant hypertensive patients. In line with the functional improvement of LV, renal denervation is reported to reduce LV hypertrophy [61] and LV mass

Fig. 22.4 Pathophysiological interactions between the brain and kidney increase total body sympathetic activity

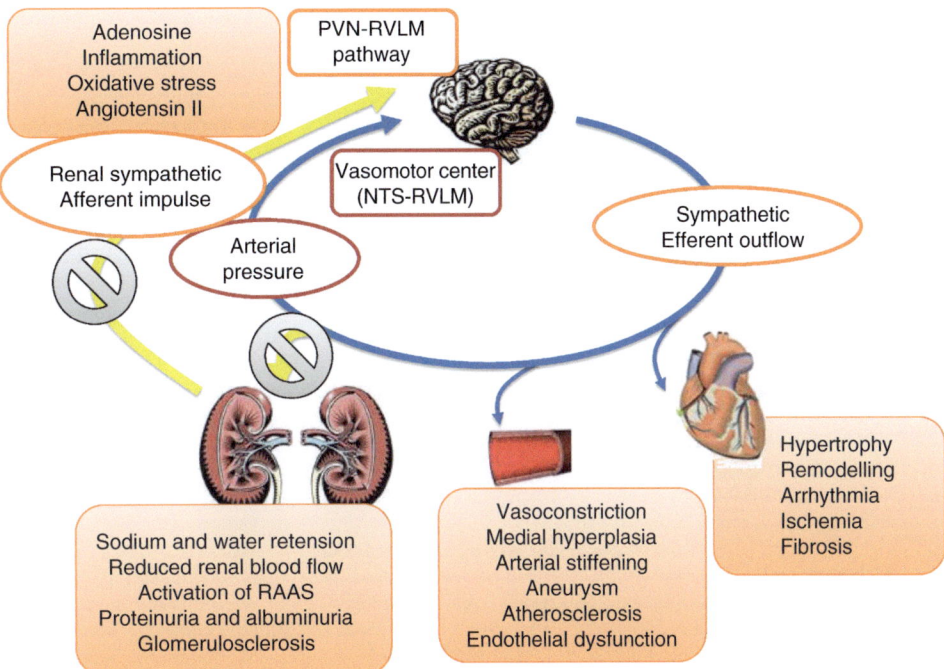

Adenosine
Inflammation
Oxidative stress
Angiotensin II

PVN-RVLM pathway

Renal sympathetic
Afferent impulse

Vasomotor center
(NTS-RVLM)

Sympathetic
Efferent outflow

Arterial
pressure

Sodium and water retension
Reduced renal blood flow
Activation of RAAS
Proteinuria and albuminuria
Glomerulosclerosis

Vasoconstriction
Medial hyperplasia
Arterial stiffening
Aneurysm
Atherosclerosis
Endothelial dysfunction

Hypertrophy
Remodelling
Arrhythmia
Ischemia
Fibrosis

index [62]. The recurrence of atrial fibrillation (AF) also seems to be reduced in hypertensive patients with chronic AF [63, 64].

The first-in-man clinical study of renal denervation in heart failure, the REACH-Pilot Study was designed to prove safety of catheter-based renal denervation for heart failure patients with reduced ejection fraction and a systolic blood pressure >120 mmHg [65]. No procedure-related complications were observed with the procedure. At 6 months follow-up, systolic and diastolic blood pressure remain unchanged (-7.1 ± 6.9 and -0.6 ± 4.0 mmHg, respectively), and a 6-min walk was significantly improved by 27.1 ± 9.7 m.

Ukena et al. reported that electrical storm was reduced after bilateral renal denervation in two patients with chronic heart failure [66]. Both patients suffered from treatment-resistant LV tachyarrhythmia and had required an implantable cardioverter defibrillator (ICD) implantation. Their etiology of heart failure was nonischemic. After renal denervation, both patients had subsequent event-free periods up to 5 months. Interestingly, blood pressure was not decreased with renal denervation in either patient.

In line with the animal studies, natriuretic effects of renal denervation might have contributed to the improvement of functional as well as electrophysiological alterations of failing myocardium in the above clinical studies of heart failure. However, given the malicious roles of sympathetic overactivity in heart failure, a reduction of sympathetic nervous activity may also have contributed but this remains to be investigated further.

Conclusion

There are preliminary albeit uncontrolled promising clinical data to suggest that renal denervation may exert beneficial effects in the context of CKD in regard to better BP control, preservation of renal function, and possible improvement of common comorbidities such as heart failure. The experimental evidence to support such notions is convincing.

In light of the results of Symplicity HTN-3 and the questions raised by this study, it will be crucial to perform properly designed randomized controlled studies applying catheter-based renal denervation in an environment with sufficient experience to better understand the potential clinical benefits of renal denervation in CKD.

References

1. Dibona GF, Kopp UC. Neural control of renal function. Physiol Rev. 1997;77:75–197.
2. Grimson KS, Orgain ES, Anderson B, Broome Jr RA, Longino FH. Results of treatment of patients with hypertension by total thoracic and partial to total lumbar sympathectomy, splanchnicectomy and celiac ganglionectomy. Ann Surg. 1949;129:850.
3. Smithwick RH, Thompson JE. Splanchnicectomy for essential hypertension; results in 1,266 cases. JAMA. 1953;152:1501–4.
4. Katholi RE, Winternitz SR, Oparil S. Decrease in peripheral sympathetic nervous system activity following renal denervation or unclipping in the one-kidney one-clip goldblatt hypertensive rat. J Clin Invest. 1982;69:55–62.
5. Bello-Reuss E, Colindres RE, Pastoriza-Munoz E, Mueller RA, Gottschalk CW. Effects of acute unilateral renal denervation in the rat. J Clin Invest. 1975;56:208–17.

6. Nozawa T, Igawa A, Fujii N, Kato B, Yoshida N, Asanoi H, Inoue H. Effects of long-term renal sympathetic denervation on heart failure after myocardial infarction in rats. Heart Vessels. 2002; 16:51–6.

7. Krum H, Schlaich M, Whitbourn R, Sobotka PA, Sadowski J, Bartus K, Kapelak B, Walton A, Sievert H, Thambar S, Abraham WT, Esler M. Catheter-based renal sympathetic denervation for resistant hypertension: a multicentre safety and proof-of-principle cohort study. Lancet. 2009;373:1275–81.

8. Symplicity HTNI. Catheter-based renal sympathetic denervation for resistant hypertension: durability of blood pressure reduction out to 24 months. Hypertension. 2011;57:911–7.

9. Krum H, Schlaich MP, Sobotka PA, Bohm M, Mahfoud F, Rocha-Singh K, Katholi R, Esler MD. Percutaneous renal denervation in patients with treatment-resistant hypertension: final 3-year report of the symplicity htn-1 study. Lancet. 2014;383:622–9.

10. Esler MD, Krum H, Sobotka PA, Schlaich MP, Schmieder RE, Bohm M. Renal sympathetic denervation in patients with treatment-resistant hypertension (the symplicity htn-2 trial): a randomised controlled trial. Lancet. 2010;376:1903–9.

11. Esler MD, Krum H, Schlaich M, Schmieder RE, Bohm M, Sobotka PA, Symplicity HTNI. Renal sympathetic denervation for treatment of drug-resistant hypertension: one-year results from the symplicity htn-2 randomized, controlled trial. Circulation. 2012;126:2976–82.

12. Bhatt DL, Kandzari DE, O'Neill WW, D'Agostino R, Flack JM, Katzen BT, Leon MB, Liu M, Mauri L, Negoita M, Cohen SA, Oparil S, Rocha-Singh K, Townsend RR, Bakris GL. A controlled trial of renal denervation for resistant hypertension. N Engl J Med. 2014;370(15):1393–401.

13. Materson BJ, Reda DJ, Cushman WC, Massie BM, Freis ED, Kochar MS, Hamburger RJ, Fye C, Lakshman R, Gottdiener J. Single-drug therapy for hypertension in men–a comparison of six antihypertensive agents with placebo. N Engl J Med. 1993;328:914–21.

14. Blake WD, Jurf AN. Renal sodium reabsorption after acute renal denervation in the rabbit. J Physiol. 1968;196:65–73.

15. Bello-Reuss E, Pastoriza-Munoz E, Colindres RE. Acute unilateral renal denervation in rats with extracellular volume expansion. Am J Physiol. 1977;232:F26–32.

16. Hering D, Lambert EA, Marusic P, Walton AS, Krum H, Lambert GW, Esler MD, Schlaich MP. Substantial reduction in single sympathetic nerve firing after renal denervation in patients with resistant hypertension. Hypertension. 2013;61:457–64.

17. Hering D, Marusic P, Walton AS, Lambert EA, Krum H, Narkiewicz K, Lambert GW, Esler MD, Schlaich MP. Sustained sympathetic and blood pressure reduction 1 year after renal denervation in patients with resistant hypertension. Hypertension. 2014;64(1): 118–24.

18. Klag MJ, Whelton PK, Randall BL, Neaton JD, Brancati FL, Ford CE, Shulman NB, Stamler J. Blood pressure and end-stage renal disease in men. N Engl J Med. 1996;334:13–8.

19. Klag MJ, Whelton PK, Randall BL, Neaton JD, Brancati FL, Stamler J. End-stage renal disease in african-american and white men. 16-year mrfit findings. Jama. 1997;277:1293–8.

20. Masuo K, Katsuya T, Sugimoto K, Kawaguchi H, Rakugi H, Ogihara T, Tuck ML. High plasma norepinephrine levels associated with beta2-adrenoceptor polymorphisms predict future renal damage in nonobese normotensive individuals. Hypertens Res. 2007; 30:503–11.

21. Masuo K, Lambert GW, Esler MD, Rakugi H, Ogihara T, Schlaich MP. The role of sympathetic nervous activity in renal injury and end-stage renal disease. Hypertens Res. 2010;33:521–8.

22. Schlaich MP, Sobotka PA, Krum H, Lambert E, Esler MD. Renal sympathetic-nerve ablation for uncontrolled hypertension. N Engl J Med. 2009;361:932–4.

23. Hering D, Mahfoud F, Walton AS, Krum H, Lambert GW, Lambert EA, Sobotka PA, Bohm M, Cremers B, Esler MD, Schlaich MP. Renal denervation in moderate to severe ckd. J Am Soc Nephrol. 2012;23:1250–7.

24. Kiuchi MG, Maia GL, de Queiroz Carreira MA, Kiuchi T, Chen S, Andrea BR, Graciano ML, Lugon JR. Effects of renal denervation with a standard irrigated cardiac ablation catheter on blood pressure and renal function in patients with chronic kidney disease and resistant hypertension. Eur Heart J. 2013;34(28):2114–21.

25. Ott C, Mahfoud F, Schmid A, Ditting T, Veelken R, Ewen S, Ukena C, Uder M, Bohm M, Schmieder RE. Improvement of albuminuria after renal denervation. Int J Cardiol. 2014;173:311–5.

26. Campese VM, Kogosov E. Renal afferent denervation prevents hypertension in rats with chronic renal failure. Hypertension. 1995;25:878–82.

27. Campese VM, Kogosov E, Koss M. Renal afferent denervation prevents the progression of renal disease in the renal ablation model of chronic renal failure in the rat. Am J Kidney Dis. 1995;26:861–5.

28. Go AS, Chertow GM, Fan D, McCulloch CE, Hsu CY. Chronic kidney disease and the risks of death, cardiovascular events, and hospitalization. N Engl J Med. 2004;351:1296–305.

29. Gerstein HC, Mann JF, Yi Q, Zinman B, Dinneen SF, Hoogwerf B, Halle JP, Young J, Rashkow A, Joyce C, Nawaz S, Yusuf S. Albuminuria and risk of cardiovascular events, death, and heart failure in diabetic and nondiabetic individuals. Jama. 2001;286:421–6.

30. de Zeeuw D, Remuzzi G, Parving HH, Keane WF, Zhang Z, Shahinfar S, Snapinn S, Cooper ME, Mitch WE, Brenner BM. Proteinuria, a target for renoprotection in patients with type 2 diabetic nephropathy: lessons from renal. Kidney Int. 2004; 65:2309–20.

31. Ibsen H, Olsen MH, Wachtell K, Borch-Johnsen K, Lindholm LH, Mogensen CE, Dahlof B, Devereux RB, de Faire U, Fyhrquist F, Julius S, Kjeldsen SE, Lederballe-Pedersen O, Nieminen MS, Omvik P, Oparil S, Wan Y. Reduction in albuminuria translates to reduction in cardiovascular events in hypertensive patients: losartan intervention for endpoint reduction in hypertension study. Hypertension. 2005;45:198–202.

32. Abramson JL, Jurkovitz CT, Vaccarino V, Weintraub WS, McClellan W. Chronic kidney disease, anemia, and incident stroke in a middle-aged, community-based population: the aric study. Kidney Int. 2003;64:610–5.

33. Koren-Morag N, Goldbourt U, Tanne D. Renal dysfunction and risk of ischemic stroke or tia in patients with cardiovascular disease. Neurology. 2006;67:224–8.

34. Sarnak MJ, Levey AS, Schoolwerth AC, Coresh J, Culleton B, Hamm LL, McCullough PA, Kasiske BL, Kelepouris E, Klag MJ. Kidney disease as a risk factor for development of cardiovascular disease a statement from the american heart association councils on kidney in cardiovascular disease, high blood pressure research, clinical cardiology, and epidemiology and prevention. Circulation. 2003;108:2154–69.

35. Ansquer J-C, Foucher C, Rattier S, Taskinen M-R, Steiner G. Fenofibrate reduces progression to microalbuminuria over 3 years in a placebo-controlled study in type 2 diabetes: results from the diabetes atherosclerosis intervention study (dais). Am J Kidney Dis. 2005;45:485–93.

36. Epstein FH, Welch GN, Loscalzo J. Homocysteine and atherothrombosis. N Engl J Med. 1998;338:1042–50.

37. Coresh J, Astor B, Sarnak MJ. Evidence for increased cardiovascular disease risk in patients with chronic kidney disease. Curr Opin Nephrol Hypertens. 2004;13:73–81.

38. Tozawa M, Iseki K, Iseki C, Kinjo K, Ikemiya Y, Takishita S. Blood pressure predicts risk of developing end-stage renal disease in men and women. Hypertension. 2003;41:1341–5.

39. Mann JF, Gerstein HC, Pogue J, Bosch J, Yusuf S. Renal insufficiency as a predictor of cardiovascular outcomes and the impact of ramipril: The hope randomized trial. Ann Intern Med. 2001; 134:629–36.

40. Böhm M, Thoenes M, Danchin N, Bramlage P, La Puerta P, Volpe M. Association of cardiovascular risk factors with micro-albuminuria in hypertensive individuals: the i-search global study. J Hypertens. 2007;25:2317–24.

41. Mancia G, Grassi G, Giannattasio C, Seravalle G. Sympathetic activation in the pathogenesis of hypertension and progression of organ damage. Hypertension. 1999;34:724–8.

42. Masuo K, Mikami H, Ogihara T, Tuck M. Hormonal mechanisms in blood pressure reduction during hemodialysis in patients with chronic renal failure. Hypertens Res. 1995;18 Suppl 1: S201–3.

43. Mena-Martin FJ, Martin-Escudero JC, Simal-Blanco F, Carretero-Ares JL, Arzua-Mouronte D, Castrodeza Sanz JJ. Influence of sympathetic activity on blood pressure and vascular damage evaluated by means of urinary albumin excretion. J Clin Hypertens (Greenwich). 2006;8:619–24.

44. Cohn JN, Levine TB, Olivari MT, Garberg V, Lura D, Francis GS, Simon AB, Rector T. Plasma norepinephrine as a guide to prognosis in patients with chronic congestive heart failure. N Engl J Med. 1984;311:819–23.

45. Rudberg S, Østerby R, Bangstad H-J, Dahlquist G, Persson B. Effect of angiotensin converting enzyme inhibitor or beta blocker on glomerular structural changes in young microalbuminuric patients with type i (insulin-dependent) diabetes mellitus. Diabetologia. 1999;42: 589–95.

46. Rao F, Wessel J, Wen G, Zhang L, Rana BK, Kennedy BP, Greenwood TA, Salem RM, Chen Y, Khandrika S, Hamilton BA, Smith DW, Holstein-Rathlou NH, Ziegler MG, Schork NJ, O'Connor DT. Renal albumin excretion: twin studies identify influences of heredity, environment, and adrenergic pathway polymorphism. Hypertension. 2007;49:1015–31.

47. Bertog SC, Sobotka PA, Sievert H. Renal denervation for hypertension. JACC Cardiovasc Interv. 2012;5:249–58.

48. Bell-Reuss E, Trevino D, Gottschalk C. Effect of renal sympathetic nerve stimulation on proximal water and sodium reabsorption. J Clin Invest. 1976;57:1104.

49. Francisco LL, Sawin LL, DiBona GF. Renal sympathetic nerve activity and the exaggerated natriuresis of the spontaneous hypertensive rat. Hypertension. 1981;3:134–8.

50. Kirchheim H, Ehmke H, Persson P. Sympathetic modulation of renal hemodynamics, renin release and sodium excretion. Klin Wochenschr. 1989;67:858–64.

51. Kopp UC, Cicha MZ, Smith LA, Mulder J, Hökfelt T. Renal sympathetic nerve activity modulates afferent renal nerve activity by pge2-dependent activation of α1-and α2-adrenoceptors on renal sensory nerve fibers. Am J Physiol-Regul Integr Comp Physiol. 2007;293:R1561–72.

52. Vecchione C, Maffei A, Colella S, Aretini A, Poulet R, Frati G, Gentile MT, Fratta L, Trimarco V, Trimarco B. Leptin effect on endothelial nitric oxide is mediated through akt–endothelial nitric oxide synthase phosphorylation pathway. Diabetes. 2002;51: 168–73.

53. Lembo G, Vecchione C, Fratta L, Marino G, Trimarco V, D'Amati G, Trimarco B. Leptin induces direct vasodilation through distinct endothelial mechanisms. Diabetes. 2000;49:293–7.

54. Kopp UC, Smith LA, DiBona GF. Renorenal reflexes: neural components of ipsilateral and contralateral renal responses. Am J Physiol-Ren Physiol. 1985;249:F507–17.

55. Kopp UC, Olson LA, DiBona GF. Renorenal reflex responses to mechano-and chemoreceptor stimulation in the dog and rat. Am J Physiol-Ren Physiol. 1984;246:F67–77.

56. Kopp UC, Smith LA, DiBona GF. Facilitatory role of efferent renal nerve activity on renal sensory receptors. Am J Physiol-Ren Physiol. 1987;253:F767–77.

57. Kopp UC, Cicha MZ, Smith LA. Dietary sodium loading increases arterial pressure in afferent renal–denervated rats. Hypertension. 2003;42:968–73.

58. Mancia G. Sympathetic activation in congestive heart failure. Eur Heart J. 1990;11:3–11.

59. Rundqvist B, Elam M, Bergmann-Sverrisdottir Y, Eisenhofer G, Friberg P. Increased cardiac adrenergic drive precedes generalized sympathetic activation in human heart failure. Circulation. 1997;95:169–75.

60. Pettersson A, Hedner J, Hedner T. Renal interaction between sympathetic activity and anp in rats with chronic ischaemic heart failure. Acta Physiol Scand. 1989;135:487–92.

61. Brandt MC, Mahfoud F, Reda S, Schirmer SH, Erdmann E, Bohm M, Hoppe UC. Renal sympathetic denervation reduces left ventricular hypertrophy and improves cardiac function in patients with resistant hypertension. J Am Coll Cardiol. 2012;59:901–9.

62. Mahfoud F, Urban D, Teller D, Linz D, Stawowy P, Hassel JH, Fries P, Dreysse S, Wellnhofer E, Schneider G, Buecker A, Schneeweis C, Doltra A, Schlaich MP, Esler MD, Fleck E, Böhm M, Kelle S. Effect of renal denervation on left ventricular mass and function in patients with resistant hypertension: data from a multicentre cardiovascular magnetic resonance imaging trial. Eur Heart J. 2014;35(33):2224–31.

63. Pokushalov E, Romanov A, Corbucci G, Artyomenko S, Baranova V, Turov A, Shirokova N, Karaskov A, Mittal S, Steinberg JS. A randomized comparison of pulmonary vein isolation with versus without concomitant renal artery denervation in patients with refractory symptomatic atrial fibrillation and resistant hypertension. J Am Coll Cardiol. 2012;60:1163–70.

64. Linz D, Mahfoud F, Schotten U, Ukena C, Neuberger H-R, Wirth K, Böhm M. Renal sympathetic denervation suppresses postapneic blood pressure rises and atrial fibrillation in a model for sleep apnea. Hypertension. 2012;60:172–8.

65. Davies JE, Manisty CH, Petraco R, Barron AJ, Unsworth B, Mayet J, Hamady M, Hughes AD, Sever PS, Sobotka PA. First-in-man safety evaluation of renal denervation for chronic systolic heart failure: primary outcome from reach-pilot study. Int J Cardiol. 2013;162:189–92.

66. Ukena C, Bauer A, Mahfoud F, Schreieck J, Neuberger HR, Eick C, Sobotka PA, Gawaz M, Bohm M. Renal sympathetic denervation for treatment of electrical storm: first-in-man experience. Clin Res Cardiol. 2012;101:63–7.

Diabetes and Metabolic Syndrome

Felix Mahfoud, Sebastian Ewen, and Michael Böhm

Introduction

Chronic activation of the sympathetic nervous system has been associated with the components of the metabolic syndrome, such as hyperinsulinemia, type 2 diabetes, and obesity [1, 2]. The metabolic syndrome, which is extremely common worldwide and can be found in approximately 30 % of patients with essential hypertension, identifying patients at high cardiovascular risk [3, 4]. Approximately 70 % of incident hypertension is associated with overweight and obesity. Over 50 % of patients with essential hypertension are hyperinsulinemic, regardless of whether they are untreated or in a stable program of treatment [5]. Elevated fasting glucose levels, impaired glucose tolerance and diabetes have been associated with an increased risk of cardiovascular disease [6–9], due to stimulation of inflammation, oxidative stress and thrombotic potential [10], as well as inhibition of vascular smooth muscle cell apoptosis [11]. Insulin resistance is involved in the pathogenesis of type 2 diabetes mellitus with a progression from impaired fasting glycaemia to impaired glucose tolerance and finally to overt diabetes. The Spanish Ambulatory Pressure Monitory registry [12] included 70,000 patients and identified 8,300 (12 %) to be resistant to drug treatment, of these 35 % were diagnosed as diabetics, representing the most common comorbidity.

Pathophysiology

Heightened central sympathetic activity is an accepted contributor to insulin resistance [13], metabolic syndrome [14], associated with central obesity, and risk of developing

F. Mahfoud, MD (✉) • S. Ewen, MD • M. Böhm, MD
Klinik für Innere Medizin III, Kardiologie, Angiologie und Internistische Intensivmedizin, Universitätsklinikum des Saarlandes, Kirrberger Str. 1, Homburg/Saar 66421, Germany
e-mail: felix.mahfoud@uks.eu; Sebastian.Ewen@uks.eu; Michael.boehm@uks.eu

diabetes [1]. Data confirms a reciprocal relation wherein heightened central sympathetic activity contributes to insulin resistance, metabolic syndrome and risk of developing diagnosed diabetes, as well as the converse, where these clinical conditions themselves contribute to central sympathetic drive [3]. The combination of essential hypertension and diabetes mellitus type 2 has been associated with the greatest sympathetic hyperactivity as measured by resting muscle sympathetic nerve activity (MSNA) compared to each condition by itself (Fig. 23.1) [1].

There is also preclinical data pointing towards a potential beneficial effect of renal denervation in metabolic syndrome. Renal denervation has been investigated in a chronically instrumented, high-fat fed dog model, which is characterized by sodium retention and increased sympathetic nervous system activation. Whilst the high fat diet resulted in a 50 % increase in body mass in both control and denervated dogs, blood pressure increased significantly only in the control but not in the denervated dogs. Furthermore, sodium retention was reduced by 50 % in the denervated dogs.

The predominant mechanism linking sympathetic drive to insulin resistance is likely related to sympathetically mediated redistribution of blood flow from insulin sensitive striated muscle, towards insulin insensitive fat tissue [3]. As such, in the human forearm, increased noradrenaline release results in a substantial reduction in forearm blood flow [15]. It has been proposed that pressure induced restriction of the microcirculation limits nutritional flow, and thereby impairs glucose uptake in the skeletal muscle [16]. There is clinical and experimental data indicating that there is (i) a direct relationship between sympathetic nerve activity to the skeletal muscle tissue and insulin resistance and (ii) that insulin resistance is inversely related to the number of open capillaries [17]. In turn, increased levels of insulin exhibit sympathoexcitatory effects [18, 19], contributing to activation of the sympathetic nervous system with its pathophysiological consequences. There is a bidirectional relationship between sympathetic overactivity inducing insulin resistance and hyperinsulinemia producing sympathetic activation, thus initiating a vicious cycle (Fig. 23.2).

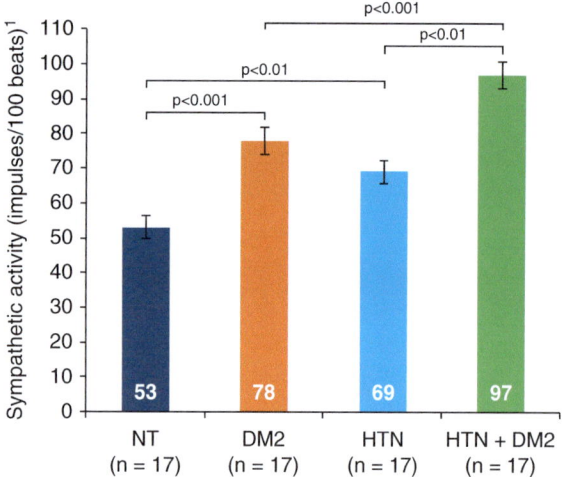

Fig. 23.1 Sympathetic activity measured by MSNA in normotensive controls (*NT*), diabetes mellitus type 2 (*DM2*), hypertension (*HTN*) and metabolic syndrome (*HTN + DM2*) (Modified from Huggett et al. [1])

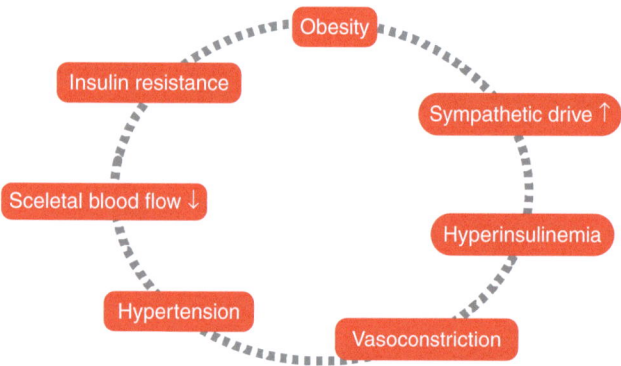

Fig. 23.2 Vicious circle initiated by increased sympathetic activity

The gold standard in diagnosing insulin resistance is the hyperinsulinemic-euglycemic clam method, but this approach is not suitable for routine clinical practice. Thus, less invasive methods for evaluation, like homeostasis model assessment (HOMA-IR = (Glucose × Insulin)/405)), were developed. HOMA-IR is an established parameter for evaluation of insulin resistance [20, 21], correlating to the results of hyperinsulinemic-euglycemic clamp [22]. There is a direct relationship between the central sympathetic activity, measured by muscle sympathetic nerve activity, and the HOMA-IR [13].

In line, inhibition of the sympathetic nervous system by moxonidine has been shown to improve glucose metabolism by decreasing glucagon secretion and increasing skeletal blood flow with less glycogenolysis and gluconeogenesis [23], which confirms the pathophysiological relation between central nervous system and insulin resistance [24]. However, the use of centrally acting sympatholytics is limited by adverse effects, leading to high non-adherence rates [25].

Effects of Renal Denervation on Glucose Metabolism

Since renal denervation has a favorable safety profile and results in marked reduction of the sympathetic activity measured by MSNA [26, 27], the benefits of the procedure may not be restricted to treat resistant hypertension. A recently published pilot study investigated the effect of renal denervation on glucose metabolism and insulin resistance in patients with resistant hypertension [28]. Fifty patients with resistant hypertension were included in the study (37 underwent renal denervation, 13 served as controls), 40 % were diabetics. Beside significant blood pressure reduction observed in the treatment group (−32/−12 mmHg; p < 0.001) after 3 months, fasting glucose (from 118 ± 3.4 mg/dl to 108 ± 3.8 mg/dl; p = 0.039), insulin levels (from 20.8 ± 3.0 to 9.3 ± 2.5 μIU/ml; p = 0.006), C-peptide levels (from 5.3 ± 0.6 ng/ml to 3.0 ± 0.9 ng/ml; p = 0.002) and the HOMA-IR improved significantly from 6.0 ± 0.9 to 2.4 ± 0.8 (p = 0.001) after 3 months (Fig. 23.3). Additionally, mean 2-h glucose levels during oral glucose tolerance test were reduced by 27 mg/dl (p = 0.012, Fig. 23.4) while there were no significant changes in blood pressure or any of the metabolic markers described above in the control group. Body mass index and antihypertensive background medication remained unchanged during the study period.

Polycystic Ovary Syndrome

These findings are supported by investigations of patients with polycystic ovary syndrome (PCOS) [29]. PCOS is characterized by obesity, insulin resistance and BP elevation related to sympathetic nervous activation. Using the hyperinsulinaemic-euglycaemic clamp methodology it was demonstrated that insulin sensitivity improved by 17.5 % in the absence of any weight change at 3 months following renal denervation. Beside the improvements in glucose metabolism authors also report a reduction in sympathetic activity measured by MSNA, urinary albumin excretion and glomerular hyperfiltration, indicating beneficial effects of renal denervation on renal structure and function. These findings are of interest as renal denervation has been shown to prevent the development of structural renal changes due to early diabetic nephropathy in an animal model [30]. Functional and anatomic studies performed 2 weeks after the onset of streptozotocin-induced diabetes in denervated rats revealed attenuation of physiologic and anatomic findings of early diabetic nephropathy. In line, studies in humans demonstrated that sympathoinhibition with the centrally acting drug moxonidine reduced microalbuminuria in normotensive patients with type 1 diabetes, in the absence of any significant blood pressure changes [31]. This is supported by

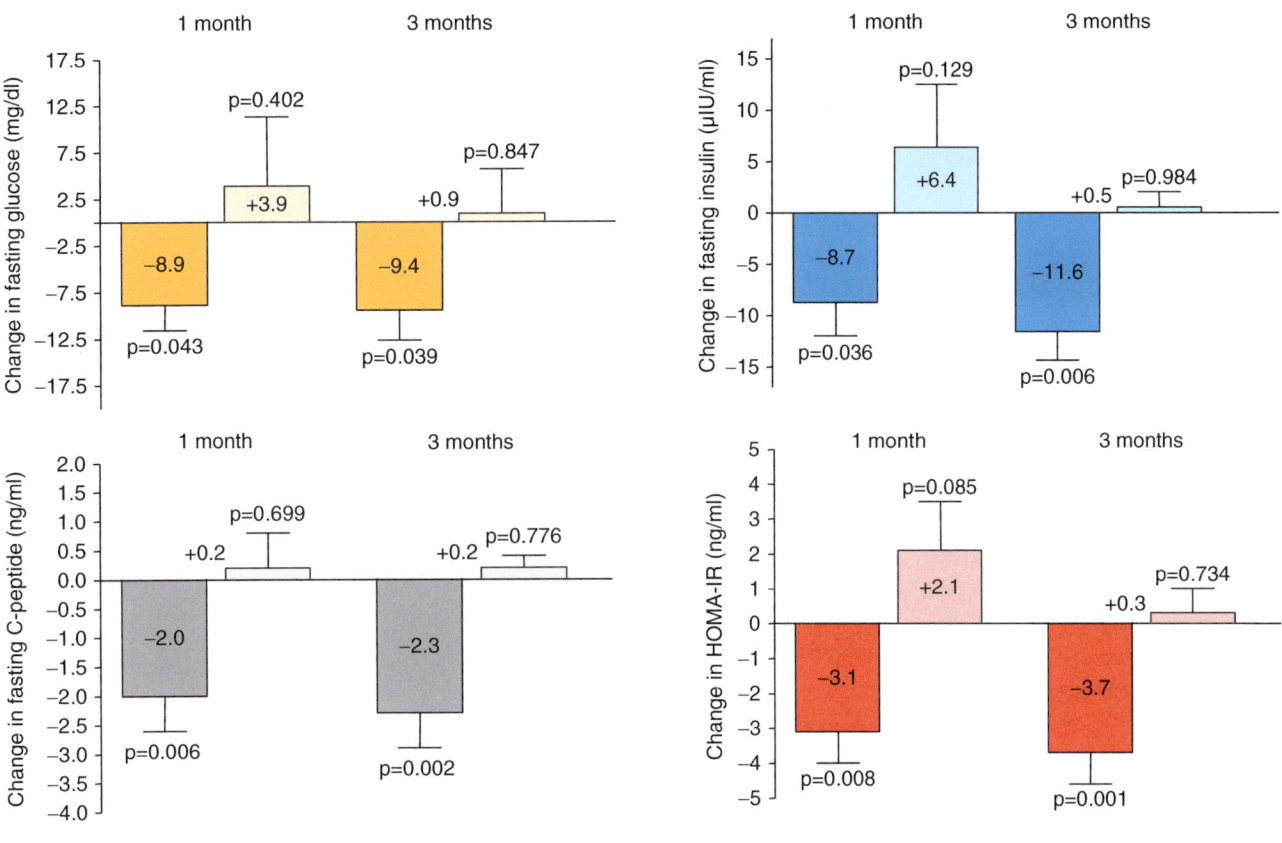

Fig. 23.3 Change in fasting glucose, insulin levels, C-peptide levels, and the HOMA-IR in patients undergoing renal denervation and in the control group (Modified from Mahfoud et al. [28])

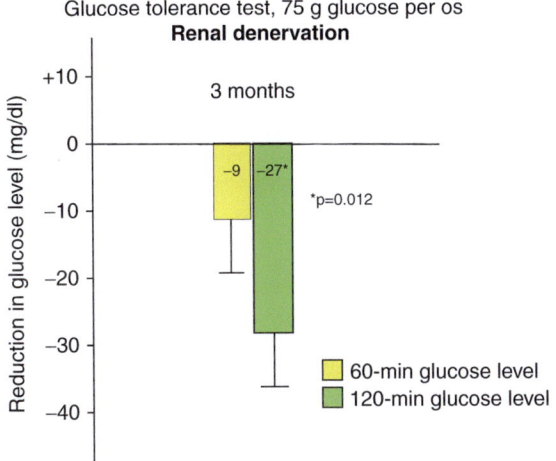

Fig. 23.4 Change in 60- and 120-min glucose level (n=37) after administration of glucose 3 months after renal denervation (Modified from Mahfoud et al. [28])

recently published data, investigating the effects of renal denervation on urinary albumin excretion in 100 patients with resistant hypertension and preserved renal function. The study demonstrated a reduced number of patients with micro- and macroalbuminuria after renal denervation and improvements in renal hemodynamics [32].

Obstructive Sleep Apnea

Individuals with obstructive sleep apnea syndrome (OSAS) are usually obese and have high prevalence of the metabolic syndrome [3]. OSAS itself is characterized by an increased sympathetic activity [33]. A recently published pilot study investigated the effects of renal denervation on OSAS severity and glucose metabolism in patients with resistant hypertension [34]. This observational series has confirmed significant reduction in blood pressure (−34/−13 mmHg; p<0.01) and improvement in the OSAS severity in eight of ten enrolled patients 6 months after renal denervation. Decreases were also observed in plasma glucose concentration 2 h after glucose administration (median: 7.0 versus 6.4 mmol/L; p=0.05) and in hemoglobin A1C level (median: 6.1 % versus 5.6 %; p<0.05) at 6 months (Table 23.1). A larger randomized controlled trial investigating the effect of renal denervation in patients with OSAS is currently ongoing (NCT01366625).

Table 23.1 Change in glucose metabolism and obstructive sleep apnea severity after renal denervation (n = 10)

	Baseline	3 months	6 months
AHI, events/h	30.7 ± 26.5	20.0 ± 25.3	16.1 ± 22.2
Epworth sleepiness scale score, points	9	6.5 (p = ns)	7 (p < 0.05)
120 min glucose level, OGTT, mmol/l	8.4 ± 3.3	6.8 ± 2.5 (p = 0.051)	6.8 ± 2.9 (p < 0.05)
HbA1C, %	6.4 ± 0.8	6.0 ± 0.7 (p < 0.05)	5.9 ± 0.7 (p < 0.05)

Created using data from Witkowski et al. [34]

Outlook

Since renal denervation in patients with resistant hypertension has been shown to reduce sympathetic activity and blood pressure [35–37], improve glucose metabolism and glucose tolerance, it may be speculated that this treatment prolongs or even prevents the progression of type 2 diabetes and associated cardiovascular complications. The estimated change in cardiovascular risk associated with blood pressure reduction and improvement in diabetic state appears to be more than additive. Preclinical observations on renal protection against diabetic glomerular sclerosis coupled with the human data on renal denervation resulting in reduced blood pressure with improved insulin sensitivity and urinary albumin excretion justify additional studies in this area. Substantial research is needed to (i) enhance the understanding on the potential retinal, renal and cardiovascular consequences of these findings and (ii) to document the durability of the results.

References

1. Huggett RJ, Scott EM, Gilbey SG, Stoker JB, Mackintosh AF, Mary DA. Impact of type 2 diabetes mellitus on sympathetic neural mechanisms in hypertension. Circulation. 2003;108(25):3097–101.
2. Vollenweider P, Tappy L, Randin D, Schneiter P, Jequier E, Nicod P, Scherrer U. Differential effects of hyperinsulinemia and carbohydrate metabolism on sympathetic nerve activity and muscle blood flow in humans. J Clin Invest. 1993;92(1):147–54.
3. Mancia G, Bousquet P, Elghozi JL, Esler M, Grassi G, Julius S, Reid J, Van Zwieten PA. The sympathetic nervous system and the metabolic syndrome. J Hypertens. 2007;25(5):909–20.
4. Kannel WB. Blood pressure as a cardiovascular risk factor: prevention and treatment. JAMA. 1996;275(20):1571–6.
5. Lima NK, Abbasi F, Lamendola C, Reaven GM. Prevalence of insulin resistance and related risk factors for cardiovascular disease in patients with essential hypertension. Am J Hypertens. 2009; 22(1):106–11.
6. Fuller JH, Shipley MJ, Rose G, Jarrett RJ, Keen H. Coronary-heart-disease risk and impaired glucose tolerance. The Whitehall study. Lancet. 1980;1(8183):1373–6.
7. Levitan EB, Song Y, Ford ES, Liu S. Is nondiabetic hyperglycemia a risk factor for cardiovascular disease? A meta-analysis of prospective studies. Arch Intern Med. 2004;164(19):2147–55.
8. The Emerging Risk Factors C. Diabetes mellitus, fasting blood glucose concentration, and risk of vascular disease: a collaborative meta-analysis of 102 prospective studies. Lancet. 2010;375 (9733):2215–22.
9. Gerstein HC. More insights on the dysglycaemia-cardiovascular connection. Lancet. 2010;375(9733):2195–6.
10. Brand-Miller J, Dickinson S, Barclay A, Celermajer D. The glycemic index and cardiovascular disease risk. Curr Atheroscler Rep. 2007;9(6):479–85.
11. Hall JL, Matter CM, Wang X, Gibbons GH. Hyperglycemia inhibits vascular smooth muscle cell apoptosis through a protein kinase C-dependent pathway. Circ Res. 2000;87(7):574–80.
12. de la Sierra A, Segura J, Banegas JR, Gorostidi M, de la Cruz JJ, Armario P, Oliveras A, Ruilope LM. Clinical features of 8295 patients with resistant hypertension classified on the basis of ambulatory blood pressure monitoring. Hypertension. 2011;57(5): 898–902.
13. Grassi G, Dell'Oro R, Facchini A, Quarti Trevano F, Bolla GB, Mancia G. Effect of central and peripheral body fat distribution on sympathetic and baroreflex function in obese normotensives. J Hypertens. 2004;22(12):2363–9.
14. Grassi G, Seravalle G, Quarti-Trevano F, Scopelliti F, Dell'Oro R, Bolla G, Mancia G. Excessive sympathetic activation in heart failure with obesity and metabolic syndrome: characteristics and mechanisms. Hypertension. 2007;49(3):535–41.
15. Jamerson KA, Julius S, Gudbrandsson T, Andersson O, Brant DO. Reflex sympathetic activation induces acute insulin resistance in the human forearm. Hypertension. 1993;21(5):618–23.
16. Julius S, Gudbrandsson T, Jamerson K, Tariq Shahab S, Andersson O. The hemodynamic link between insulin resistance and hypertension. J Hypertens. 1991;9(11):983–6.
17. Schlaich MP, Hering D, Sobotka P, Krum H, Lambert GW, Lambert E, Esler MD. Effects of renal denervation on sympathetic activation, blood pressure, and glucose metabolism in patients with resistant hypertension. Front Physiol. 2012;3:10.
18. Scherrer U, Sartori C. Insulin as a vascular and sympathoexcitatory hormone: implications for blood pressure regulation, insulin sensitivity, and cardiovascular morbidity. Circulation. 1997;96(11): 4104–13.
19. Bardgett ME, McCarthy JJ, Stocker SD. Glutamatergic receptor activation in the rostral ventrolateral medulla mediates the sympathoexcitatory response to hyperinsulinemia. Hypertension. 2010;55(2):284–90.
20. Katz A, Nambi SS, Mather K, Baron AD, Follmann DA, Sullivan G, Quon MJ. Quantitative insulin sensitivity check index: a simple, accurate method for assessing insulin sensitivity in humans. J Clin Endocrinol Metab. 2000;85(7):2402–10.
21. Matthews DR, Hosker JP, Rudenski AS, Naylor BA, Treacher DF, Turner RC. Homeostasis model assessment: insulin resistance and beta-cell function from fasting plasma glucose and insulin concentrations in man. Diabetologia. 1985;28(7):412–9.
22. Chen H, Sullivan G, Yue LQ, Katz A, Quon MJ. QUICKI is a useful index of insulin sensitivity in subjects with hypertension. Am J Physiol Endocrinol Metab. 2003;284(4):E804–12.
23. Yakubu-Madus FE, Johnson WT, Zimmerman KM, Dananberg J, Steinberg MI. Metabolic and hemodynamic effects of moxonidine in the Zucker diabetic fatty rat model of type 2 diabetes. Diabetes. 1999;48(5):1093–100.

24. Rocchini AP, Mao HZ, Babu K, Marker P, Rocchini AJ. Clonidine prevents insulin resistance and hypertension in obese dogs. Hypertension. 1999;33(1 Pt 2):548–53.

25. Prichard BN, Jager BA, Luszick JH, Kuster LJ, Verboom CN, Hughes PR, Sauermann W, Kuppers HE. Placebo-controlled comparison of the efficacy and tolerability of once-daily moxonidine and enalapril in mild to moderate essential hypertension. Blood Press. 2002;11(3):166–72.

26. Lenski M, Mahfoud F, Razouk A, Ukena C, Lenski D, Barth C, Linz D, Laufs U, Kindermann I, Böhm M. Orthostatic function after renal sympathetic denervation in patients with resistant hypertension. Int J Cardiol 2013;169:418–24.

27. Hering D, Lambert EA, Marusic P, Walton AS, Krum H, Lambert GW, Esler MD, Schlaich MP. Substantial reduction in single sympathetic nerve firing after renal denervation in patients with resistant hypertension. Hypertension. 2013;61(2):457–64.

28. Mahfoud F, Schlaich M, Kindermann I, Ukena C, Cremers B, Brandt MC, Hoppe UC, Vonend O, Rump LC, Sobotka PA, Krum H, Esler M, Böhm M. Effect of renal sympathetic denervation on glucose metabolism in patients with resistant hypertension: a pilot study. Circulation. 2011;123(18):1940–6.

29. Schlaich MP, Straznicky N, Grima M, Ika-Sari C, Dawood T, Mahfoud F, Lambert E, Chopra R, Socratous F, Hennebry S, Eikelis N, Böhm M, Krum H, Lambert G, Esler MD, Sobotka PA. Renal denervation: a potential new treatment modality for polycystic ovary syndrome? J Hypertens. 2011;29(5):991–6.

30. Luippold G, Beilharz M, Muhlbauer B. Chronic renal denervation prevents glomerular hyperfiltration in diabetic rats. NDT. 2004; 19(2):342–7.

31. Strojek K, Grzeszczak W, Gorska J, Leschinger MI, Ritz E. Lowering of microalbuminuria in diabetic patients by a sympathicoplegic agent: novel approach to prevent progression of diabetic nephropathy? J Am Soc Nephrol. 2001;12(3):602–5.

32. Mahfoud F, Cremers B, Janker J, Link B, Vonend O, Ukena C, Linz D, Schmieder R, Rump LC, Kindermann I, Sobotka PA, Krum H, Scheller B, Schlaich M, Laufs U, Böhm M. Renal hemodynamics and renal function after catheter-based renal sympathetic denervation in patients with resistant hypertension. Hypertension. 2012;60(2):419–24.

33. Narkiewicz K, van de Borne PJ, Cooley RL, Dyken ME, Somers VK. Sympathetic activity in obese subjects with and without obstructive sleep apnea. Circulation. 1998;98(8):772–6.

34. Witkowski A, Prejbisz A, Florczak E, Kadziela J, Sliwinski P, Bielen P, Michalowska I, Kabat M, Warchol E, Januszewicz M, Narkiewicz K, Somers VK, Sobotka PA, Januszewicz A. Effects of renal sympathetic denervation on blood pressure, sleep apnea course, and glycemic control in patients with resistant hypertension and sleep apnea. Hypertension. 2011;58(4):559–65.

35. Krum H, Barman N, Schlaich M, Sobotka P, Esler M, Mahfoud F, Böhm M, Dunlap M. Catheter-based renal sympathetic denervation for resistant hypertension: durability of blood pressure reduction out to 24 months. Hypertension. 2011;57(5):911–7.

36. Esler MD, Krum H, Sobotka PA, Schlaich MP, Schmieder RE, Böhm M. Renal sympathetic denervation in patients with treatment-resistant hypertension (The Symplicity HTN-2 Trial): a randomised controlled trial. Lancet. 2010;376(9756):1903–9.

37. Schlaich MP, Sobotka PA, Krum H, Lambert E, Esler MD. Renal sympathetic-nerve ablation for uncontrolled hypertension. N Engl J Med. 2009;361(9):932–4.

Obstructive Sleep Apnea

Adam Witkowski and Jacek Kądziela

Epidemiology of Obstructive Sleep Apnea

The prevalence of sleep apnea in general population varies from 5 to 10 % [1]. In general population and in patients with cardiovascular diseases, obstructive sleep apnea (OSA) is two to three times more common in men than in women and in older than in the young [2]. In hypertensive subjects the diagnosis of OSA is based on polysomnography – it is confirmed when apnea-hypopnea index (AHI) exceeds 15 events/h [3]. OSA is the most common disease associated with resistant hypertension – according to abovementioned definition it was diagnosed in 64 % of patients. In hypertensive patients OSA is associated with obesity. However in patients with heart failure and stroke direct relationship between body mass index and OSA severity was not firmly proved [4–6].

OSA is considered independent risk factor for cardiovascular events, including ischemic heart disease, heart failure, stroke and death [7]. Several mechanisms as inflammation, oxidative stress, and endothelial dysfunction underlie the association between OSA and cardiovascular diseases [8, 9]. Continuous positive airway pressure (CPAP) is a treatment of choice to reverse severe OSA and its consequences [2, 10].

Pathophysiology of Obstructive Sleep Apnea

OSA is characterized by recurrent episodes of complete or partial upper airway obstruction during sleep [11]. OSA occurs when sleep-related inhibition of respiratory drive to the upper airway dilator muscles is superimposed on previ-

Conflict of Interest Statement
Professor Adam Witkowski – consultancy and proctoring fees from Medtronic
Dr Jacek Kądziela – consultancy and proctoring fees from Medtronic

A. Witkowski, MD, PhD, FESC (✉) • J. Kądziela, MD, PhD
Department of Interventional Cardiology and Angiology, Institute of Cardiology, 42 Alpejska Street, Warsaw 04-628, Poland
e-mail: witkowski@hbz.pl; Kadziela@ikard.pl

ously narrowed airway [2]. The upper airway may be narrowed due to macroglossia, tonsillar hypertrophy or increased fatty deposits in surrounding neck tissues. In addition, peripharyngeal fluid retention and its rostral nocturnal shift while sleeping was postulated as a reason for increasing of peripahryngeal tissue mass. Recumbent position provokes neck veins distension and edema of surrounding soft tissue that increases the upper airway resistance and facilitates its obstruction. In different scenarios (heart failure, chronic kidney disease, hypertension, obesity) increased sodium and water retention may be dietary [12], neurogenic – resulting from increased sympathetic activity leading to renin release [13], or humoral – as a consequence of activation of the renin-angiotensin-aldosteron axis [14]. It has been demonstrated that in response to the application of lower body positive pressure, neck circumference increases and the pharyngeal cross-sectional area decreases resulting in higher pharyngeal resistance and collapsibility [15, 16]. Simultaneously, leg fluid volume is reduced confirming that changes of upper airway resistance are secondary to the fluid shift towards the peripharyngeal area. In other study including non-obese healthy subject, direct relationship between the volume of the nocturnal fluid shift and the change of neck circumference and severity of OSA was reported [17]. Moreover, in patients with chronic venous insufficiency, the use of compression stockings diminished daytime fluid accumulation in the legs and overnight fluid shift and, by consequence, reduced AHI by 35 % [18]. The another evidence that nocturnal rostral fluid shift can cause OSA was provided by two studies, demonstrating that fluid removal using overnight peritoneal dialysis in patients with chronic renal failure increased pharyngeal upper airway diameter and alleviated OSA severity as compared to the removal of the same amount of fluid with continuous 24-h dialysis [19, 20]. Similar improvement was confirmed by the conversion of hemodialysis from daytime to overnight procedure [21].

Another potential mechanism linking OSA and fluid retention is hyperaldosteronism that is very common in subjects with resistant hypertension. Aldosterone-mediated chronic fluid retention may influence OSA severity in patients with resistant hypertension. In one study treatment with a mineralocorticoid receptor antagonist substantially reduced the severity of OSA [14].

Relationship Between Hypertension and Obstructive Sleep Apnea

It is known that intermittent hypoxia or experimentally induced OSA can cause persistent daytime hypertension in rats and dogs [22, 23]. In one study it was demonstrated that subjects with an AHI ≥15 had almost threefold greater likelihood of developing hypertension than those with an AHI of zero [24], however other studies did not confirmed this association [25, 26]. Nevertheless, the remarkable finding that OSA is by far the most common disease associated with drug resistant hypertension and that its treatment may lower blood pressure suggest that OSA plays a provocative role in the hypertension pathogenesis [27].

Sympathetic Neural Mechanisms in Resistant Hypertension and Obstructive Sleep Apnea

Increased sympathetic activity, consistently evident in OSA patients, likely plays a key role in the development of resistant hypertension. Autonomic and hemodynamic responses to obstructive sleep apnea are very complex and include the effects of apnea, hypoxia, hypercapnia, the Mueller maneuver (inspiration against a closed glottis), and arousal [28]. Hypoxia and hypercapnia act synergistically in increasing sympathetic activity and this increase is especially marked during apnea [29–32]. The role of sympathetic activation in OSA patients was further elucidated in a study by Somers et al. [33]. Patients with OSA had high sympathetic activity when awake, with further increment in blood pressure and sympathetic activity during sleep. These increases are attenuated by treatment with CPAP, indicating that OSA induces sympathetic activation and facilitates blood pressure rises during sleep. Sympathetic over-activation in OSA patients also acts to increase heart rate [34] and can worsen the prognosis of patients with cardiovascular diseases, specifically by causing cardiac ß-adrenoreceptor desensitization, arrhythmias, myocyte injury and necrosis and peripheral vasoconstriction [35]. It may also promote renal sodium retention, both directly and through stimulation of the renin-angiotensin-aldosterone axis.

Renal Denervation in Resistant Hypertension and Obstructive Sleep Apnea

Animal Studies

In an experimental study by Linz et al. renal denervation (RDN) but not treatment with ß-blocker inhibited post-apneic blood pressure rises in pigs [36]. RDN also induced antiarrhythmic effect by reducing atrial fibrillation inducibility by modulation of the autonomic nervous system. In another paper RDN induced elevation of urine volume and sodium excretion in rats with acute total obstructive apnea [37]. This suggests that the increase of the renal sympathetic nerve activity during apnea episodes does prevent the elevation of renal excretory function in non-denervated animals. It supports the hypothesis that renal sympathetic nerves play an important role in sodium homeostasis, with renal nerve activation enhancing sodium retention and suppression the sympathetic activity by RDN may impose opposite effect.

Human Experience

The potential impact of renal sympathetic denervation on sleep apnea course was reported in one human study [38]. The study included ten patients with resistant hypertension (defined as systolic office blood pressure greater than 160 mmHg despite the treatment with three or more antihypertensive drugs including diuretic) and sleep apnea. OSA was diagnosed in eight patients and mixed sleep apnea (obstructive and central) in two. There were five patients with mild sleep apnea (AHI 5–15 events/h) and five patients with moderate-to-severe apnea (AHI >15 events/h). Two patients were treated with CPAP before RDN and maintained this treatment during follow-up period. All patients underwent catheter-based radiofrequency RDN (Symplicity, Medtronic, Minneapolis, MN, USA) The median reduction of systolic blood pressure was 22 mmHg (p<0.01) and 34 mmHg (p<0.01) at 3 and 6 months after RDN, respectively (Fig. 24.1), with no differences between the patients with mild and moderate-to-severe sleep apnea.

Decreases in AHI at 3 months (non-significant) and at 6 months (with a tendency towards significance) after RDN were noted (median 16.3 events/h before RDN versus median 4.5 events/h after 6 months; p=0.059). Also decreases in oxygen desaturation indices (ODI) at 6 months (median 13.0 events/h before RDN versus median 8.7 events/h; p=0.11) and decreases in median Epworth Sleepiness Scale score at 6 months (9.00 points versus 7.00 points; p<0.05) were also reported. In summary, in eight of ten patients an improvement in AHI was observed at 6 month (Fig. 24.2). There were two patients with mixed sleep apnea. In one of them, a reduction in sleep apnea indices was also observed with a change in AHI −30.5 events per hour at 6 months. In patients with improvement in AHI, a significant decrease in 24-h, daytime, and nighttime ambulatory Blood pressure monitoring (ABPM) levels was observed, the latter being most pronounced (median: −8/−4 mmHg, −12/−5 mmHg and −10/−8 mmHg for 24-h, daytime, and nighttime, respectively; p<0.05 for all).

Along with blood pressure reduction and sleep apnea course improvement significant decreases in plasma glucose

Fig. 24.1 Median systolic and diastolic BP changes after renal sympathetic denervation procedure at 3 and at 6 months of follow-up. Error bars represent interquartile range

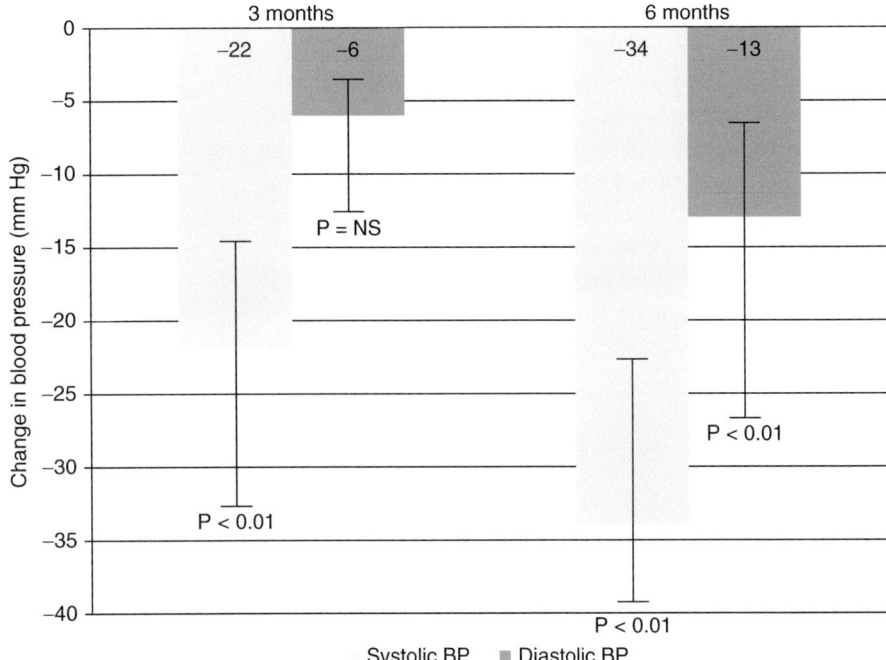

Fig. 24.2 Changes of AHI at 3 and 6 months after denervation. Data of individual cases

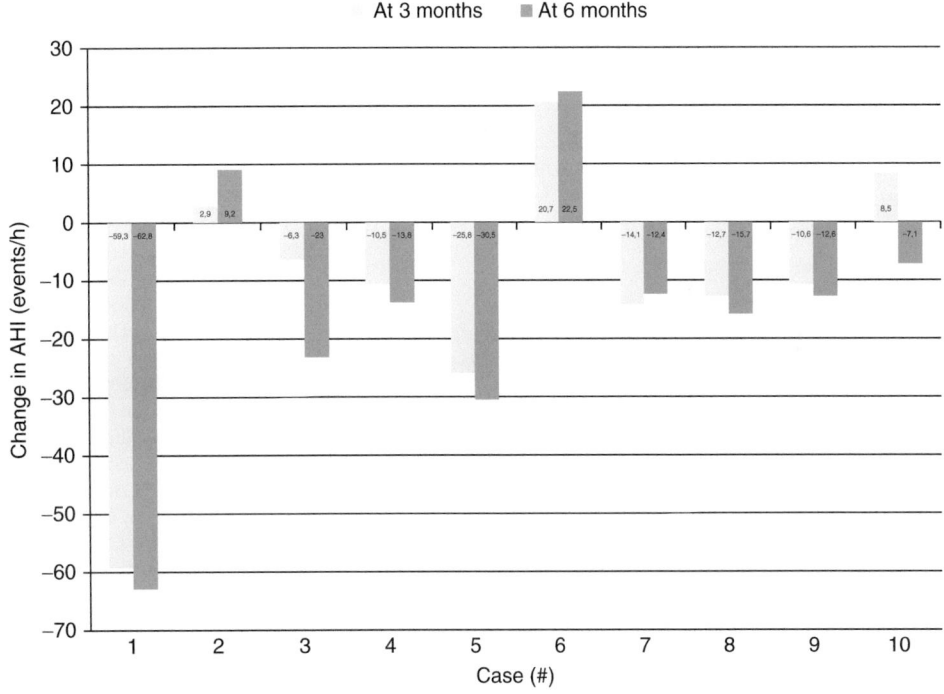

concentration 2 h after glucose administration at 3 and at 6 months (median 7.0 mmol/dL versus median 6.4 mmol/dL at 6 months; p<0.05) and in hemoglobin A1C level at 6 months (median 6.1 % versus median 5.6 %; p<0.05) were demonstrated.

This study confirmed that RDN lowers blood pressure in patients with resistant hypertension [39, 40] and endorsed the work of Mahfoud et al. documenting that RDN in humans improves indices of insulin action and glucose metabolism [41]. However, this publication extended previous work by

documenting that the blood pressure and metabolic benefits of renal denervation include patients with sleep apnea and improve the course of the disease. Because these data were observational, the study could not identify the exact mechanism responsible for any amelioration of sleep apnea. Nonetheless, it should be emphasized that RDN influences key mechanisms regulating sympathetic activation. The efferent sympathetic renal nerves can affect control of renal vascular resistance, increase renin release, and regulate sodium and water excretion [12]. The afferent renal nerves enhance the activity of the sympathetic nervous system. It has been also suggested that, in conditions of high-sodium dietary intake, activation of the afferent renal nerves contributes to the arterial baroreceptor-mediated suppression of efferent sympathetic renal nerves in the overall goal of preventing sodium retention and maintaining water and sodium homeostasis [12, 42]. Therefore, RDN in patients with resistant hypertension and OSA might attenuate the effects of sympathoactivation additionally and independently of CPAP treatment. Lastly, it need to be considered that the fall in blood pressure may itself contribute to the attenuation of sleep apnea.

Summary

Obstructive sleep apnea is potential independent risk factor for cardiovascular events, including ischemic heart disease, heart failure, stroke and death. Obstructive sleep apnea is also the most common disease associated with resistant hypertension. As both hypoxia and hypercapnia result in increased sympathetic activity, sympathetic nervous system plays a key role in the development of resistant hypertension in patients with obstructive sleep apnea. Sympathetic overactivation in OSA patients can worsen the prognosis of those patients with cardiovascular diseases, specifically by causing arrhythmias, myocyte injury and necrosis, peripheral vasoconstriction and the promotion of renal sodium retention, both directly and through stimulation of the renin-angiotensin-aldosterone axis. Preliminary results show that catheter-based renal sympathetic denervation may not only lower systolic blood pressure by $\approx$30 mmHg in resistant hypertensive patients with sleep disordered breathing but also improve sleep apnea severity. In eight of ten patients an improvement in apnea-hypopnea index was observed at 6 months after procedure. Along with blood pressure reduction and sleep apnea course improvement significant decreases in plasma glucose concentration 2 h after glucose administration in hemoglobin A1C level were observed.

Renal sympathetic denervation may conceivably be a potentially useful therapeutic option for this subset of patients; however large randomized controlled clinical trials are needed to confirm these initial proof-of-concept data.

References

1. Punjabi NM. The epidemiology of adult obstructive sleep apnea. Proc Am Thorac Soc. 2008;5:136–43.
2. Kasai T, Floras JS, Bradley TD. Sleep apnea and cardiovascular disease: a bidirectional relationship. Circulation. 2012;126:1495–510.
3. Pedrosa RP, Drager LF, Gonzaga CC, Sousa MG, de Paula LKG, Amaro ACS, Amodeo C, Bortolotto LA, Krieger EM, Bradley TD, Lorenzi-Filho G. Obstructive sleep apnea. The most common cause of hypertension associated with resistant hypertension. Hypertension. 2011;58:811–7.
4. Yumino D, Wang H, Floras JS, Newton GE, Mak S, Ruttanaumpawan P, Parker JD, Bradley TD. Prevalence and physiological predictors of sleep apnea in patients with heart failure and systolic dysfunction. J Card Fail. 2009;15:279–85.
5. Bassetti CL, Milanova M, Gugger M. Sleep-disordered breathing and acute ischemic stroke: diagnosis, risk factors, treatment, evolution, and long-term clinical outcome. Stroke. 2006;37:967–72.
6. Arzt M, Young T, Peppard PE, Finn L, Ryan CM, Bayley M, Bradley TD. Dissociation of obstructive sleep apnea from hypersomnolence and obesity in patients with stroke. Stroke. 2010;41:e129–34.
7. Logan AG, Perlikowski SM, Mente A, Tisler A, Tkacova R, Niroumand M, Leung RS, Bradley TD. High prevalence of unrecognized sleep apnea in drug-resistant hypertension. J Hypertens. 2001;19:2271–7.
8. Kohler M, Stradling JR. Mechanisms of vascular damage in obstructive sleep apnea. Nat Rev Cardiol. 2010;7:677–85.
9. Alonso-Fernandez A, Garcia-Rio F, Arias MA, Hernanz A, de la Pena M, Pierola J, Barcelo A, Lopez-Collazo E, Agusti A. Effects of CPAP on oxidative stress and nitrate efficiency in sleep apnoea: a randomized trial. Thorax. 2009;64:581–6.
10. Marin JM, Carrizo SJ, Vicente E, Agusti AG. Long-term cardiovascular outcomes in men with obstructive sleep apnoea-hypopnoea with or without treatment with continuous positive airway pressure: an observational study. Lancet. 2005;365:1046–53.
11. Bradley TD, Floras JS. Obstructive sleep apnea and its cardiovascular consequences. Lancet. 2009;373:82–93.
12. Kasai T, Arcand J, Allard JP, Mak S, Azevedo ER, Newton GE, Bradley TD. Relationship between sodium intake and sleep apnea in patients with heart failure. J Am Coll Cardiol. 2011;58:1970–4.
13. DiBona GF, Esler M. Translational medicine: the antihypertensive effect of renal denervation. Am J Physiol Regul Integr Comp Physiol. 2010;298:R245–53.
14. Gaddam K, Pimenta E, Thomas SJ, Cofield SS, Oparil S, Harding SM, Calhoun DA. Spironolactone reduces severity of obstructive sleep apnea in patients with resistant hypertension: a preliminary report. J Hum Hypertens. 2010;24:532–7.
15. Chiu KL, Ryan CM, Shiota S, Ruttanaumpawan P, Arzt M, Haight JS, Chan CT, Floras JS, Bradley TD. Fluid shift by lower body positive pressure increases pharyngeal resistance in healthy subjects. Am J Respir Crit Care Med. 2006;174:1378–83.
16. Shiota S, Ryan CM, Chiu KL, Ruttanaumpawan P, Haight J, Arzt M, Floras JS, Chan C, Bradley TD. Alterations in upper airway cross-sectional area in response to lower body positive pressure in healthy subjects. Thorax. 2007;62:868–72.
17. Redolfi S, Yumino D, Ruttanaumpawan P, Yau B, Su MC, Lam J, Bradley TD. Relationship between overnight rostral fluid shift and obstructive sleep apnea in nonobese men. Am J Respir Crit Care Med. 2009;179:241–6.
18. Redolfi S, Arnulf I, Pottier M, Lajou J, Koskas I, Bradley TD, Similowski T. Attenuation of obstructive sleep apnea by compression stockings in subjects with venous insufficiency. Am J Respir Crit Care Med. 2012;184:1062–6.
19. Tang SC, Lam B, Ku PP, Leung WS, Chu CM, Ho YW, Ip MS, Lai KN. Alleviation of sleep apnea in patients with chronic renal failure by nocturnal cycler-assisted peritoneal dialysis compared with conventional continuous ambulatory peritoneal dialysis. J Am Soc Nephrol. 2006;17:2607–16.
20. Tang SC, Lam B, Lai AS, Pang CB, Tso WK, Khong PL, Ip MS, Lai KN. Improvement in sleep apnea during nocturnal peritoneal

dialysis is associated with reduced airway congestion and better uremic clearance. Clin J Am Soc Nephrol. 2009;4:410–8.

21. Hanly PJ, Pierratos A. Improvement of sleep apnea in patients with chronic renal failure who undergo nocturnal hemodialysis. N Engl J Med. 2001;344:102–7.

22. Brooks D, Horner RL, Kozar LF, Render-Teixeira CL, Phillipson EA. Obstructive sleep apnea as a cause of systemic hypertension. Evidence from a canine model. J Clin Invest. 1997;99:106–9.

23. Fletcher EC, Lesske J, Behm R, Miller III CC, Stauss H, Unger T. Carotid chemoreceptors, systemic blood pressure, and chronic episodic hypoxia mimicking sleep apnea. J Appl Physiol. 1992;72:1978–84.

24. Peppard PE, Young T, Palta M, Skatrud J. Prospective study of the association between sleep-disordered breathing and hypertension. N Engl J Med. 2000;342:1378–84.

25. O'Connor GT, Caffo B, Newman AB, Quan SF, Rapoport DM, Redline S, Resnick HE, Samet J, Shahar E. Prospective study of sleep-disordered breathing and hypertension: the Sleep Heart Health Study. Am J Respir Crit Care Med. 2009;179:1159–64.

26. Cano-Pumarega I, Duran-Cantolla J, Aizpuru F, Miranda-Serrano E, Rubio R, Martinez-Null C, de Miguel J, Egea C, Cancelo L, Alvarez A, Fernandez-Bolanos M, Barbe F. Obstructive sleep apnea and systemic hypertension: longitudinal study in the general population: the Vitoria sleep cohort. Am J Respir Crit Care Med. 2012;184:1299–304.

27. Sjostrom C, Lindberg E, Elmasry A, Hagg A, Svardsudd K, Janson C. Prevalence of sleep apnoea and snoring in hypertensive men: a population based study. Thorax. 2002;57:602–7.

28. Shepard Jr JW. Cardiopulmonary consequence of obstructive sleep apnea. Mayo Clin Proc. 1990;65:1250–9.

29. Somers VK, Zavala DC, Mark AL, Abboud FM. Influence of ventilation and hypocapnia on sympathetic nerve responses to hypoxia in normal humans. J Appl Physiol. 1989;67:2095–100.

30. Somers VK, Zavala DC, Mark AL, Abboud FM. Contrasting effects of hypoxia and hypercapnia on ventilation and sympathetic activity in humans. J Appl Physiol. 1989;67:2101–6.

31. Somers VK, Mark AL, Abboud FM. Potentiation of sympathetic nerve responses to hypoxia in borderline hypertensive subjects. Hypertension (Dallas). 1988;11:608–12.

32. Somers VK, Mark AL, Abboud FM. Sympathetic activation by hypoxia and hypercapnia-implications for sleep apnea. Clin Exp Hypertens Part A Theory Pract. 1988;A10 Suppl 1:413–22.

33. Somers VK, Dyken ME, Clary MP, Abboud FM. Sympathetic neural mechanisms in obstructive sleep apnea. J Clin Invest. 1995;96:1897–904.

34. Nauman J, Janszky I, Vatten LJ, Wisloff U. Temporal changes in resting heart rate and deaths from ischemic heart disease. JAMA. 2011;306:2579–87.

35. Floras JS. Sympathetic nervous system activation in human heart failure: clinical implications of an updated model. J Am Coll Cardiol. 2009;54:375–85.

36. Linz D, Mahfoud F, Schotten U, Ukena C, Neuberger H-R, Wirth K, Böhm M. Renal sympathetic denervation suppresses postapneic blood pressure rises and atrial fibrillation in a model for sleep apnea. Hypertension. 2012;60:172–8.

37. Franquini JVM, Medeiros ARS, Andrade TU, Araújo MTM, Moysés MR, Abreu GR, Vasquez EC, Bissoli NS. Influence of renal denervation on blood pressure, sodium and water excretion in acute total obstructive apnea in rats. Braz J Med Biol Res. 2009;42(2):214–9.

38. Witkowski A, Prejbisz A, Florczak E, Kądziela J, Śliwiński P, Bieleń P, Michałowska I, Kabat M, Warchoł E, Januszewicz M, Narkiewicz K, Somers VK, Sobotka PA, Januszewicz A. Effects of renal sympathetic denervation on blood pressure, sleep apnea course, and glycemic control in patients with resistant hypertension and sleep apnea. Hypertension. 2011;58:559–65.

39. Krum H, Schlaich M, Whitbourn R, Sobotka PA, Sadowski J, Bartus K, Kapelak B, Walton A, Sievert H, Thambar S, Abraham WT, Esler M. Catheter-based renal sympathetic denervation for resistant hypertension: a multicentre safety and proof-of-principle cohort study. Lancet. 2009;373:1275–81.

40. Esler MD, Krum H, Sobotka PA, Schlaich MP, Schmieder RE, Bohm M. Renal sympathetic denervation in patients with treatment-resistant hypertension (the symplicity HTN-2 trial): a randomised controlled trial. Lancet. 2010;376:1903–9.

41. Mahfoud F, Schlaich M, Kindermann I, Ukena C, Cremers B, Brandt MC, Hoppe UC, Vonend O, Rump LC, Sobotka PA, Krum H, Esler M, Bohm M. Effect of renal sympathetic denervation on glucose metabolism in patients with resistant hypertension: a pilot study. Circulation. 2011;123:940–1946.

42. Kopp UC, Jones SY, DiBona GF. Afferent renal denervation impairs baroreflex control of efferent renal sympathetic nerve activity. Am J Physiol Regul Integr Comp Physiol. 2008;295:R1882–90.

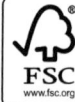